Strange Harvest

Strange Harvest

Organ Transplants, Denatured Bodies, and the Transformed Self

LESLEY A. SHARP

University of California Press

BERKELEY   LOS ANGELES   LONDON

University of California Press, one of the most distinguished university presses in the United States, enriches lives around the world by advancing scholarship in the humanities, social sciences, and natural sciences. Its activities are supported by the UC Press Foundation and by philanthropic contributions from individuals and institutions. For more information, visit www.ucpress.edu.

University of California Press
Berkeley and Los Angeles, California

University of California Press, Ltd.
London, England

© 2006 by The Regents of the University of California

Library of Congress Cataloging-in-Publication Data

Sharp, Lesley Alexandra.
    Strange harvest : organ transplants, denatured bodies, and the transformed self / Lesley A. Sharp.
        p.   cm.
    Includes bibliographical references and index.
    ISBN 978-0-520-24784-0 (cloth : alk. paper)
    ISBN 978-0-520-24786-4 (pbk. : alk. paper)
        1. Transplantation of organs, tissues, etc.—Social aspects—United States.   2. Medical anthropology—United States.   3. Ethnology—United States.   4. Funeral rites and ceremonies—United States.   5. Death—United States.   6. Mourning customs—United States.   7. Memorials—United States.   8. Kinship—United States.   I. Title.
    [DNLM: 1. Organ Transplantation.   2. Tissue and Organ Procurement.   3. Attitude to Death.   4. Funeral Rites.   5. Anthropology, Cultural.   WO 660 S531s   2006]
    RD120.7.S49 2006
    306.4'61—dc22   2005032838

Manufactured in the United States of America
15 14 13 12 11 10 9 08 07
10 9 8 7 6 5 4 3 2

For my mother, Rosemary Cochran Sharp
(1929–2002), gifted iconographer, shrewd diagnostician,
intrepid globe-trotter

Contents

Illustrations

Acknowledgments

When I first conceived of this project in 1991, I could not have predicted that it would hold my interest for so long. As this book goes to press, I remain captivated by the internal workings—and future—of human organ transfer. I am intrigued not only by the ethos that drives and legitimates so complex a medical realm but by an inherent dynamism, too, one that always insists on innovation and further perfection. What this means, of course, is that each time I describe, for instance, surgical techniques, donor recruitment methods, or bureaucratic or clinical practices, I may need to acknowledge that other often recent statements have become outdated only a few years following publication. Thus, I continue to be driven by a desire to remain involved as an inquisitive ethnographer.

The stamina such work entails derives its energy in large part from the unflagging support offered by a wide range of colleagues, friends, and family, many of whom, I suspect, may be unaware of how much their interest and encouragement have meant to me over the years. Within the all too often ingrown circles of academia, I have consistently encountered warmth and support, even among those who would not count themselves as medical anthropologists. Some of these people I know, for instance, through my work in Madagascar, rather than American clinics and the like. Long-term, persistent support from Elizabeth Colson, Nancy Scheper-Hughes, Stephen Foster, Burton Benedict, Frederick Dunn, Gillian Feeley-Harnik, Paula Rubel, Abe Rosman, and Morton Klass has made me realize how fortunate I am to have had so precious a collection of mentors as these. Their inquisitiveness about human nature, paired with rigorous method and theoretical interrogation, are qualities I attempt to model daily in my own pursuits. Still others, through their administrative capacities at Butler University, Barnard College, and Columbia University, have made my work possible and enjoyable—at times because of financial support, at others simply because their enthusiasm for my work gave me the shot in the arm I sometimes needed to continue with my research. Paul Yu, Geoff Bannister, Flora Davidson, Elizabeth Boylan, Judith Shapiro, and Richard Parker have been especially supportive. I am deeply appreciative, too, of the many hours of formal and informal discussion with a range of invaluable colleagues. I cannot possibly name them all, but here I wish at the very least to thank Brian Larkin, Nan Rothschild, Paige West, Maxine Weisgrau, Paul Silverstein, Jason James, and Karen Seeley at Barnard College; Brink Messick, Neni Panourgia, Sherry Ortner, Robert Sember, and Carole Vance, as well as members of the Seminar on Death, at Columbia University; and, elsewhere, Nancy Chen, Margaret Clark, Kata Chillig, Linda Green, Cecil Helman, Renée Fox, Linda Hogle, Sharon Kaufman, Joshua Lederberg, Margaret Lock, Patty Marshall, Emily Martin, Mary Beth Mills, Eleni Papagaroufali, Rayna Rapp, Carolyn Rouse, Janelle Taylor, and Dorothy Nelkin. Lynn Morgan, Helen Gremellion, and Megan Crowley-Matoka offered detailed and insightful comments on the manuscript itself.

A virtual phalanx of extraordinarily talented students has lent invaluable support, often wending their way into domains I could not reach because of time and other constraints. I simply could not have learned as much as I have without the assistance and involvement of Marcy Assalone, Marcie Brink, Heather Fisher, Katie Kilroy-Marac, Sarah Muir, Evi Rivera, Sonya Rubin, and Thurka Sangaramoorthy. Kari Hodges and Scott Michener provided invaluable technical expertise and humor, too. Other close friends have offered good cheer, keeping me laughing even during the worst of times. I am especially grateful for the friendship (and accompanying insights, clinical and otherwise!) of Maureen Hickey, Michael Grider, Vinita Seghal, Elan Louis, Lisa Tiersten, Tovah Klein, Linda Beck, Susie Blalock, Robin Rudell, Annie Raherisoanjato, and Hanta and Chris Rideout. Erika Doss has been an exceptional source of inspiration during various road trips and other serious or silly pursuits.

Among the greatest frustrations an ethnographer encounters is the inability to thank the many people by name who have made one's research possible—this stems not only from the sheer number of people involved but also from the promise of anonymity during interviews and other activities. Nevertheless, I must express my heartfelt thanks to the many people who have so willingly given of themselves; their generosity is astounding, for not once did anyone refuse a request for an interview or turn me away from an event. I am deeply indebted to the many organ recipients who described their experiences and shared their thoughts; the donor kin who so willingly opened their homes to me and offered such intimate details of their personal lives; the staff from a range of hospitals, research labs, and conferences who granted me time—and access—during hectic daily schedules; and the many employees and volunteers based throughout the country's organ procurement agencies who have taught me so much about the difficulties of compassionate work. Still other organizations, including LOLA, MOTTEP, NATCO, NDFC, NKF, TRIO, and UNOS have enriched my work in ways I find difficult to describe in words. Quite a number of people have been important guides and teachers, often serving as valuable sources when I have required clarification on some of the more intricate aspects of organ transfer. Still others have encouraged my work through invitations to present my findings to involved audiences; thus, I wish to thank by name Arlene Barnett, Henry Broadbent, Maggie Coolican, Larraine DePasquale, Chris Gilmore, Kenny Hudson, Greg Holman, Shanon Moser, Barbara Musto, Miriam Perez, Leo Trevino, Susan Stoops Watson, and, most of all, Christine Wilson. Any errors that remain within this text are, of course, mine alone.

The research from which *Strange Harvest* emerges would never have come to fruition were it not for an unending stream of support from a range of generous institutions. These include the Project on Death in America of the Soros Foundation's Open Society Institute, The Wenner-Gren Foundation for Anthropological Research (grant 7017), a range of faculty research grants made available through Barnard College, including several that were funded by the Mellon Foundation, and an academic grant from Butler University that launched the initial project back in the early 1990s. Two separate residencies at the Hastings Center for Bioethics, where I was a Visiting North American Scholar during the summer of 2002, and later at the Russell Sage Foundation throughout the 2003–4 academic year, enabled me to gather my thoughts in wonderfully peaceful settings that allowed me to write this book. A year's sabbatical from Barnard College was also essential to this project. I have been fortunate to have been able to work with Randy Heyman, Jacqueline Volin, and Susan Ecklund at the University of California Press. Eugene Kain and Bill Nelson deserve special praise for their artwork. I am also deeply indebted to Stan Holwitz, who has offered unwavering support on every project I pursue. One could not wish for a kinder and more encouraging editor.

Finally, I am deeply thankful for the haven provided by my family. In a sense, it is for them that I have pursued this work for so long. This book is dedicated to my mother, whose intelligence, hilarious wit, and intellectual presence I miss terribly. My father, who read this manuscript with meticulous care, has proved subsequently to be a reliable source of lively discussion and a firm anchor as well. Erik and Paula have similarly stimulated me to rethink some of my questions, although it is their love that has mattered the most. Similarly, Ross, Julio, Emily, Ruthie and Wally, and Mary and Frank have all, in their own unique ways, kept me going and laughing, too. Most important of all is Andy's love and support, and the joy that Alex brings daily to my life. My work is secondary to such happiness as this.

Introduction

Strange Harvest

Organ transplantation in the United States has entered a state of crisis, albeit one of its own design. The boldness of this statement rests on the supposition that transplantation simultaneously epitomizes technical genius and medical hubris in this country. Specialized surgeons now understand the function of highly sophisticated organs so well that they routinely remove these organs from the recently deceased, using them in turn to replenish life in their ailing patients. Nevertheless, even after fifty years of practice and refinement, transplantation looms as a troubling realm of medicine, especially within the lay imagination. Although it stands as an icon of medical accomplishment—and in some quarters may even be considered a routine response to a range of severe health problems—it nevertheless generates a host of perplexing questions about healing and illness, medical versus social definitions of death, the hybridization of human bodies, and nonmedicalized constructions of personhood, individuality, and the embodied self.

As a widespread surgical technique and lucrative arm of medicine, transplantation has generated a plethora of literature: its persistent ability to fascinate ensures its recurrent treatment within the mainstream press (early developments were featured on the cover of *Life* magazine). Organ transplants also provide rich fodder for plots in a wide range of media, including thriller fiction, television dramas, and film. Further, transplantation, as an icon of medical accomplishment, defines a regular subject of scientific inquiry in such flagship medical publications as the *Journal of the American Medical Association*, the *New England Journal of Medicine*, and the *Lancet*. It also lays claim to a range of specialized periodicals, including *Transplantation*, *Transplantation Proceedings*, the *American Journal of Transplantation*, *Clinical Transplantation*, *Liver Transplantation and Surgery*, *Pediatric Transplantation*, *Transplant Immunology*, and *Transplantation Interna-*

tional, to name but a few. Numerous social scientists also have worked on the subject of transplantation: early studies date back to the first kidney transplants of the 1950s, attempts that were facilitated by the advent of hemodialysis a decade earlier. Organ transplantation indisputably generates an unusual combination of curiosity, celebration, and anxiety. As such, it defines a highly problematic and fascinating realm of medicine in America.[1]

Through ethnographic investigation, *Strange Harvest* strives to decipher the problematic status of organ transplantation in this country. As an anthropologist I approach transplantation as an exotic branch of medical culture, with its own particular ethos that guides the behavior, thinking, and embodied practices of involved professional and lay parties. In applying the label *exotic,* I have no intention of demeaning the transplant profession. Rather, I concur with Micaela di Leonardo, who asserts the need to consider "exotics at home" and posits that the anthropological stance initiates an examination of cultural phenomena that are "hidden in plain sight around us" (1998: 10). My purpose is to identify and rethink much of what is taken for granted about organ transplants in the United States. In turn, I seek to uncover essential elements of an intriguing medical realm that remain unseen or unspoken, either because they seem far too mundane to warrant consideration or because professional policy imposes taboos that ultimately obscure such key elements from plain sight.

The mode of questioning that drives this work is characteristic of anthropology; the great beauty of the discipline is its persistent devotion to shifting frames of reference, a process that inevitably renders the strange familiar and the familiar strange (Geertz 1973: 215, after Percy 1958; also Malinowski 1961 [1922]). In addition, ethnographic research involves a special form of witnessing (Geertz 1983: 73–101), the ethnographer assuming an odd combined stance of both professional stranger and friend among research participants (Agar 1996; Powdermaker 1966). The anthropological fieldworker always aspires to the role of keen observer, one who nevertheless struggles to maintain a relativist position. When successful, the process of "being there" enables the anthropologist to observe, translate, order, and then interpret systems of local knowledge, and even at times to offer alternative readings of cultural truths (Geertz 1988: 1–24). An assumption that underlies this book is that organ transplantation defines an intriguing and exotic milieu in which to explore a highly specialized array of medicalized behaviors and associated ideological premises.

This book is first and foremost an ethnography; on a very basic level, it insists on the power of vivid description as an illuminative technique. As such, this book augments a puny yet sophisticated collection of detailed research authored by social scientists working in the postindustrial settings of the United States, Canada, Japan, and Germany. Nevertheless, it marks an important break by exploring a wider range of activities than those that typify existing studies. Most important, the word *transplantation* is regularly employed in the literature as an umbrella term and is applied to a wide range of activities. In contrast, I assert the need to recognize organ transplantation's dependency on two other domains of medical practice: organ procurement and organ donation. My point is that existing book-length research overwhelmingly privileges transplantation alone and may even treat it without any discussion of these other two domains. Renée Fox and Judith Swazey's long-term work in the United States on living donors who offer one of two functioning kidneys to kin in need, Linda Hogle's examination of organ procurement in unified Germany and the United States, and Margaret Lock's comparative study of brain death in Japan and North America are laudable exceptions to current trends (Fox and Swazey 1978, 1992; Hogle 1999; Lock 2002).[2] The privileging of transplantation elsewhere occurs in large part because hospital transplant units are more readily accessible to medical investigators, and transplantation as a research concern is a far less emotionally trying subject than organ procurement or donation, both of which are inevitably morbid in focus. Researchers who study transplantation most certainly must confront the suffering and even the deaths of patients, yet medical successes often render their work joyfully rewarding. I assert, however, that death and suffering frame much of the research within the other two domains because critically ill patients, who are rapidly relabeled as *brain-dead cadaveric donors*, are so frequently involved.

As I will explain in greater detail, the overwhelming attention given to transplantation is what eventually drove me to work successively within all three domains. As a result of my range of activities, I have come to view transplantation, procurement, and donation as inextricably intertwined. Transplants, for instance, could not occur as frequently as they do in the United States if organ donation and procurement were illegal. Likewise, families would never be approached about donation in hospital intensive care units (ICUs) were there no patients elsewhere awaiting transplants, nor would organ procurement be considered a medical necessity or important specialized profession. Throughout this book I employ the expression *organ transfer* as a unifying term intended to underscore the interdependency of these three domains, thus also avoiding the assumption that one domain is more important than the other two. This study nevertheless privileges the experiences of donor kin and procurement specialists as a means to offset another strong focus within the current literature, specifically that on organ recipients' lives. As will soon become clear, however, the lives of donor kin and recipients are elaborately intertwined as well, in such intriguing ways that a discussion of one necessitates making reference to the other.

As Gregory Bateson once argued (1958), careful anthropological investigation can illuminate the hidden complexity and grace of a cultural ethos—that is, an unconscious moral code that guides human actions, thoughts, and language within a particular social group. In my study of organ transfer, descriptions of medical techniques, key settings, and subjects are essential if readers, especially those who are not medically trained, are to follow my purpose. This work is driven by a desire to translate the deeper meanings associated with organ transfer as a sociomedical process. When research is set squarely within the realm of organ transfer, such anthropological probing emerges as an epistemological enterprise (see Scheper-Hughes and Lock 1987), one framed by especially pronounced concerns for such themes as the symbolics of the human body, physical suffering, medical expertise and public trust, competing definitions of death, and proper forms of mourning. Against these interests, certain key issues define the parameters of this book.

Strange Harvest is concerned exclusively with cadaveric donation. That is, it focuses on contexts where transplantable organs are acquired from the bodies of deceased hospitalized patients, the vast majority of whom are declared brain dead and are maintained on respirators in anticipation of organ procurement surgery. Donors are peculiarly liminal beings, caught somewhere between patient and cadaver status. Early in my research I was struck by the pervasiveness of language designed to depersonalize these donor-patients and, further, by the ways in which involved professional and lay parties struggled to make sense of this process while nevertheless embracing donation, procurement, and transplantation as laudable and necessary social acts. I also soon came to learn that a host of intriguing social relationships emerge among these parties in direct response to the presence of the cadaveric donor. As we shall see, even the donor body itself may be reanimated in the minds of recipients and donor kin who share the understanding that transplanted organs can retain the life essence of their donors. Organ transfer mitigates these peculiar and fascinating social relationships and associated symbolic constructions precisely because it relies on retrieving organs from donors who are considered legally and medically dead and who, at least at the outset, are anonymous to transplant recipients.

A brief contrast with other forms of organ donation will help clarify the importance of my exclusive focus on the cadaveric body. Kidneys, for instance, can be transferred legally and with relative medical ease from living kin; recent news accounts also indicate a rise in the national incidence of kidneys offered by friends and even strangers to patients in need. This sort of organ transfer is referred to as *living donation* and involves two tandem surgeries. An assumption that renders this medical procedure possible is the widely accepted view that it poses relatively little harm to a healthy donor, who continues to thrive because he or she retains a second kidney.[3] Much has been written on living kidney donation in the United States, with pronounced interest in the long-term survival rates of donors and recipients, as well as the nature of their social relationships (see especially Fox and Swazey 1992). The United States as a research context shapes these dominant concerns, for as one moves into the global arena, the focus shifts rapidly to investigations of both legal and clandestine forms of trafficking in human body parts, with organs taken from donors who, unlike recipients, lack access to quality health care.[4] My decision to limit my focus to the United States is in part a matter of scale. The United States has long stood as a world leader for organ transplants, both in terms of the innovative use of biotechnologies and because of the sheer volume of surgeries performed each year. Today many American cities can boast of at least one hospital with a transplant unit, and as other researchers have found, it can be difficult to avoid comparison with the United States when writing about transplants elsewhere (Hogle 1999; Lock 2002). I therefore leave living donation, tissue (that is, non-organ) procurement, and global trends for others to explore.

As the chapters in this book detail, highly complex social relationships arise in response to cadaveric donation. These relationships can be difficult to uncover because of the strict taboos imposed by involved health professionals, many of whom, for example, insist that donor bodies be viewed as mere corpses that generate reusable parts; that recipients should neither identify with or idealize their donors nor humanize their organs; and that surviving donor kin and recipients should not communicate with one another but instead move on with their separate lives. Nevertheless, many health professionals wrestle privately with highly medicalized constructions of donors' deaths. Further, recipients do in fact imagine a donor's identity in all sorts of ways and frequently integrate this unknown Other as an intrinsic part of their subjective sense of self. Finally, organ recipients and their donors' surviving kin may long to encounter one another, and they may go to great lengths to do so, even when blocked by transplant professionals who hold records of their respective identities, addresses, and histories.[5] Among the great ironies of organ transfer in the United States is that it generates a host of new social relationships that at first may seem altogether strange to the uninitiated, yet which are in fact common and, I argue, culturally generated and thus *naturalized* responses to the peculiar qualities of cadaveric organ donation.

With this in mind, I am most intrigued by the manner in which medicalized definitions of death affect how involved parties think about organ donors, transplanted organs, and donors' deaths. Key to understanding cadaveric organ donation is that it relies overwhelmingly on donors who have sustained sudden, unexpected head traumas and who are declared brain dead within hospital settings (most frequently by staff neurologists in hospital ICUs). Because the shadow of death pervades this form of organ transfer, I argue that very particular and peculiar responses emerge that stand in contrast to those associated with living donation. Donor death is highly problematic: for transplants to be socially acceptable, all involved parties must embrace legal definitions of brain death as legitimate in medical, physiological, and spiritual terms. Nevertheless, careful probing reveals that there is tremendous disjunction between expressed public (or official) and private understandings of brain death criteria. For these reasons, throughout this book I will refer to *cadaveric* (that is, of or like a cadaver) forms of donation while avoiding the label *cadaver* when speaking specifically of the organ donor (that is, the donor-patient). Also, the logistics of donor care inevitably force involved parties to struggle with conflicting messages about death and suffering. This remains true regardless of whether one is a transplant specialist who works with patients on a transplant ward; a procurement professional who talks to kin about donation as a loved one lies dying in an ICU, and who may later assist, too, in the surgical procurement of organs; a patient who becomes an organ recipient through transplant surgery; or a donor's surviving kin who have granted permission so that a donor-patient's organs can be taken and transplanted in recipients elsewhere. The unusual form of death so intrinsic to organ transfer's success generates deeply personal responses, which persist long after donation, procurement, and transplantation occur. These responses may stand in stark contrast to what is currently represented in the literature as transplant dogma.

As an in-depth exploration of the ethos of organ transfer, this book is structured around conundrums or nagging questions that I will refer to as *transplant paradoxes*. These paradoxes spring from a set of ideological premises that guide research participants' everyday actions and speech, as well as the tenor and focus of both specialized professional publications and promotional literature on organ transfer written for general audiences. As I shall illustrate throughout, a wealth of knowledge is embedded in the ways professional and lay parties behave and talk about organ transfer in a variety of settings, including transplant wards; professionally orchestrated events such as conferences, annual commemorative celebrations, and patient support group meetings; and interviewees' private homes. I am especially sensitive to dominant narrative genres—that is, the particular ways in which participants learn how to speak of or write about their experiences with organ transfer. Most intriguing is the fact that responses offered in public venues may differ radically from the private thoughts individuals share only with trusted friends, close colleagues, and, at times, the anthropologist. Applied carefully, the methodological approaches that define ethnographic research reveal insider understandings of transplant decorum, exposing those moments when involved parties defy scripted forms of behavior, or when they question dominant ways of thinking about organ transfer. Surprisingly, these moments of disjunction are hardly rare. My ultimate goal is to uncover these paradoxical moments and then decode their significance as a means for understanding organ transfer as a dominant, albeit troubled, sociomedical process in America.

THE IDEOLOGICAL UNDERPINNINGS OF ORGAN TRANSFER

The cadaveric organ donor offers an especially rich site for exploring the paradoxical nature of organ transfer in the United States, where discussions of this unusual category of patient rapidly shift to a questioning mode. First, when considering cadaveric donors, do all parties think of and respond to them as a social category? For instance, how do donor kin, on the one hand, and hospital staff, on the other, talk about brain dead donors or behave when in their presence? What sorts of ideas about donors do transplant recipients and their surgeons, nurses, and social workers share, and where might their ideas diverge? Second, is it possible to speak of a collective understanding of the cadaveric donor body itself, or can conflicting ideas coexist? Can the donor be viewed simultaneously as a deceased loved one, a source of exchangeable parts, and the repository of an unusual kind of social gift? Third, does the presence of the organ donor clarify or confound understandings of death? And when precisely does a donor's death occur? Do all parties concur? Is it at the moment when a neurologist declares a patient brain dead, or during surgery when a donor's organs are removed? Is death lodged in the brain, the body, a soul, or a combination of these or other possible sites? Fourth, do brain death and organ donation confirm, confound, or enhance cultural understandings of personhood and social worth? Where does the donor-as-person dwell before, during, and after the surgical removal of transplantable organs? What issues are at stake when donors' identities remain anonymous? Finally, does it make sense to ask who owns the donor body and its parts? Can anyone claim rights to the donor's transplanted organs? If so, following transplantation, do organs belong exclusively to their recipients? If others lay claim, at what point should they relinquish their hold?

These overlapping philosophical, ethical, and cultural dilemmas shape this investigation as a whole. At one level, such questions define the parameters for debates considered regularly by medical ethicists. My purpose, however, is neither to offer definitive answers nor even to negotiate conflicts so that a compromise might be reached that would satisfy both the emotional and the practical demands of involved parties. Rather, from an anthropological standpoint, I view such debates as generating valuable data that ultimately expose troubled yet culturally driven concerns about organ transfer in this country. Such concerns are also linked to larger problems that plague medical practice more generally, especially regarding the medical versus social worth of patients; the social significance of the hospital death; the importance of altruism and kindness in medical contexts; and perplexing questions about death and proper forms of mourning. Thus, my work is most heavily invested in exploring the subject and tenor of these debates to broaden medical policy discussions and to stimulate frank and open public consideration of the social value of organ transfer.

As I will explain here and illustrate in subsequent chapters, transplantation rests on a paradoxical set of ideological or moral premises that guide medical conduct, professional public outreach efforts, and dominant lay understandings of death, the body, and gift giving. The tenuous nature of the assumptions driving organ transfer also contributes to the current transplant crisis in America. In this regard, transplant ideology relies on the following set of premises: (1) the concept of transplantation as a medical miracle; (2) the denial of transplantation as a form of body commodification; (3) the perception of transplantable organs as precious things; (4) the dependence on brain death criteria for generating transplantable parts; (5) the assertion that organs of human origin are becoming increasingly scarce in our society and require radical solutions; (6) an insistence that the melding of disparate bodies is part of a natural progression in a medical realm predicated on technological expertise; and, finally, (7) the imperative that compassion and trust remain central to the care of dying patients, even when a new corporate style of medicine demands an increasing number of transplantable organs. I will now consider the paradoxical nature of each of these premises.

The Miracle of Technocratic Medicine

Transplantation is regularly hailed as one of the great miracles of modern science. As such, it might very well be viewed as the quintessential example of millennial medicine, for we have remained in awe of its accomplishments since the mid–twentieth century and into the twenty-first. In one sense, labeling transplantation as miraculous is justified: it is truly astonishing that surgeons can save lives by replacing failing organs in their patients with those taken from other humans' bodies. Nevertheless, this passion for the miraculous can obstruct our view of a problematic underside.

The social construction specifically of transplant surgery as a miraculous procedure draws on the successful development of an elaborate array of sophisticated technologies intrinsic to American medicine. For instance, medical progress in this country is frequently tracked along timelines that trace the experimental design and implementation of a host of complex machines (for a recent example, see Maeder and Ross 2002). A quick glance at the history of visual technologies alone underscores this remarkable progress, as one moves, say, from the X-ray to the sonogram, CAT scan (or CT scan, for computed axial tomography imaging), magnetic resonance imagery (MRI), and fiber-optic devices.[6] Of great relevance to organ transfer's success is the development of "life support" devices, a history marked by the development of the iron lung (invented in 1929 and in common use by the 1940s to sustain polio victims) to the routinized hospital use of the respiratory ventilator, the latter now essential to sustaining brain dead organ donors prior to and during procurement surgery. Other crucial technologies range from hemodialysis to heart-lung bypass devices. Pharmaceuticals represent yet another important thrust of medical success that renders posttransplant survival possible. Among the most significant developments involved the creation in the 1980s of the powerful immunosuppressant cyclosporine, which prevents the body from rejecting an organ of foreign origin. Cyclosporine and other immunosuppressants, paired with powerful steroids, are the mainstay of daily transplant survival for many patients.[7] This array of technological developments has enabled organ transplantation to make phenomenal strides, so that it now epitomizes medical possibility within the collective American imagination.

The miracle of transplant surgery also underscores the impressive capabilities of mainstream cosmopolitan medicine in this country. For one, American medicine is overwhelmingly allopathic: in other words, it assumes a heavily biomedical approach to the human body and to suffering. In the healing encounter the patient is generally approached as an individual and, thus, as a discrete entity, where treatment is possible without considering the significance of a larger social milieu. This is because the body itself is viewed as a sophisticated organism whose splendor stems from its physiological complexity. The biomedical model is wed to the rationale of disease theory; as such, a progression from diagnosis to treatment and cure is essential to the paradigm. Allopathic practices can be highly invasive, driven by an overwhelming concern for the body's inner workings (marked, for example, by the displacement of general practitioners by internists in recent decades). As a result, the surgical ability to alter, remove, and replace body parts ranks among biomedicine's most impressive accomplishments to date. Through such practices the human body is rapidly transformed into a highly medicalized system of interdependent parts and processes.

Transplantation signifies the zenith of medical skill, albeit for a small minority it heralds the dangers of technological medicine run amok (Illich 1976). More generally, mainstream American medicine is wed to a technocratic model, argues Robbie Davis-Floyd (1994), relying increasingly on specialized diagnostic methods, technical procedures, mechanical implants, and a vast array of potent pharmaceuticals as a means to alter, cure, and improve the human body. At the high end of technocratic medicine, patients may emerge as little more than medically manipulated cyborgs, hooked up to an array of machines, their functions sustained by powerful drug regimens (Davis-Floyd and Dumit 1998; Downey, Dumit, and Traweek 1997; C. Gray 1995).

The United States is hardly unique here; it does, however, offer an unavoidable benchmark for comparison. Technocratic practices are part and parcel of capitalist medicine in this country. More so than in any other nation, American medical decisions are driven by private insurance responses to market trends, where high-end technologies are increasingly vilified in discussions on the rising cost of medicine (Neumann and Weinstein 1991: 1). Health care costs in the United States totaled $1.3 trillion in 2000, jumping 6.9 percent from the previous year (Alliance for Health Reform 2003), and by 2002, these accounted for fourteen cents of every dollar spent in this country (PBS 2002). American consumers are drawn to technological innovation, too, a fact facilitated by legal marketing strategies, such as direct-to-consumer advertising of pharmaceuticals (Hogle 2001, 2002). Against these developments, transplantation defines a multibillion-dollar industry in America, and more transplants are performed in the United States each year than in any other country. In 1997, for instance, a national total of 20,297 transplant surgeries fell only 194 short of the 20,491 for all of Europe (ITCS 1997; UNOS 2003b).[8] The technocratic approach to healing—as epitomized by organ transfer, and even more so by transplant surgery—is a medical fact of life in America.

The Commodification of Human Body Parts

Transplantation's ascent to iconic status as a miraculous medical procedure has generated a number of other troubling consequences. Among these is an overwhelming commodification of the human body (Scheper-Hughes and Wacquant 2003; Sharp 2000b). Today the human body is a treasure trove of reusable parts, including the major organs (lungs, heart, liver, kidneys, pancreas, intestine, and bowel); tissue (a category that includes bone, bone marrow, ligaments, corneas, and skin); reproductive fragments (sperm, ova, placenta, and fetal tissue); as well as blood, plasma, hair, and even the whole body (Hogshire 1992; Roach 2003). In 1978, *Forbes* estimated the worth of the full range of the human spare parts industry in the United States at $700 million, with a projected annual growth rate of 15 percent (Solomon 1978). Furthermore, by 1998 the country could boast more than one thousand biotechnology firms that manufactured products from bodily materials (Nelkin and Andrews 1998: 30–31). Today the trade in body parts has expanded well beyond this nation's boundaries, such that the international tissue market alone is worth at least $500 million annually (AP 2000).

Clearly, the cadaveric human body has become a highly lucrative entity: as many as 150 parts can be reused, and an individual body alone is worth more than $230,000 on the open market (Hedges and Gaines 2000; *Pantagraph* 1991). The manner in which body parts are categorized also affects their value. Long-standing legislation within the United States renders illegal the direct buying and selling of human organs so that their retrieval, distribution, and placement are managed solely by nonprofit organizations. These exchanges are strictly controlled at both state and national levels, as dictated by the 1984 National Organ Transplant Act (NOTA) and the Uniform Anatomical Gift Act, which was passed by all fifty states by 1973 (Maeder and Ross 2002: 44). Furthermore, organ procurement and placement are overseen by the United Network for Organ Sharing (UNOS) in Richmond, Virginia, under contract through the U.S. Department of Health and Human Services (HHS). UNOS administers the Organ Procurement and Transplantation Network (OPTN), established under NOTA and funded by Congress. Tissues, on the other hand, have encountered significantly less regulation and are handled largely by a wide array of for-profit national and international firms. Beyond the boundaries of organ transplantation, the reuse of human skin can be crucial to survival for persons who have been severely burned; other tissues are employed regularly for such purposes as dental and orthopedic reconstruction, cornea transplantation, and a wide assortment of cosmetic surgeries. When taken as a whole, the human "body shop" (Andrews and Nelkin 2001; Kimbrell 1993; Nelkin and Andrews 1998; Rothman 1997) shapes a significant portion of high-end millennial medical practice in America.

As Paul Brodwin (2000c) has argued, the intensity of ethical debates surrounding radical biotechnologies is evident in the levels of anxiety they generate, and organ transfer is no exception. Among the strongest ideological underpinnings of transplant medicine is the adamant denial of body commodification. The collective horror Americans share for the utilitarian use of human bodies is apparent in our folklore. Negative associations link the reuse of body parts with Hollywood's original rendering of Frankenstein's monster. A persistent theme within futuristic Anglophone fiction is the routine and frequently clandestine medical or industrial use of human bodies to sustain society and feed individual or corporate greed. Classics include Harry Harrison's *Make Room! Make Room!* (1964; the basis for the film *Soylent Green*, in which the general populace is fed recycled humans without its knowledge); Robin Cook's *Coma* (1977; in which healthy people are drugged and held in comatose states until their organs can be removed for sale); and the darkly comical rendering found in *Monty Python's the Meaning of Life* (wherein procurement officials arrive at a man's home and assert their rights to retrieve his organs while he is still very much alive, all because he has signed his donor card). The corporate preying on the body stands as a symbolic form of necrophagy—or what Youngner has dubbed "nonoral cannibalism"—where a chilling utilitarian ethos drives villains to harvest body parts without guilt (Youngner 1996: 35; for similar language, see Fox 1993; Lindenbaum 2004; Scheper-Hughes 1998b). In these tales only sensitive heroes can still recognize the humanity of captured or discarded souls.

What such fictional stories (and parodies) reveal is that body commodification—especially within the highly celebrated arena of organ transplantation—quickly erodes an already shaky public investment in medical trust. In response to such deep concerns, the transplant industry has generated an elaborate array of powerful euphemistic devices that obscure the commodification of cadaveric donors and their parts.

Precious Things

The most elaborate and pervasive rhetoric involves the shrouding of body commodification in the language of a gift economy. This language is evident in early bureaucratized form in the wording of NOTA, or the 1984 National Organ Transplant Act. Today the language of the gift permeates nearly all discussions of organ transfer, which is defined as a very particular kind of social giving in America. Most important, organs are nearly always described as "gifts of life," a turn of phrase that has long been used within the blood industry (and especially by the American Red Cross) and now in reference to ova donation (Ragoné 1999). Both realms differ from organ transfer in that they are marked by histories of direct agency-to-donor monetary compensation. In the specific context of cadaveric donation, the vast majority of organs are offered by donors' surviving kin to anonymous strangers; procurement specialists help negotiate the transfer of these body parts to surgeons, who will then transplant them in their own ailing patients. Without question, much money is exchanged, but payments made by insurance companies, individual patients, transplant hospitals, and procurement agencies are typically described as covering technical, transportation, and other support services, rather than being linked directly to the cost of the organ itself. An important shared understanding within transplant circles is that taboos surround discussions of the financial worth of organs. Furthermore, strict moral sanctions insist that donor kin should receive no direct payment for a gift offered as an ultimate form of altruistic sacrifice.

Nevertheless, I have seen on rare occasions itemized price sheets for various organs. In one hospital where I conducted research, staff regularly distributed detailed price information directly to potential recipients so that they would know the enormous costs entailed in acquiring a kidney, heart, lung, or liver. Staff saw no reason to be secretive about this. Nevertheless, because such procedures are rare, they emerge as subversive acts. Perhaps more obvious is the fact that a transplant unit defines a tremendously prestigious program for any hospital, both assuming a high community profile and generating significant income for surgeons and for the institution itself. Procurement offices, too, though nonprofit firms, operate on impressive annual budgets dispensed by UNOS. Inherent tension underlying the daily struggle to maintain transplantation's credibility arises from the fact that transplantation is as lucrative as it is medically miraculous. One dominant solution to this conundrum involves the deliberate and ceaseless denial of even the more obvious forms of body commodification.

Cadaveric donation further complicates this configuration. Whereas a vast percentage of kidney transplants in this country involve living pairs of relatives, friends, or colleagues, in nearly all cadaveric cases the donor is an anonymous stranger to the respective set of organ recipients. In those situations where living donor and kidney recipient know one another, both parties understand the kidney as being a special kind of gift to which no monetary value can be assigned.[9] This initial shared understanding eventually may become a source of either increased mutual love or insurmountable conflict. As Renée Fox and Judith Swazey explain, the "tyranny of the gift" springs from the sense that the giving of so precious a thing—a part of oneself—can never be fully reciprocated (1992: 39–42). A different configuration arises in the context of anonymous cadaveric donation, where recipients are generally told only the age of their donors, their family status, the region of the country from which they came, and sometimes their cause of death. Recipients find it difficult to shake the sense that someone else had to die so that they could live, their anxieties exacerbated if they imagine how close kin—typically the donor's spouse, offspring, or parents—must have suffered when faced with the donor's sudden and unexpected death.

As a result, donated cadaveric organs simultaneously emerge as interchangeable parts, as precious gifts, and as harboring the transmigrated souls of the dead. Whereas transplant recipients are encouraged by hospital staff to depersonalize their new organs and speak of them in terms that can sometimes even approximate car repair, procurement staff regularly tell donor kin that transplantation enables the donor's essence to persist in others who are thereby offered a second chance at life. These competing messages offer evidence of what I refer to as a form of *ideological disjunction*, a pervasive characteristic of transplant ideology that inevitably drives professionals to become powerful gatekeepers who work aggressively to prevent communication between recipients and donor kin (Sharp 1994). Whereas these professionals may deliver contradictory messages to different people about the symbolic nature of transplanted organs, all parties are nevertheless united in the revulsion they feel for blatant forms of body commodification.

As Robert Coombs and his colleagues have illustrated, within hospital contexts, and especially in emergency wards, one encounters a rich array of medical slang, where death and dying patients define prominent foci. Indeed, organ transfer generates a specialized category of insider slang: common labels applied to patients include *GPO* (good [for] parts only), *organ donor* (a motorcycle rider or an accident victim with little chance of survival), and *bone* (bone marrow transplant) (Coombs et al. 1993). Within transplant wards and procurement offices, and during celebratory organ transplant events, one encounters an even richer panoply of symbolic expressions that specifically obscure references to death, human suffering, and body commodification. Donors' bodies, for instance, are frequently transformed metaphorically and visually into an array of greenery, including trees and flowers, a set of images that play off the idea that organs are transplanted in or grafted on to new bodies. Context also proves crucial for determining the appropriateness of various terms. For instance, those awaiting transplants are readily referred to as "patients" by all hospital staff, whereas potential donors, whether declared brain dead or not, are rapidly dehumanized. Procurement staff may even correct one another's language if someone refers to potential donors as "patients" or even as living individuals. Donor kin, however, insist on humanizing and personifying their loved ones throughout donation and procurement: personal names are always used, and a label such as "donor" is abhorrent.

Competing forms of euphemistic wordplay also serve to mystify the procurement process. Surgeons frequently employ the expression "organ harvesting," viewing this as an unproblematic way to underscore the act of reaping life to assist others in need. Other professionals, however (and especially those who work with donor kin), are repulsed by this phrase because it offers an all too graphic reference to the physical destruction of the donor body. Agricultural imagery in other forms nevertheless abounds in all domains of organ transfer, marked by what I refer to as the systematic "greening of the body" (Sharp 2001), where even the most basic term *transplantation* inspires images of renewal and rebirth, rather than extraction, death, and decay. Thus, just as nature renews itself, so, too, does the human body, albeit through the assistance of sophisticated medical techniques. In contrast, all parties despise depictions of procurement as the mining of the body for its parts because of the horrific suggestion that this is a profit-making enterprise that preys on the bodies of the dead. Further, such commercial language simultaneously defies the purpose of NOTA, challenges the miraculous quality of body repair, and discredits the selfless love that enables grief-stricken kin to give to anonymous strangers. As we shall see, particularly pronounced is the current (though rapidly eroding) understanding that a precious gift economy drives transplantation's success, because newly acquired body parts enable organ recipients to undergo a radical transformation, often referred to as a "second life" or "rebirth."

Bodies, Persons, and Things

Cadaveric donation inescapably places a heavy emotional toll on all concerned parties because of death's inevitable presence. Recipients, donor kin, and transplant and procurement professionals alike must make sense of transplantation as a lifesaving technique that nevertheless relies on donors' deaths and the surgical removal of their organs. For such epistemological constructions to work, all involved parties must embrace the legitimacy of brain death criteria, for head injury—be it from an auto accident, gunshot wound, or massive cerebral hemorrhage—is the overwhelming cause of organ donors' deaths in this country. Brain death is a relatively new medical construction, stemming initially from recommendations put forth in 1968 by the Ad Hoc Committee at Harvard Medical School (HMS and Beecher 1968; Ramsey 1968). The committee's recommendations shaped national policy and subsequent state-by-state legislation. Today medical historians and ethicists generally agree that the committee's actions were driven by the surgical desire for organ donors. As Stuart Youngner explains, discussions surrounding newly conceived brain death criteria "were quite rational" and were driven by two key factors: "to facilitate organ procurement and . . . to avoid legal concerns about turning off ventilators" (1996: 41).

Today organ transfer remains highly dependent on ventilator use (or what is referred to in other contexts as "life support"), because this now ubiquitous machine enables staff to maintain a donor in physiological stasis before, during, and after brain death is declared. Each breath of air forced into the lungs in turn stimulates the heart, which then sustains other vital organs by supplying them with a steady flow of oxygenated blood. Without the technological assistance of the ventilator, human tissue rapidly deteriorates, rendering the organs useless for transplant. When the body is denied a regular flow of oxygenated blood, a process known as warm ischemia sets in, which threatens the later graft survival of transplanted organs in recipients. Sepsis is yet another constant threat. Without medical intervention, human organs are quickly lost. In the United States various drugs are also administered to facilitate physiological stasis in the donor prior to procurement (Fox, DeVita, and Ritchie 1998; Hogle 1995b). It is important to understand that a (potential) donor remains connected to a ventilator both before and after brain death is declared, while consent is being acquired from kin, and during initial surgery stages, when the donor is anesthetized so that the organs can be removed without the body going into shock. Such practices are considered medically essential, yet they can trigger feelings of great unease among kin and professionals alike, who may struggle to accept brain death criteria as proof of absolute death (Sanner 1994; Sharp 2001; Youngner et al. 1989).

Within this ideological framework, the maintenance of brain dead donors is carefully orchestrated by a range of health professionals whose actions radically transform the organ donor into an extraordinary category of person. It is accepted as medical fact that brain dead patients will never regain consciousness, unlike cases involving patients who are comatose or in persistent vegetative states (Kaufman 2000, 2005). Further, because their level of brain damage is so severe, organ donors lack personhood as it is understood and valued in this culture; that is, brain dead patients have irretrievably lost their subjectivity and thus can no longer assert themselves in social contexts. This construction of personhood rests firmly on the medicalized assumption that the self is lodged in the brain: with severe and irreversible head trauma, we cease to be who we are, we are no longer human, and thus we cease to exist. The brain dead donor, then, is but a human shell, a body that functions physiologically but no longer thinks or senses the surrounding world. By medicolegal definition these donors are dead: whereas the ventilated brain-dead body appears to be alive to lay parties and health professionals alike, each breath taken is technologically dependent. The bodies of such donors maintain their natural coloring and remain warm to the touch, and they may even manifest what are understood as involuntary movements that result from residual nervous system activity. Such contradictions render them inherently strange.

Transplantable organs, too, are peculiar things. Because of their unusual origins, they are steeped in elaborate symbolic imagery. Their preciousness may lead to a displacement of the donor-as-person, once medical (or certainly procurement) attention is riveted on retrieving organs in time to save dying patients elsewhere. It is no wonder, then, that even after more than half a century of practice, organ transfer continues to be described simultaneously as a remarkable medical miracle, the giving of life, a legalized form of body commodification, and a medical process circumscribed by an unusual form of death.

Scarcity Anxiety

One of the great ironies of organ transfer is that its remarkable technological success has engendered a national crisis of supply and demand. Because the surgical transfer of organs strikes us as unmistakably wondrous, it has produced an ever-growing need for new surgical techniques, pharmaceuticals, and clinical subspecialties that then further perfect the medical ability to sustain life in this way. The intense desire to prolong life and cure disease has spawned as well an ever-increasing national list of patients for whom transplantation is deemed a basic medical right. Today the national list is an urgent topic of debate: heated discussions are spurred on by fears associated with the assumed shortage of transplantable organs and, thus, the dire need to increase the supply of willing donors. For more than a decade I have watched how proposals designed to enhance donation have shifted from casual, what-if scenarios to a pronounced level of alarm and even desperation. Thus, although concerns over supply and demand have always pervaded transplantation, the intensity of organ scarcity anxiety is new.

Significantly, much attention is given to the growing number of patients in need, set against either an assumed leveling or, at most, a sluggish climb in the annual number of donors. The urgency expressed in a recent story from the *Boston Globe* typifies current phrasing (the data and wording nearly always supplied by UNOS):

> The waiting list for organs, now at about 82,000 people, keeps growing, and nothing has succeeded in significantly increasing the number of donations. Almost 60 percent of those on the list are expected to die waiting. . . . The transplant community has tried various initiatives. . . . But the gap keeps growing. Overall, the waiting list has been increasing by about 12 percent a year, while the number of brain-dead donors has been rising by under 3 percent, to about 6,000 a year. A recent study estimated that the number of potential donors each year is about 17,000. (Goldberg 2003)

The UNOS Web page has at times displayed a clock alongside an up-to-date report on the number of candidates on the national waiting list, recorded to the minute, stressing, too, that "for each person who receives a transplant, two more are added to that list."[10] As these examples illustrate, scarcity anxiety is focused squarely on the short supply of organs as transplant's great dilemma. In contrast, little is said about the responsibility the transplant industry bears in generating its own patients, a process that in turn increases the national demand for organs. Transplantation is in essence the capitalist's dream because the supply can never answer the pressing and ever-increasing social desire for these coveted goods.

When I first entered this field of research in 1991, innovative proposals designed to stave off the organ shortage were generally dismissed because they defied dominant assertions that linked bodily integrity to a respect for the dead. In short, professionals collectively expressed open disgust for blatant forms of body commodification, a stance guided in large part by the medical imperative to do no harm. Today, all involved parties embrace the need for ever more diligent public education campaigns; nevertheless, within the last five years financial incentives have surfaced as the most popularly proposed solutions. The momentum of this approach is evident in recent policy statements issued by the American Medical Association (AMA), which, in partnership with UNOS, now advocates investigating the viability of financial reward programs. Proposals include offering to donor kin a maximum ten-thousand-dollar tax credit, a funeral expense supplement, a charitable donation credit, direct payment, or a donor family medal of honor.[11] A dominant assumption today, then, is that Americans will respond more quickly to monetary rewards than to more basic requests of altruism. Such proposals nevertheless require delicate semantic massaging (Richardson 1996) for fear that financial incentives will be interpreted as offering direct payment for human organs.

A decade later, these proposals have advanced to an entirely new level of understanding and debate, illustrated by recent testimony delivered by the AMA before the House Energy and Commerce Subcommittee (AMA 2003). Some of these new policy initiatives have moved to the pilot phase of experimentation. The state of Pennsylvania (which houses several of the nation's most prestigious transplant centers) provides a case in point. Its State Act 102, which became effective in March 1995, was initiated under the late governor Robert Casey, who himself was a liver and heart recipient. This legislation offers a comprehensive approach to public outreach and donor motivation, strategies that other states and federal agencies have duplicated. An earlier and controversial component proposed offering partial financial assistance to donor kin for funeral costs (Nathan 2000). Although this section of the act failed to win full support in the legislature, it evolved at one point into a proposal for a three-year pilot project designed to test the effectiveness of three thousand dollars in funeral assistance to donor kin.[12] This sort of cash payment remains a highly experimental strategy (and one that to date has failed to evolve into official practice); this proposed component of Act 102 nevertheless marks an important watershed in policy responses to organ scarcity anxiety. More recently, Wisconsin passed legislation that reimburses living donors for travel expenses and lost wages, an example other states are certain to follow.

States have tried a variety of other approaches to increase organ donation within their own borders. Many currently use donor card campaigns as a means to raise donor awareness; the most common strategy entails offering this card when residents register for or renew a driver's license. This approach targets especially the nation's youth, thus capturing the attention of the very segment of the population that defines the ideal donor category. More specifically, these are young people whose organs are free from diseases associated with advanced age, and for whom the incidence of deaths from automobile, motorcycle, and bicycle accidents is particularly high (such accidents often result in head traumas and, thus, potentially, brain death).[13] What most Americans fail to realize, however, is that the donor card has long served merely as a reflection of a desire, not the promise, to donate, for it is surviving kin who ultimately decide whether or not a loved one's organs will be offered for transplantation. In response, recently many states have also passed legislation that transforms the donor card into an advanced directive so that procurement staff can legally override the desires of surviving kin. Also, nearly all states have long-established laws that require hospital personnel to report all cases of potential brain death to their local procurement offices (but enforcing these laws is another matter entirely). In such instances, health care workers may fail to comply because they are unaware of the law, they do not embrace the definition of brain death, or they are too deeply disturbed by the idea of shifting their attention from keeping a patient alive to monitoring the physiological status of a brain dead donor.

In response to these sorts of limitations, some reformers now advocate for presumed consent laws: such legislation means that unless one has registered one's opposition to organ donation, one can be categorized automatically by hospital personnel as a donor, thus bypassing the objections of kin (AMA Council on Ethical and Judicial Affairs 1994; C. Cohen 1992). As evidence of the great potential of presumed consent, advocates point to Spain, where this approach is believed to have altered radically the size of the nation's donor pool.[14] As the foregoing discussion makes clear, however, the United States presents significant barriers to such reforms, perhaps the most significant being that, unlike a country with socialized medical care, each of the fifty states passes its own legislation relevant to donor registration and brain death criteria. Thus, one can become an organ donor more rapidly in Pennsylvania (which houses several of the nation's largest transplant centers and among the most active organ procurement organizations [OPOs]) than in, say, Idaho (a predominantly rural state far less involved in organ transfer).[15]

A more mundane approach—mundane because it has required no specific legislation to bring it into effect—involves a loosening of medical criteria that allow a larger pool of dying hospitalized patients to qualify for donor status. In the context of my own research I have watched how procurement staff have shifted various medicalized boundaries so that those who might have been excluded ten years ago are now considered viable candidates for donation. For instance, in the early 1990s brain dead patients greater than seventy years of age were categorized as too old to donate, their organs considered too spent for safe reuse.[16] A commonsense approach dictated, too, that it would be unfair to transplant into an already chronically ill person an old and thus inferior organ. By 1995, however, procurement professionals had begun to take aged donors more seriously, the argument being that an old organ was better than none at all. As Gretchen Reynolds explains, an ever-increasing demand for organs "has led transplant specialists to quietly begin to relax the standards of who can donate . . . [such that] the transplanting of what doctors refer to as 'marginal' or 'extended criteria' organs, organs that once would have been considered unusable, has increased considerably in the last several years" (2005: 38). Formerly, prisoners, for instance, were automatically excluded because of fears of incipient HIV and hepatitis infections, yet by the mid-1990s I witnessed discussions of their viability as donors, and the procurement staff whom I observed had begun to make special efforts to collect reliable social and medical histories on some dying prisoners. The new value placed on prisoners' bodies has been extended in turn to include arguments that those willing to donate kidneys might then receive shortened sentences or death-row clemency as a reward for this act of goodwill (Ayres 1998; Bartz 2003; Bell 1998; Guttmann 1992; cf. Waldby 2000).

An even more unsettling intervention within the realm of organ transfer involves a recent, albeit still limited, shift to obtaining organs from what are referred to as "non-heartbeating cadavers" or "non-heartbeating donors" (NHBDs), and the procedure itself as "donation after cardiac death" (DCD).[17] This protocol, which has expanded the boundaries of death, concerns specifically those patients who are maintained on ventilators yet who fall outside the criteria for brain death, their failing health instead indicating signs of imminent cardiac arrest. Their potential donor status is dependent on there being a do not resuscitate (DNR) order entered in their medical chart. At the moment the heart stops beating (either on its own or after the patient is disconnected from a ventilator), medical staff make no attempt to restimulate it but, rather, rapidly prepare the patient-turned-donor for the surgical removal of his or her organs (DuBois 1999; Greenberg 2001; Institute of Medicine 1997). One of the most publicized cases to date involved fourteen-year-old Nicholas Breach, a child under the care of staff at Children's Hospital in Philadelphia, who suffered from an inoperable brain tumor and had declared his desire to be an organ donor. As Nick's family explained to a reporter for the *New Yorker*, in order for Nick "to become a donor, it was not enough for their son to die with his body more or less intact. He would have to have the right kind of death, with the systems in his body shutting down in a particular order" (Greenberg 2001: 36). The understanding was that his ultimate demise had to be carefully orchestrated if his organs were to remain viable for transplantation. During his final days at home, Nick's parents kept a death watch over him; when he stopped breathing, they initiated cardiopulmonary resuscitation (CPR) to maintain their son in a condition that would then allow hospital staff to deliver him to surgery. (Their efforts failed, however, and so only Nick's corneas could be retrieved; Greenberg 2003.) This procedure is moving rapidly from the experimental to the routine. As noted by Renée Fox, this unsettling approach to organ retrieval can transform the dying patient prematurely into a source of transplantable parts (Fox 1993; Fox, DeVita, and Ritchie 1998; cf. Lynn

1993). This new protocol also raises serious questions about the role that health care providers should play in facilitating death versus prolonging a patient's life (not to mention the ethical problems associated with slotting minors to NHBD status). Ultimately, this new protocol runs great risk of eroding an already shaky public trust in hospital care in this country.

Final examples of responses to scarcity anxiety involve new forms of medical research and experimentation. These ultimately rely on new hybrids of the human body that extend well beyond allotransplantation, or the melding of human-to-human bodies and parts. Briefly, these sorts of hybrids include the development of mechanical and organic alternatives, which could either help bridge the gap while patients await organs of human origin or sidestep the human organ donor entirely. Among the most celebrated examples is the development of several models of mechanical heart, including the Jarvik-7 in the 1980s and, currently, the AbioCor and other recent total artificial heart (TAH) prototypes (ABC 1996; Gil 1989; Hamilton 2001; Plough 1986; Rowland 2001). Currently such devices ensure only very short-term success rates for patients who, as little more than human guinea pigs, inevitably die from a cascading set of serious medical complications. In short, at present medical science is unable to duplicate the long-term workings of our sophisticated organs. Implantable devices that help drive a failing heart, most notably left ventricular assist devices (LVADs) currently bear more promise. Yet another highly experimental domain of research is the realm of xenotransplantation, or the creation of hybrid animal species (especially simian and porcine) that bear human genetic material and might one day define a source of organs for human use. The obstacles to creating such viable designer creatures are immense, and the research is plagued by the immunological dangers associated with cross-species infection. Such dangers have defined a focus for heated debates within this country and even more so in England (Bach, Ivinson, and Weeramantry 2001; Birmingham 1999; Butler 1999a, 1999b; Clark 1999; Vanderpool 1999). Nevertheless, within the transplant community, experimental mechanical and organic alternatives are imagined as potentially viable—and highly profitable—solutions to the current scarcity of organs (Maeder and Ross 2002). The desire for alternatives that would eliminate the problem of organ scarcity is so strong in some professional quarters that discussions may skirt ethical and other inherent dangers associated with radical proposals.

Natural and Denatured Bodies

As noted earlier, the miracle of organ transfer rests largely on surgical prowess and technological sophistication. In this sense, the range of medical expertise associated with the retrieval, preservation, and replacement of human organs represents the zenith of biomedical accomplishment in a nation that celebrates biotechnological solutions to human health problems. When framed by this dominant cultural ethos, the transfer of human parts between disparate bodies is conceived of as a natural progression within medicine. A new, experimental procedure may quickly become routine, spreading in practice from one surgeon or hospital unit to others throughout the country (and beyond) once described in published form or demonstrated with slides and videos at professional conferences.

If innovation defines a natural progression of knowledge and technique in transplant medicine, then the bodies of organ donors and transplant recipients become naturalized through this process, too. Much is made over this phenomenon within the realm of organ transfer, and this understanding is expressed through several rhetorical forms. Common assertions are that there is nothing odd, strange, or unnatural about organ transfer as a sociomedical process; nor in the ways that organs are retrieved from the dead; nor even in the fact that a surgeon can remove a patient's heart, support the body temporarily on a bypass device, and then restart a new heart once it has been properly implanted in the patient's chest (and all this without killing the patient in the process).

From the point of view of a range of lay parties—and even among recipients—the medical miracle of organ transfer is a strange act indeed. The strange and unnatural qualities of organ transfer together define a troublesome and seemingly unstoppable undercurrent. Most pronounced is the sense that the recipient body is a hybrid one because its viability as a living organism relies on its being made up of parts from at least two human beings. In contrast, a widespread understanding within anthropology and other social sciences is that hybridization is part and parcel of human existence, especially within postindustrial contexts. As Van Wolputte explains, "We are all Creoles of sorts: hybrid, divided, polyphonic, and parodic—a pastiche of our Selves. The contemporary body-self is fragmentary, often incoherent and inconsistent, precisely because it arises from contradictory and paradoxical experiences, social tensions, and conflicts" (2004: 263; cf. Haraway 1989, 1991; Latour 1993). Within the highly medicalized realm of organ transfer, however, talk of a multiple, disparate, or fragmented self is evidence of pathological thinking and requires therapeutic intervention. Lurking in the darker corners, it seems, is the specter of Frankenstein's monster (J. Cohen 1996; Shildrick 2002). Transplant recipients who openly express the sense that another person dwells within them may well acquire medical labels that draw on monstrous imagery, such as "Frankenstein syndrome"

(Beidel 1987; Rollin 1995). In an effort to quell the potential unease associated with the hybrid body, transplant professionals regularly describe body parts as inert objects. In this way, the surgeon's craft centers on the repair of a complex and fragile *machine*. Further, when members of the lay public express unease or more blatant distaste for organ transfer, such sentiments are considered evidence of superstitious or misguided religious thoughts that can be redirected especially by procurement staff through aggressive public education campaigns.

Regardless of this professional stance, both organ recipients and donor kin regularly consider and even embrace the idea that the recipient body is a hybrid one. Although their opinions are generally voiced out of earshot of professionals, many recipients understand their new lives as dependent on the workings of parts derived from others. In this sense, both the dead donor and once ailing recipient are rejuvenated through the melding of their bodies. Donor kin may similarly embrace this idea, understanding the deceased donor as living on in the bodies of recipients. At work here, then, is an altogether different idea of the composite human form, now redefined as a gestalt composed of once disparate human parts. Such responses, rather than being pathological, naturalize the recipient body in an altogether different sense. In essence, by "embodying the monster" (Shildrick 2002), an action so feared in professional circles, organ recipients naturalize hybridity.

A key component of this process of naturalization is the manner in which numerous donor kin and recipients seek out each other, transforming one another from anonymous strangers to intimate friends and even kin. Socialization in this sense similarly defies dominant professional premises that assert that transplanted organs are inert and, thus, denaturalized parts incapable of harboring traces of their once human origins. This resocialization of the deceased donor (now understood as an integral part of the living recipient) also flies in the face of the seemingly inevitable commodification of bodies-as-parts within the transplant industry. Transplanted organs are perceived instead as fragments of beloved individuals who live on within and grant new life to others.

The Corporate Body

A final premise crucial to this study involves professional concerns over the corporate restructuring of organ transfer. This shift characterizes medicine more generally in the United States, yet, as described earlier, in the realm of organ transfer it is driven especially by anxieties over organ scarcity. Amid this shift, involved professionals may express distress over changing labor requirements and the restructuring of the workplace itself. As one longtime procurement professional lamented, her agency began twenty years ago as a mere "shoe box operation," where a small collective of employees worked elbow to elbow in a cramped, one-room office, sharing all duties. Today this same agency is housed in an impressive suite with a large and highly specialized staff who are divided into a range of divisions. Such developments are hardly confined to the transplant industry: Lorna Rhodes (1991), for instance, recorded similar sentiments among mental health care specialists who began as community activists working the streets on foot or from the back of a van.

Of special concern to transplant and procurement professionals is the constant demand from superiors to increase the number of successful outcomes. A team of transplant surgeons can qualify for transplant unit status under hospital and UNOS guidelines only by performing a minimum number of surgeries per year; even greater numbers are required to merit additional funds and staffing necessary for experimental research. Throughout the nation, hospitals proclaim their success through the actual number of transplant surgeries they perform, and certain organs, such as hearts and livers, bear more cultural capital than do others, such as kidneys. Procurement specialists in turn are under great pressure to increase their number of successful donations. It is not enough, however, simply to identify donors or acquire consent; only the actual number of organs transplanted in the end matters. As frustrated procurement staff explain, how can they predetermine the quantity of organs they acquire when the supply is beyond their control? Such demands inevitably facilitate the rapid dehumanization of patients and undermine staff morale. Under the worst circumstances, sloppy work or employee corruption may result.[18]

Such developments clearly generate serious dilemmas. As organ transplantation shifts to the corporate model, organ transfer is driven increasingly by market forces that discourage health professionals' compassionate and courageous acts. This in turn affects the social value of the *potential* donor, who may be transformed even more rapidly from a dying patient to a body capable of supplying society with highly coveted, reusable parts.

The Paradoxical Premises of Organ Transfer

In the preceding discussion, I do not mean to imply that the world of organ transfer is jaded and callous. Without exception, all participants who have assisted me with my research care deeply about the well-being of hospitalized patients, regardless of whether they are potential donors or organ recipients. Nevertheless, as transplant and procurement professionals succumb to demands for more donations, they risk undermining even further an already shaky public trust in American medical practices. Organ transfer is especially vulnerable because it must always struggle against public perceptions that this highly specialized branch of medicine preys on the bodies of dying patients. Nevertheless, the current demands associated with organ transfer may drive professionals to overlook the moral dangers of their work. To underscore the complexity of such dangers, I wish to conclude with a review of how the paradoxes just described intersect with one another and define an ethos inherent in organ transfer in America, one that guides the thoughts and actions of both professional and lay participants.

For half a century, although transplant medicine has borne the aura of the miraculous, its success has been dependent on a highly technocratic approach to healing. As noted, transplantation is driven by increasingly sophisticated diagnostic, surgical, pharmaceutical, and ultimately life-sustaining technologies that potentially dehumanize both transplant patients and potential donors as little more than medicalized cyborgs. From a purely utilitarian perspective, transplant medicine is extraordinarily expensive by virtue of its technological dependency. Although veiled in a complex array of euphemistic constructions, organ transfer and, in turn, the donor body are sites of lucrative medical practices sustained by an ever-expanding demand for technological expertise.

Set against this "technological imperative" (Davis-Floyd 1994) of transplant medicine, the donor body emerges as a site mired in contradictions. Among the most troubling is the denial of the dehumanizing force of organ transfer. Whereas a host of tissues is readily bought and sold, long-standing legislation, spearheaded by the National Organ Transplant Act of 1984, renders it illegal specifically to market transplantable organs. In response, organ transfer relies heavily on euphemistic terms that deny body commodification: organs are not bought or sold but donated; through transactions steeped in the language of a gift economy, organs are gifts offered to needy patients through great acts of kindness by anonymous Samaritans. Nevertheless, transplant patients (or, most frequently, their insurers) pay enormous sums for their surgeries; and procurement offices, though nonprofit in status, are hardly driven by volunteer labor. The symbolic rhetoric of organ transfer insists that transplantable human organs are extraordinarily precious things, yet their value is understood in radically different ways by different categories of involved parties. Whereas official rhetoric insists that organs are gifts of life, some still consider them as little more than replaceable parts, and others view them as harboring the lost souls of the dead. This array of competing constructions arises in response to the contradictory messages professionals supply to recipients versus donor kin. This ultimately leads professionals to block communication between these two sets of parties because their encounters would uncover the depth of ideological disjunction intrinsic to their work.

An even more troubling aspect of organ transfer's ideological underpinnings involves the necessity of embracing brain death criteria as evidence of absolute death. Organ transfer as a medical reality is bolstered by life-sustaining technologies, for without the respiratory ventilator, for instance, hospital and procurement staff could not maintain potential donors prior to and during the surgical removal of their organs. All involved parties must accept that these donor-patients are dead, even though they are warm to the touch, breathe (albeit with technological assistance), and can move. As we shall see, publicly expressed acceptance among all sets of involved parties may be contradicted by their more private musings over brain death criteria.

The growing anxiety over organ scarcity problematizes the assumed miraculous qualities of this unusual gift economy of death. As noted, responses now under serious consideration call largely for financial incentives for organ donation, a development that only further commodifies organs and the donor body, reducing these "precious things" to little more than coveted goods that can be acquired for a price from surviving kin. This bald-faced approach threatens the very stability of the gift economy, the linchpin of organ transfer's success to date. Other radical solutions undermine the sanctity of the medical imperative to do no harm through the NHBD protocol, or through radical forms of mechanical and xenographic experimentation. In essence, then, the miracle of transplantation may quickly dissolve into a dollar-driven medical nightmare.

Finally, the ever-increasing corporate structure of organ transfer—driven by the pairing of medical success and organ scarcity anxiety—marks the further dehumanization of its practices. Procurement and transplant professionals alike express deep frustration over demands from their superiors that they acquire, transfer, and transplant more organs every year. In some centers, staff are now confronted with monthly and annual quotas, and their inability to meet these puts their own jobs at risk. Of even greater concern are the dangers associated with corporate greed: one need only consider the science fiction tales that loom in the collective American consciousness to grasp the tenuousness of public faith in organ transfer as a medical miracle.

Anthropology and Bioethics

Against this set of paradoxical premises and accompanying anxieties, bioethicists provide an important and growing set of critical voices. Of particular interest to me is the manner in which their own critiques have shifted over the course of the last decade in tandem with growing concerns in transplant medicine. Commentaries in the early 1990s frequently bore the tone of the playful gadfly, notably expressed, for instance, in Arthur Caplan's book title *If I Were a Rich Man Could I Buy a Pancreas?* (1992). Most ethicists assumed a relativist stance, seeking primarily to expose conflicts inherent in competing positions, thus encouraging open debate among involved parties. Yet another dominant approach involved labeling or categorizing various arguments: for instance, ethicists deliberated whether calls for further commodification fit utilitarian or patient autonomy paradigms. Within the past three or so years, however, I have observed that ethicists have become more brazen in their critiques, a shift generated in large part by current proposals that so blatantly commodify the body. Thus, Caplan himself is quoted in the *Wall Street Journal* as stating that the market demand in human body parts "has created a kind of eBay of the body."[19] Likewise, Jeffrey Kahn acknowledges that the euphemistic language of organ transfer is merely "a semantic difference. . . . What's really being sold isn't the time and energy, but the material itself" (Saranow 2003).

In response, bioethicists and anthropologists can form a compelling partnership; of special interest to me are the moments of disjunction exposed by a merging of ethical and ethnographic thinking.[20] As anthropologists have long known, human actions and words may defy what a society's members claim to do or what they embrace as cultural truths. In the medical realm of transplantation, this is especially evident in the language employed in public versus private venues for speaking about reusable organs, death, and donors' bodies. The ultimate questions generated by such disjunction are: What are the perceived (and hidden) ethical ramifications of transplant's technocratic miracle? Of the reworking of the donor body? Of the denial of body commodification? Of redefinitions of death? Of the unending demands placed on involved professionals in response to anxieties over organ scarcity? As I shall illustrate throughout this book, these questions bear heavily on the medical imperative to prevent physical suffering, prolong life, and preserve the sanctity of the body when working against the demands of technocratic and capitalist medical practices (Davis-Floyd 1994; Davis-Floyd and St. John 1998; Lock, Young, and Cambrosio 2000; Zola 1978). Organ transfer is guided by its own particular ethos, within which the most troubling elements involve an ever-increasing desire for human body parts. As transplant medicine embraces more blatant forms of body commodification, it risks permanent association in the public mind with avaricious corporate willingness to plunder the helpless bodies of the dead and dying.

STUDYING TRANSPLANTATION IN AMERICAN CONTEXTS

Such imagined national horrors are of anthropological interest because they uncover a public uncertainty about the legitimacy of cadaveric donation policies.[21] Anthropological analysis offers a means for sorting out the imagined from the very real possibilities that characterize this astonishing realm of medicine. Following Brodwin (2000c), I argue that those regions marked by the most pronounced anxieties often generate the richest data—precisely because they are so problematic.

A study of transplantation in America is facilitated by the fact that nearly everyone within our society has an opinion on it; further, such opinions are frequently marked by conflicting ideas about its relevance, viability, and social worth. For instance, most people support the premise that no one should have to suffer or die prematurely, and we regularly embrace the assumption that a primary role of biomedicine is to alleviate pain, prolong the joy of life, and stave off death whenever possible. But what if solutions require intense medical scrutiny, prolonged hospitalization, a medically orchestrated death, the fragmentation of the human body, or someone else's demise so that another can live? There are no clear-cut answers to which all involved parties agree. It is for these reasons that I, as a medical anthropologist, have been drawn to this arena of research for the last decade and a half.

Set against the peculiar paradoxes I describe here, my remarks run the risk of being perceived as a condemnation of organ transfer by those most intimately associated with this medical realm. This is far from my intent: rather, I argue as a social scientist with the goal of constructive critique. As asserted earlier, the methodologies of the anthropological enterprise offer ways to question and thus reexamine what is taken for granted within a social group about legitimate forms of thought, belief, and action. How, then, might we step back and consider the relevance of what is left unsaid? In response to my work, others occasionally ask me why I oppose transplantation (a question that always startles me). Such questioning merely exposes my failure to communicate the full complexity of the topic at hand. Organ transfer is clearly beneficial, its technological accomplishments saving and sustaining an inordinate number of lives in the United States. Many people I have met through this research would be long dead were it not for transplantation; thus, on a more visceral level, a condemnation of organ transfer would mean that individuals whom I cherish would no longer walk this earth. Thoughts of, for instance, a moratorium on transplantation, or an active campaign to discourage procurement, disturb me deeply.

My long-term fascination with transplantation's possibilities drove me initially to explore this research subject. As a child I was captivated by a televised broadcast about Christiaan Barnard's attempt to transplant a human heart in 1967, which was rendered all the more moving—and surreal—on our family's color television, acquired by my father. The broadcast in living color of this event, as well as other televised surgeries (I recall another riveting program on an eye operation) confirmed the brilliance of my father's seemingly extravagant purchase once and for all. Similarly, for many years I coveted our family's copy of *Life* magazine that contained a photographic essay on Barnard (*Life* 1967); when it was lost in one of the many moves that marked my childhood, I never ceased to long for a duplicate (which I subsequently acquired). Throughout my childhood my parents supplied me with a steady flow of transparent model kits of various bodies with removable parts. I painstakingly constructed and painted a "Visible Man" and "Visible Woman" (the latter could become instantly pregnant if so desired), a skeleton, a horse, and a human eyeball, displaying these together on a single shelf in my bedroom. I imagined myself one day occupying the glorified role of a surgeon who might indeed follow in Barnard's footsteps.[22] Thus, the inner workings of the human body were familiar to me well before the age of ten, feeding my profound respect for an acclaimed surgeon who clearly knew it so intimately (cf. Selzer 1974). Although my interests later shifted away from physiology to the mode of social critique intrinsic to the anthropological enterprise, I have nevertheless maintained a profound interest in the human body, a focus central to my training as a medical anthropologist. It thus troubles me to read retroactive assaults on Barnard's professional character (Scheper-Hughes 1998a), or accounts that fail to question the preposterousness of some reports of body snatching (for impressive treatments of such folklore, see Campion-Vincent 1992, 1997). As I have learned through my own research efforts, biomedicine in the United States is indisputably experimental, invasive, and technocratic, with transplantation merely offering an especially high-profile example.

Writing about Transplantation in America

There is no paucity of material on transplantation in the United States. So much has been published, in fact, that one can now speak of particular genres of style, or dominant narrative forms. These include strictly clinical treatments of organ function and patient survival outcomes; personal histories and journalistic patient biographies; and a burgeoning literature in the social sciences, initiated several decades ago by sociologists Renée Fox and Judith Swazey. My own agenda differs from the existing literature in several ways. As explained in the opening of this introduction, I draw heavily on the ethnographic method, my research to date spanning fifteen years (1991–2006) of work linking the three interdependent realms of organ transfer. My presentation is framed specifically by a set of paradoxical premises outlined here that hamper the ongoing success of transplant medicine. Such a focus facilitates a deep questioning of the often hidden assumptions that drive organ transfer, allowing in turn for a critical analysis of a range of interrelated symbolic, philosophical, and ethical constructions. The remainder of this book is composed of four essays, each of which focuses on an unusual, and thus remarkable, set of social relationships between donor kin and organ recipients that arise specifically in response to the presence (or absence) of the cadaveric organ donor.

These strangely original social responses to donors' deaths and their transferable body parts are rarely described in the literature precisely because, as I will argue, they are considered pathological or they defy the premises underlying transplant ideology and associated rules of daily decorum. In other words, acknowledging social relationships between donor kin and organ recipients as legitimate would require questioning the very foundation on which organ transfer rests in this country. In preview, I will offer a few brief examples. For instance, organ recipients are dissuaded consistently from thinking of their transplanted organs as being anything more than bits of flesh and blood. At times their organs are even described as if they were replaceable mechanical parts, in an effort to dehumanize their origins. In addition, transplant professionals often tell organ recipients that their thoughts should not dwell on their organ donors; for this reason recipients are given only minimal information about their donors' backgrounds. Recipients nevertheless regularly defy these directives, identifying psychologically in a host of creative ways with their imagined anonymous donors, integrating them into their newly formed sense of posttransplant self. Organ kin in turn are persuaded to donate the organs of lost loved ones through careful counseling from procurement professionals who emphasize the finality of brain death. Procurement staff may also promote the contradictory message that donors can live on in the bodies of others, a construction widely embraced by donor kin long after donation has occurred. Such contradictory messages have a profound effect on how donor kin grieve lost donors: as I will argue, the construction of the transmigrated donor soul can initiate a period of ceaseless mourning.

As they enter the world of organ transfer, members of each of these involved categories of participants are bound by a sanctioned set of behaviors; they nevertheless regularly defy associated taboos. Communication between donor kin and organ recipients still stands as among the most subversive acts, although efforts to restrict encounters are eroding. Many people now attempt to locate one another: recipients are driven by the desire to encounter the families that saved their lives, while surviving donor kin long to track the destinations of their lost loved ones, whose essences are embodied in transplanted body parts. An extraordinary array of complex—and frequently long-term—relationships are established as a result of these encounters. Whereas these relationships may seem strange and unsettling to the uninitiated, within the realm of organ transfer they are natural responses to an extraordinary form of death, to the medical ability to revive human life, and to the fact that organ transfer is about sharing hidden parts of oneself with a community of anonymous strangers.

A Comparative Approach to Organ Transfer: Field, Methods, Scope

A sociocultural and medical anthropologist by training, I am wed to ethnographic approaches to data collection, those that, more specifically, frequently demand long-term immersion in a cultural milieu. My earlier anthropological projects, set within a radically different context in tropical Africa, focused on aspects of suffering and healing in a cosmopolitan migrant community in Madagascar (Sharp 1993, 2002c). Although some readers may be troubled by the disruption such a reference generates, my work in Madagascar has proved essential to much of my thinking about organ transfer in the United States. Anthropology is by definition a comparative science, the discipline driven by the assumption that one may glean more of a given culture through comparison with others. Thus, my knowledge of healing in Madagascar has been enriched by medical anthropological studies set elsewhere. Likewise, cultural bases of health and suffering that are peculiar to Madagascar throw American assumptions into high relief. Among the most striking are Malagasy people's beliefs about death, for this is an island known for its elaborate mortuary rituals. I have long remarked that anyone who conducts anthropological research on this island is destined to write about death, for the majority of Malagasy devote great emotional and financial attention to determining where their bodies will be placed once they die (Bloch 1971; Feeley-Harnik 1984, 1991; cf. Evers 2002).

Personal concerns—as well as research set in other cultures—may well shape the thrust of an ethnographic investigation, where encounters in one context "bleed" into another (cf. Rapp 2000: 1). As Rayna Rapp comments, "The boundaries between self and other, or more properly, several selves . . . are inherently blurry. Beyond the rich research materials generated" by the requirements of a specific project "lies another realm of informant collection . . . that I would describe as 'serendipitous' or 'karmic'" (2000: 14). This most certainly has been my experience during this extraordinary journey within the realm of organ transfer. The greatest inspiration for this work in fact springs from an event that occurred one night when I was in Madagascar: I had been invited to dinner by my dear friend Dr. Annie so that I might visit with her father, the historian Raherisoanjato Daniel (Papan'i'Annie). Papan'i'Annie, a senior among his Betsileo kin, is a marvelous storyteller whose gift for gab in quotidian circumstances transforms him into a legendary orator in ritualized contexts.[23] Midway through this family meal I left for the kitchen to bring out more food; when I returned, Papan'i'Annie was sitting before a captivated audience, recounting a grisly tale of body snatching set in the United States. I found that I could not hold my tongue, and I seized the first opportunity to insist that such things did not occur in my homeland. In response, everyone at the table fell silent, but then Annie, in her wonderful way, burst out laughing, patted me on the arm, and explained that her father was simply recounting one of his favorite science fiction stories.

Papan'i'Annie's tale inevitably stimulated my own thinking on the subject. At the time, my work in Madagascar focused on the symbolics of the body and local understandings of commoner and royal death. I knew of Malagasy fears of heart- and blood-thieves (*mpaka-fo, mpaka-raha*) and their deadly association with sorcery practices, and, as a result of conversations with Annie and a host of other Malagasy health professionals, I perceived how impossible national blood drives could be on this island, because doctors would quickly be viewed as having nefarious goals in mind (cf. White 2000). I pondered this stance from a comparative perspective, making note of its possible relevance for a future research project set within the United States. Later, while writing my dissertation in California, I had the great fortune of being able to work as a research assistant to Margaret Clark, who was writing about the ethics of transplantation from an anthropological perspective (Clark 1993, 1999). This experience roused my curiosity even further.

My opportunity to explore questions of organ transplantation arose during my first teaching position in Indianapolis, where in 1990 I joined the staff of a small urban-based university as its first full-time anthropologist. I had spent my high school years in a small midwestern town, and so I knew that international travel would be a rare experience for most of the young people whom I would teach. In fact, the majority of my students had never ventured beyond the state's boundaries; as a result, my tales of Madagascar were outrageously exotic, and thus I sought to illustrate to them (and to some of my colleagues) that anthropology could be practiced in one's own backyard. I had read that Indianapolis was an important regional transplant center, and preliminary probing uncovered the fact that no fewer than four separate hospitals in this city of approximately one million had transplant units. (A few years later the number would shrink as hospital centers consolidated.) Taking my chances, I made an appointment to speak with a transplant social worker based at one of the city's largest units. By the end of the month, I had worked my way through a hierarchy of specialists whose consistently warm welcome quickly enabled me to become a participant observer on their ward. This marked the beginning of a truly remarkable journey.

Ethnographic research is heavily qualitative in its approach, and thus the bulk of the data reported here is generated from one-on-one, open-ended interviewing techniques and through participant observation in a host of settings. Such work is complemented by additional data collected through group interviews, survey work, and archival research. Interviews themselves have targeted all three domains of organ transfer and have involved thousands of hours spent with transplant surgeons, neurologists, transplant nurses, social workers, and hospital chaplains; organ recipients and their kin; the surviving kin of organ donors; organ procurement specialists; public relations staff who promote organ donation; mortuary technicians; medical ethicists; and research scientists involved in experimental research.

My research on organ transfer falls into four phases of activity. The first phase (1991–94) focused on transplantation, the most popularly researched—as well as most accessible—domain (Sharp 1994). This work was based primarily in a major transplant hospital in the Midwest whose unit performed kidney, heart, lung, and liver transplants. The bulk of my time was spent in the company of organ recipients, patients awaiting transplants, their respective kin, and the nurses and social workers who assisted them with an array of medical, insurance, family, and daily survival needs. Here I conducted one-on-one interviews with a dozen transplant patients and, in two cases, their kin; six nurses and social workers who assisted them; a hospital chaplain; and two procurement professionals from the local OPO. I was also welcomed as an integral member of a monthly support group meeting for patients who awaited or who had received transplants. Participant observation was an integral activity, and I attended meetings regularly for more than two years. I also attended three separate memorial services hosted by hospital professionals and staff of the state's OPO; these were designed to enable organ recipients or donor kin to pay tribute to the city's annual roster of organ donors. Complementary data on patients' experiences with kidney transplantation formed the core of a research project conducted by my student assistant Marcy Assalone who interviewed a handful of patients and three health professionals in addition to conducting participant observation on a dialysis ward. Marcy also helped distribute and analyze a survey on local attitudes on donation within the university community where I taught.

In addition to primarily locally based activities, in summer 1992 I accompanied the hospital's team to the Transplant Olympics in Los Angeles, a biannual event hosted by the National Kidney Foundation, where organ recipients from around the country compete in various athletic events, promoting a public image of transplant's medical success. Here I interviewed another eight transplant patients from around the country. I also attended (and, over time, was invited to make presentations at) three national transplant conferences.[24] At these venues I also learned more of the regional differences in medical practices and transplant ideology, and I was able to expand my contacts beyond the Midwest. In subsequent years I conducted another dozen interviews with recipients and professionals from a wide range of national locations. I also ventured to Richmond, Virginia, to visit UNOS, the organization that oversees the distribution of organs in this country. Here I interviewed two staff members and witnessed firsthand how they reported and managed donor cases and how they allocated organs locally, regionally, and nationally. Finally, I traveled to Washington, D.C., on three occasions specifically to consult with a half dozen health professionals and a small cohort of transplant recipients who are advocates for minority transplant needs.

The second phase (1994–96) began when I moved to New York City to assume my current teaching post at Barnard College. As a result of the sporadic attention I gave to donation in the Midwest, I had become sensitized to the professional split between those who worked with transplant recipients versus organ donor kin. This split became especially apparent to me when I was invited to give a presentation at a national meeting: as I soon learned, the membership was so divided that transplant and procurement professionals typically sat on opposite sides of the aisle when attending an event in the main conference hall. Especially striking was the fact that procurement specialists were regarded as a necessary evil of sorts among members from the hospital-based transplant community; moreover, it was not unusual for them to self-identify as "vultures" and "ambulance chasers." Given the obvious privileging of transplant medicine, I was troubled by the absence of descriptions of procurement activities in the literature, the compelling work of Linda Hogle (1995a, 1995b) soon emerging as a remarkable exception.

My research during this period (and beyond) focused on the lives of professionals employed in three East Coast OPOs. Thanks to the grace and trust of the managing staff of one office, I was allowed to track the comings and goings of staff, shadowing them as they followed donor cases; for nearly a year (February–December 1995), I attended monthly staff meetings at which all donor cases were systematically discussed. From early 1995 until early 1996, I interviewed thirteen employees; half of these involved second and sometimes third or fourth follow-up interviews. Between 1999 and 2004, I interviewed five additional staff and conducted follow-up interviews with several from the original cohort. To test for regional differences in attitudes, training, and work activities, I paid on-site visits to an additional seven OPOs, interviewing staff based in the East, South, West, Southwest, Central Mountain region, and Midwest. Complementary data were generated through additional experiences at conferences and other transplant-related events where I encountered staff from an additional five OPOs representative of these same national regions. In short, over the course of fifteen years, I have interviewed and worked among staff from fourteen separate OPOs. Of key concern to me have been professionally guided understandings of brain death and how OPO employees think and talk about donor bodies, donor kin, and the social ramifications of organ procurement.

Early in my research I became aware of the ubiquitousness of donor memorial events, and so during this second phase of my work I began attending these on a regular basis. (Three separate organizations in New York City host their own large-scale annual event.) These memorials are staged primarily for either organ recipients or donor kin, offering attendees a means for honoring donors (and their kin). Although a primary goal is to offer a safe and open context in which to grieve, organizers are nevertheless fearful of excessive emotional outbursts among participants. As a result, these events are tightly orchestrated by health professionals and administrative staff. Typically, too, they are rife with symbolic imagery that emphasizes transplantation's life-giving mission: often they involve the planting of trees in donor gardens located on hospital grounds or in public parks. Regular memorial services are also held in local churches or cathedrals in some parts of the country, as are elaborate banquets with a host of high-profile speakers. Given the Christian overtones of many of these events (and related imagery in the transplant literature), I became intrigued by what might be left unsaid about how various faiths understood the sanctity of the body and its disruption by organ procurement. To date I have attended fourteen of these memorial events (three in Indianapolis, eight in New York City, one in Washington, D.C., and two at separate Transplant Olympic events), as well as two Transplant Walks staged in New York City, all organized to raise public awareness about organ donation. Throughout much of my work during this second phase, I was greatly assisted by Sarah Muir, who conducted interviews with religious practitioners in New York City as well as with morticians who prepare the dead from an array of faiths for burial. In addition to my own participation in the arenas described here, Sarah regularly attended two sets of organ recipient support groups whose members were of radically different ethnic, religious, and class backgrounds.

Each time I attended donor memorial events in the early 1990s, I was struck by the absence of donor kin; or, if they attended, I perceived deliberate attempts to silence them or script their presentations. Early in the course of my research I voiced this concern to a woman who had organized such an event in Indianapolis. Rather than rebuking me, she explained in a hushed voice that she herself had been dissuaded by hospital staff from including donor kin as speakers. I wanted to know why, and, thus, I eventually turned my attention to this question during the third phase of my research (1996–2001). This period focused on the long-term effects that organ donation has on the lives of surviving donor kin, a social category about which, again, very little has been written. Several key concerns became important here. How might donor kin's perspectives on death differ from those expressed by recipients and procurement specialists? How did surviving kin respond to professionally orchestrated memorials? How did they mourn their dead in private arenas? What were their reactions to the insistence that they remain anonymous to organ recipients? Under what circumstances might they defy taboos on communication with recipients? At this point I became aware of subversive memorial sites where donor kin could speak publicly of donors and their deaths devoid of professional control. Among the most visible was the production of a national donor quilt (one modeled after the AIDS quilt). My student assistant Marcy Brink also thankfully drew my attention to virtual cemeteries located on the World Wide Web; her initial analysis of these Web entries helped to stimulate my later thoughts on their significance.

At this time I conducted on-site observations and interviews with the founder and three staff members at a recently formed donor advocacy group; these individuals also allowed me to consult their files and make use of material generated from a nationwide survey that targeted donor kin. This work was further enhanced by the adroit skills of graduate student Katie Kilroy-Marac, who was allowed to join this group as an intern as part of my ongoing research. Among the most striking accomplishments of this group was their insistence that the Transplant Olympics become a more inclusive event that welcomed donor kin. In summer 1998, Katie and I attended yet another

Transplant Olympics, this time in Columbus, Ohio, where she spent much of her time working alongside staff who coordinated donor kin activities (and solving myriad logistical and individual participants' problems). In addition to attending six events and workshops designed specifically for donor kin, I conducted a series of open-ended interviews with fifteen individual donor kin, two family members of recipients, and two paired (that is, simultaneous) interviews, where a donor family member and a recipient spoke with me together about the history of their relationship. At the invitation of the donor advocacy group, Katie and I also ran a focus group of fourteen, its membership restricted to donor kin who had met their respective organ recipients. I conducted additional interviews with four donor kin at various conferences or in the privacy of their own homes; these data are complemented by approximately ten additional personal stories I have heard over the years as recounted by speakers at various transplant events.

Finally, the fourth phase of my research (2002–present) focuses on the relevance of organ scarcity anxiety in shaping a range of experimental realms of organ transplant medicine. A major concern involves the search for alternative sources of transplantable parts, which currently include mechanical devices, animal parts, and organs grown from cell cultures (sometimes referred to as "organogenesis"). Within this book I will focus specifically on data generated from my research on xenotransplantation, or the creation of transgenic animals (simian and porcine) that might one day supply organs for human implantation. I am especially interested in how scientists imagine xenotransplantation's possibilities as a miraculous medical frontier, and how the potential hybrid melding of humans with animals may generate a new set of lay and professional anxieties. This most recent work is complemented by a survey I distributed to fifty students during the first phase of my research, and an additional, much smaller set to faculty and staff at the university where I taught in Indianapolis (all returned completed questionnaires). This survey focused on respondents' reactions to the possibility of receiving replacement parts of human, simian, porcine, and mechanical origins. Xenotransplantation marks a radically new approach to the human body; of greatest interest to me are highly contentious debates over definitions of human nature, species integrity, and deliberate evolutionary change, as well as the manner in which involved research scientists imagine its possibilities. Xenotransplantation also underscores constant—and now intensified—forms of body commodification as the demand for organs increases and, thus, renders them scarce and highly coveted goods of human origin. My ethnographic work during this final phase has involved interviews with four research scientists, two neurologists, and four medical ethicists and attendance at numerous international and national conferences specifically to gather data on new experimental efforts. I remain deeply indebted, too, to Thurka Sangaramoorthy, whose earlier work as a research assistant later shaped her ideas for a senior thesis project in anthropology at Barnard College (Sangaramoorthy 1998).

My long-term involvement in this medical realm has inevitably led to encounters with an array of extraordinary individuals. Professionals and lay participants alike have willingly offered their candid remarks, heartfelt sentiments, and personal reflections on the significance of organ transfer in their lives. I am deeply grateful to the many individuals who have, without exception, welcomed me so warmly to the workplace, into their homes, to support groups, and to celebratory and commemorative events. As the data reported throughout this work reveal, the realm of organ transfer is troubled by the contradictory nature of public versus private experience. More specifically, sanctioned, and thus often bureaucratized, policies and behaviors frequently serve to deny, mask, and silence the thoughts of those whose lives have been affected so intimately by organ transfer. A question that arises, then, concerns the ethics of reporting, especially in instances where interviewees' statements offer direct challenges to transplant ideology.

Anthropology as a discipline has long insisted on the importance of protecting the personal identities of research participants. From the onset of my research I have made assurances to participants that they would remain anonymous in my writings and that their statements would remain confidential. Thus, all names reported here are pseudonyms; further, as explained to participants during the process of obtaining informed consent, minor, and thus relatively insignificant, details have been altered to ensure even further that the speaker or organization described remains obscure. (Typically, such details consist of a person's hair color or age, or an organization's name or location within the country.) I trust that participants will not be disappointed, then, if indeed they cannot locate themselves within the text. One point of exception involves references to five nationally known organizations—the United Network for Organ Sharing (UNOS), the National Kidney Foundation (NKF), the Transplant Recipients International Organization (TRIO), the National Donor Family Council (NDFC), and LifeNet of Virginia. Their publications and public activities are so well known and central to organ transfer that it would be impossible to obscure their identities. Specific employees' identities nevertheless remain obscure, except in instances where I quote published work (in print or Web-based form).

Organization of the Study

This book is organized as four essays, each of which focuses on a specific set of social practices and relationships peculiar to the world of organ transfer in America. Each is mitigated by the presence—or, more appropriately put, the necessity—of the cadaveric organ donor. In chapter 1, I analyze the paradoxical nature of brain death criteria, exploring in turn the significance of scarcity anxiety in shaping how transplant and procurement professionals think of and speak about donors' deaths and their body parts. Especially intriguing are the elaborate ways in which dead bodies are transformed symbolically so as to render them simultaneously inert yet life-giving. Chapter 2 then turns to dominant forms of "memory work": these projects—both public and private—commemorate selfless acts of giving that are intrinsic to organ transfer's success. An astounding aspect of such projects is the radical difference between how transplant-related organizations commemorate donors' lives and deaths, versus how surviving kin understand memory work. Among the more pronounced differences is the professional desire to protect donor anonymity, whereas donor kin struggle openly to proclaim highly personalized histories of individual donors. Surviving donor kin have grown increasingly wary of professionally orchestrated events because such efforts silence public grief and deny the individual identities of their beloved.

Chapter 3 pursues other facets of themes found in chapter 2, analyzing specifically the peculiar nature of sociality as it is conceived of in the realm of organ transfer. This chapter looks specifically at those instances where donor kin and organ recipients break down the barriers of anonymity and seek out one another, not unlike the process of adoptees finding their biological parents. Face-to-face encounters between donor kin and organ recipients inevitably develop into long-standing bonds of intimacy, where terms of fictive kinship define and legitimate these deeply peculiar new forms of association. Chapter 4 extends questions about sociality even further by examining the implications of highly experimental research contexts, where genetically altered nonhuman simian and porcine species bear the promise of generating organs for human use. Of key importance here are the ways in which medical and research scientists versus organ recipients view the ethical quandaries involved in melding human and animal bodies.

As argued throughout this introduction, organ transplant surgery has acquired iconic status within the American imagination as a simultaneously wondrous and disquieting medical field. It is frequently argued that technological innovations are always disturbing, especially when new (Vanderpool 1999). A striking facet of transplantation, however, is its persistent ability both to produce wonder and to disturb, even after half a century of astounding medical success. As Barbara Koenig (1988) explains, ethical debates over medical techniques are most pronounced at their onset; once their use become routinized, concerns subside or altogether disappear. Most interesting is the failure of organ transfer to become routinized within the collective lay imagination in the United States even after half a century of practice.

As a means for exploring the significance of this peculiar development, I offer alternative methods of seeing and knowing, with data generated from long-term ethnographic involvement in the field. In utilizing anthropological forms of analysis, I hope to broaden social understandings of hidden aspects of this highly lucrative and astonishingly skillful branch of American medicine. Anthropology (and medical anthropology more specifically) offers a compelling array of theory from which to draw, with its strong concern for the symbolics of the human body, transcultural sensitivity to modes of death and mourning, and burgeoning interest in bioethics. As we shall see, transplant medicine defines a nexus for a complicated array of medical, social, and economic practices. Through culturally informed critique I strive to generate more open discussion and debate, and perhaps stimulate the transformation of medical policies that concern technological innovation, public trust, patient care, and the handling of cadaveric bodies. With this in mind, let us begin with the peculiar subject of the brain dead organ donor.

1   We Are the Dead Men

Mind over Matter

The human body is a fascinatingly peculiar thing: its size can range from under twenty inches at birth to an adult stature of more than six feet, and as it matures it masters the ability to move through the world, first by rolling over, then later, perhaps, by progressing on all fours in anticipation of a life-long bipedal stride. It can propel itself on a bicycle or in a wheelchair, or run at breakneck speed. Beneath the skin one encounters a dizzying array of systems that together enable the body to survive as well as perform astonishing tasks. As the artful renderings of anatomist Andreas Vesalius (1973) illustrate so vividly, the body's inner workings include the web of the nervous system, an interlocking musculature complex, an extensive vascular network, an elegant skeletal framework, and a sophisticated amalgamation of internal organs that can draw oxygen from the atmosphere, pump and maintain blood at a stable volume and temperature, and filter and expel inhaled, ingested, and absorbed toxins.

The brain is frequently described as the nexus of control for this body complex. This single organ drives the inner workings in exquisitely complex ways, enabling us to move, breathe, and sense the world around us. Whereas the brain, as the control center, governs bodily functions, the mind is its abstract counterpart, serving as the seat of learning, the emotional center, and the locus of the self. The mind, understood as such, enables us to create, preserve, and recall memories, and to form words into speech, manual signs, and written text; it also generates dreams. We are thus simultaneously organic creatures, cognitive beings, social persons, and private selves, categories of existence that are all inextricably linked to this mind-brain complex. The mind-brain is always at work, regardless of whether we occupy conscious or slumbering states. This sophisticated complex defines

42

us as alive, as functioning, and, ultimately, as human beings (Damasio 1994; 1999: 3–31, 317–55; Sacks 1973, 1985).[1]

This exercise in describing ourselves in reference to the mind-brain may seem truly odd; my attempt to do so certainly strikes *me* as such. For one, it is shaped by an extreme form of biological reductionism; for another, it is an exclusively secular vision, allowing no room for musings on the soul, for instance. My intention is to underscore the ease with which we comprehend this view of our bodies. (Whether we embrace it is another matter, of course.) American culture is permeated by scientific reasoning, represented quite obviously by the pervasiveness of biomedicine as a dominant system of thought. Indeed, we frequently allow ourselves to be described in terms derived from biology, physiology, and anatomy, permitting internists, pulmonologists, cardiologists, and neurologists to probe and ponder us when all is not right with our health.

As philosopher Drew Leder reminds us, it is precisely at those moments when the body breaks down that we become painfully aware of its existence (Leder 1990; Sacks 1998), and biomedicine provides a framework for comprehending bodily disorder. At moments of sickness we typically ask, "What is wrong with me?" (cf. Zola 1978), and the answers are supplied most frequently by physicians, nurses, or other specialists who explain, "You have a lung infection," "You've broken your leg in two places," or "You've sustained a concussion." Thus, within medical parlance we are frequently reduced to our functioning body parts. More important, we might accept this model of the body unquestionably and embrace such diagnoses and their associated treatments with gratitude.

Medical anthropologists have long argued that a pervasive weakness within biomedicine is the insistent separation of the body and mind in clinical discourse and treatment. Biomedicine privileges knowledge concerned with the body's biomechanics, often to the exclusion of both the inner workings of the self, or emotions, and the individual's place within larger social or ecological milieus. For instance, surgery occupies a more prestigious position in the biomedical hierarchy than does psychiatry, and psychosomatic disorders may quickly be dismissed as patients' fantasies rather than being read as embodied, covert forms of protest and misery (Kleinman, Das, and Lock 1997; Sawday 1995; Scheper-Hughes 1992; A. Young 1997). Today even psychotherapy is rapidly being displaced by approaches that favor drug therapies designed to tackle problems in brain chemistry (Luhrmann 2000). In contrast, within medical anthropology one encounters an established tradition of arguing for greater mind-body harmony in medicine, with propo-

nents frequently drawing on cross-cultural data to illustrate how other healing traditions reflect more holistic approaches to human suffering (Murphy 1987; Scheper-Hughes and Lock 1987).

Nevertheless, a dominant cultural logic insists on the primacy of the
mind-brain as a defining principle of our humanity. We are certain, after all,
that we most definitely are not chimps, or dolphins, or lizards. This sense of
difference not only springs from our morphological uniqueness but is driven,
too, by a widely accepted premise within American culture that our brains
are radically more sophisticated than those of all other creatures in the animal kingdom. The success of anthropology as a social science is certainly
driven by such principles. Our uniqueness as a species is marked by our ability to generate complex social systems, sophisticated forms of symbolic communication, and creative technological innovations that enable us to transform hostile environments into habitable ones. In addition, arguments
about our special abilities are phrased in evolutionary terms, and they rest
heavily on assumptions concerning the primacy of the human mind. As
René Descartes so famously asserted, *cogito, ergo sum* ("I think, therefore
I am"; Descartes 1999 [1637]). Within a host of other specialized fields—
such as sociolinguistics, cognitive psychology, neuroscience, and artificial
intelligence—it is possible to argue that the mind-brain complex defines
how unique we truly are.

Against such premises, organ transfer emerges as an intriguing realm of
medical practice because it insists on these forms of mind-body bracketing,
yet specialists in the field still struggle to maintain a stable boundary between the two. Consider these sorts of contradictory circumstances. On the
one hand, the identities of organ recipients are often reduced to their transplanted parts, so that at transplant events recipients are relegated to such
categories as "the hearts," "the lungs," or "the kidneys."[2] Organ donors, too,
are rapidly reduced to the status of bodies or body parts because both procurement professionals and transplant surgeons may conceive of them primarily as repositories of reusable organs. On the other hand, cadaveric organ donation in the United States is possible because we legally sanction
brain death as true death. The label of death is applied even though the
artificially ventilated donor-patient remains warm to the touch, appears to
breathe, and has a heart that continues to beat within its own chest. Even
more bewildering is the fact that brain dead organ donors are routinely anesthetized at the onset of procurement surgery.

When we accept brain death criteria, as defined within a clinical framework, it is because we recognize that what matters is whether the mind, not
the body, has ceased to function. In other words, we care greatly whether

the essence of the individual person is no longer there, and thus the body's significance in defining the self slips away. A comatose patient, while assisted by "life support," might thus be described as a broken mind-brain inhabiting a dormant body. In contrast, a brain dead individual (and, thus, an organ donor) is a mindless and dead—yet artificially maintained and thus temporarily functioning—body. The conundrum posed by brain death criteria problematizes certain assumptions about our selfhood, our humanity, and our social worth as (non)sentient human beings. It also uncovers subtle forms of medical unease over what we are certain of, versus what we can never truly know, about human death. Particularly troubling for all concerned parties are questions about the timing and detection of death, questions that quickly degenerate into existential quandaries. This is most clearly marked by the tension created between brain death and cardiac death as markers of true or absolute death. Are organ donors dead once they cease to be sentient beings, or does everyone secretly believe that true death occurs only when the body itself expires?

Such questions arise because of a flawed logic that insists on death as an either-or category of (non)existence. As we shall see, a range of involved parties understands death in more creative and flexible ways, although opinions remain muted, because to voice them publicly and openly is regarded as a dangerously transgressive act. Alternative visions defy a dominant ideological premise of organ transfer, where death occurs at a precise moment in time, coinciding with the legal declaration of the cessation of brain function at, say, Tuesday, March 9, at 5:06 P.M. If one embraces organ transfer as a social good, then one should accept, unquestionably, that brain death is a marker of true or absolute death. Nevertheless, subsequent cardiac death, or the death of the body, creeps in as contradictory evidence for nearly all concerned parties.

In response to these troublesome contradictions, Margaret Lock (2002), in her comprehensive study of brain death in North America and Japan, has described organ donors as a category of the "twice dead" (cf. Savulescu 2002; Shrader 1986). As she illustrates, this model of the double death, so to speak, is pervasive in transplant contexts: first declared brain dead, the organ donor later experiences biological death when his or her organs are removed during procurement surgery. As Lock demonstrates, historicized cross-cultural comparison proves especially helpful for underscoring that this is a Euro-American biomedical construction (or struggle). In contrast, in Japan, proponents of brain death criteria (and, thus, transplantation) have encountered especially hostile resistance from the lay public precisely because of the widespread understanding that the body houses an individual's spirit or essence, and to remove body parts (particularly the heart) threatens a spirit by trapping it in a dangerously liminal state between life and death (Lock 1995: 7). Unlike in the United States, where key legislation supporting organ transfer spans the 1960s to the 1980s, Japan's Organ Transplantation Law took effect only in 1997. In an effort to recognize a plurality of voices, this law (inspired by the "conscience clause" of New Jersey's Declaration of Death Act) allows self-designated donors to "choose between brain death and traditional death by writing their preference on their donor cards" (Morioka 2001). In essence, Japanese citizens can designate what form of death they consider legitimate. The Japanese public nevertheless remains skeptical of brain death and critical of transplantation in general (Lock 2002), which frustrates Japanese transplant surgeons, a few of whom may have received some training in American medical or research institutions.

In contrast, within North America (and, more particularly, the United States), brain death criteria overcame legal hurdles much earlier because of a more widespread acceptance of mind-body dualism, which stresses that the self resides in the mind. As Lock and Christina Honde (1990) illustrate, the arenas that circumscribe ethical debates over medical practices expose important cross-cultural differences. Whereas in the United States ethical discussions that shape transplant policy have involved overwhelmingly those working within the clinical realm, national health decisions in Japan are regularly subjected to heated debate in the larger public sphere.

In the United States, *official* medicolegal rhetoric precludes the possibility that one can die twice. As a result, challenges are quickly silenced, a phenomenon that is especially pronounced in the realm of organ transfer. Nevertheless, anthropologists have long known that normative assumptions are regularly accompanied by unconventional thoughts and actions. Anthropologists know, too, that cross-culturally there are many ways to die. As data from a range of societies attest, death is not understood universally as the moment when a person permanently loses consciousness, or has no pulse, or when a body turns cold and gray. Instead, death encompasses a range of other possibilities far less biologically deterministic in their outlook. Separating definitions of death per se from what are often extraordinarily complicated ritualized forms of mourning may be difficult (Bloch and Parry 1982; Metcalf and Huntington 1991). The cross-cultural perspective reveals the limitations of the clinical assertion that the threshold between life and death is clearly marked by the measurable cessation of brain or bodily functions. Rather, anthropologically speaking, death should be viewed more broadly as a social process that allows for the possibility that a person may gradually slip away.

This is, however, a dangerous assertion within the realm of organ transfer because it ultimately destabilizes a key component of transplant ideology. In official contexts—ranging from clinical to forensic—great care is taken to identify the exact moment when death occurs. More specifically in reference to organ donors, a shift to considering death as a gradual process would inevitably generate questions about how a donor died and, potentially, who might be responsible. Such questions would expose hospital, procurement, and transplant staff to relentless lawsuits driven by accusations that these professionals orchestrate the deaths of vulnerable patients under the guise of ICU care in anticipation of the subsequent surgical removal of vital organs.

Such accusations in fact shaped the first legislative initiatives generated as protective measures in response to early instances in which transplant surgeons faced criminal charges for murdering donors for their organs (Starzl 1992: 148). I regard as absurdly simplistic the assertion that organ procurement is a medically sanctioned form of murder. As an anthropologist, I am nevertheless intrigued by the paradoxes that arise in response to this particular form of hospital death. Among the most striking developments is the manner in which transplant ideology most certainly shapes sanctioned, public sentiments and actions. Thus, I have learned to listen carefully to what people express privately as their personal perceptions, and how these may at times coincide with, and at others challenge, medicolegal rhetoric specifically about brain death. What if, instead of insisting that death can (or must) be linked to a specific, timed event, we allow it to occur incrementally, its progress marked by discrete episodes detectible sometimes by clinical tests, and at others through heartfelt sentiments of love and loss? As I will show, if we indeed pay close attention to this seepage of covert sentiments, beliefs, and turns of phrase, we discover a wondrous counterreality to the official rhetoric and public face of organ transfer in America.

A MOST PECULIAR DEATH

A Brief History of Donation

Brain death is a truly peculiar category of human experience because its mere definition dictates that professional and lay parties alike must embrace medical criteria that contradict commonsense understandings of the evidence of life. Brain death was first supported by medical specialists who, by the 1960s, were increasingly confronted with the conundrum of dying patients who were nevertheless sustained artificially on respirators. Such specialists' recommendations later shaped federal policy and state-by-state legislative initiatives that render the practice of acquiring organs from patients diagnosed as "brain dead" both legally and socially acceptable. A relatively unchallenged opinion voiced within medical circles today is that brain death criteria were most certainly developed to produce a supply of transplantable organs (see, for instance, Cowan et al. 1987; Fox and Swazey 1978, 1992; Lock 2002; Starzl 1992; P. Young and Matta 2000).

The sanctioning of brain death criteria, alongside the surgical harvesting of organs, initiated a significant ideological shift in twentieth-century medicine. This shift is reflected quite clearly in the language offered by liver surgeon Thomas Starzl, who twenty years ago explained it thus in his memoir *The Puzzle People*: "With the wide acceptance of brain death in the Western world, all injured patients who come to the hospital in a helpless condition could have a fair trial at resuscitation. Then, in an orderly way, it can be determined whether these people already were dead but with functioning hearts and lungs, or if they had a chance of restoration of brain function. The quality of care and the discriminate application of such care to terribly damaged people was one of the great fringe benefits of transplantation" (1992: 148). Although Starzl's language may strike the reader as calculating or macabre, it nevertheless exposes a seasoned surgeon's willingness to speak frankly about the early years of transplantation. Among the most revealing developments is the manner in which ventilator use marks a clear watershed. Not only could this new technology sustain brain-damaged patients, but, when paired with cardiopulmonary resuscitation, the ventilator permitted health professionals to *revive* the dead, assess their subsequent status, and then, through an unusual form of triage, ultimately determine whether subsequent care should focus on healing or in preparation for organ procurement as yet another form of death. Although organ procurement is never described in these terms by involved professionals, such conditions have in fact become the mainstay of contemporary practices in the realm of organ transfer.

Thus, some patients might well be described as the "thrice dead" because they die, first, from a head injury, accompanied by cardiac and/or pulmonary crisis, only to be resuscitated by emergency medical technicians (EMTs) through CPR and then placed on a ventilator. These patients' second deaths, so to speak, occur when they are pronounced brain dead while still sustained by machines. The third (and final cardiac) death, or death of the body, occurs during procurement surgery. The importance of CPR was underscored by a statement made during an interview in 2003 with Octavia Zamora, who works for an organ procurement organization based in a western state. In

Octavia's area, the speed limit had been raised from fifty-five to seventy-five miles per hour only a few years before we met; local EMTs linked subsequent drops in donation levels to the fact that victims of high-speed car accidents typically are so badly injured as to render CPR impossible. Under earlier limits of fifty-five miles per hour, there was a greater possibility of saving accident victims, who might then be declared brain dead in the ICU.

Body Trades

Much has been written on the history of transplantation in the United States, and thus I mention only the significant legislative strides that have rendered procurement a medical reality in this country.[3] The advent of American transplant medicine is frequently traced to the first successful attempts at kidney transfer between identical twins in 1954. Many Americans (particularly if they are in their late forties or older) are most familiar with the highly publicized story involving South African surgeon Christiaan Barnard, who in 1967 removed a healthy heart from the body of Denise Darvall and transplanted it in Louis Washkansky, who survived for eighteen days. Within the United States, the growing desire to harvest organs from patients sustained on ventilators provided the impetus for the Harvard Ad Hoc Committee, which argued in 1968 for "irreversible coma" as a new category of death. The committee's recommendations formed the basis for the Uniform Anatomical Gift Act of 1968, which stipulated how anatomical gifts—including transplantable organs and whole bodies bound for medical research—could be offered either by oneself or one's surviving kin. As such, the act simultaneously sanctioned brain death criteria and early donor campaigns and criminalized the selling of human organs for profit.[4]

The development and marketing of the potent immunosuppressant cyclosporine by the early 1980s subsequently ensured transplant's success, enabling patients to stave off the short- and long-term effects of graft rejection.[5] Yet, again, legislation trailed medical accomplishment. In 1982, Congress passed the Uniform Determination of Death Act, whose central purpose was to standardize the "proliferation" (CUSL 1980) of criteria found in an array of states' statutes; of particular importance was the goal to define brain death in legal terms. By 1987 this act was adopted in some form in nearly all states. The regulatory aspects of organ transfer were defined in 1984 by yet another key piece of legislation, the National Organ Transplantation Act (NOTA). Organs were to be distributed through the Organ Procurement and Transplant Network (OPTN), a contract that has been managed since 1986 by the United Network for Organ Sharing (UNOS), which is currently based in Richmond, Virginia.

Today, nearly all states—and even most major cities—can boast a transplant unit stationed within at least one of their largest hospitals. Currently, all such units are linked to a network of fifty-nine OPOs throughout the United States and Puerto Rico.[6] These are grouped, in turn, into eleven geographic regions. UNOS, as a federally funded regulatory agency, oversees the activities of the nation's OPOs, maintaining waiting lists and establishing national guidelines designed to ensure that organs are distributed fairly throughout the country. The logistics of placement are complex; briefly, as explained by the Association of Organ Procurement Organizations (AOPO), a set of predetermined guidelines is based, for instance, on patients' levels of medical urgency, length of time on the relevant waiting list, body and/or organ size, and blood type.[7] Organ transfer in the United States has taken on an international character, too: some patients hail from other nations; organs are at times procured from noncitizens who die in U.S. hospitals; and procured tissues and, to a lesser extent, transplantable organs may sometimes travel to other countries.

There is a national trade in transplantable human organs in the United States and, once procured, organs are most certainly transformed into precious commodities. Although buying and selling solid human organs is illegal, transplant medicine is among the most lucrative forms of medical practice within this country.[8] The movements of transplantable organs, as precious goods, are tracked with extraordinary care. Although most organs stay within the region in which they were procured, UNOS ultimately dictates their placement. Thus, if UNOS determines that the best match for a heart procured from a midwestern region is a patient based in a Southern California hospital, the midwestern OPO cannot override this decision. Southern California, however, then assumes the debt of a heart that must later be repaid to the region of origin. OPOs, with assistance from UNOS, tally such organ exchanges and debts with great care. In short, organ transfer defines a peculiar segment of interstate trade in America.

The rhetoric of organ transfer serves to deny and even disguise the fact that transplantable organs are highly valued medical commodities. Surviving kin receive no financial recompense for the organs they "donate" as "gifts of life." Nevertheless, all parties understand on some level that organ transfer is driven in part by the desire for profit. In the words of a long-standing director of a midwestern OPO, "Health care is a business . . . let's not fool ourselves." Although they are nonprofit organizations, OPOs certainly charge for their services (at the very least this covers donor care prior to, during, and following procurement). These costs are then passed on to transplant recipients, who are also billed for their respective surgeries, as well as for pre- and postoperative care. It is a public myth, however, that transplants are an option available only to the nation's wealthiest individuals. Few people in this country can afford to pay for a transplant out of pocket; nevertheless, with the assistance of savvy transplant social workers, patients from a wide range of backgrounds acquire support either through employer insurance plans (if not their own, then that of a parent or spouse), or by liquidating their assets, or by qualifying for disability and Medicaid coverage. The most destitute patients sometimes acquire support from private foundations or even from their own surgeons, who may dip into pools of research funds to help improve or save the lives of their most financially desperate patients.

Donor Histories

The human body is a tremendously profitable source of reusable parts. Together with the major organs (heart, liver, lungs, kidneys, pancreas, and small intestine), a range of others, categorized as tissues, include approximately fifty regularly salvaged body parts.[9] Surviving donor kin quickly become aware of the complexity of this economy of the body, for by law they must work their way through a complicated checklist of reusable parts once they have consented to donation. The process of donation, however, is far more complicated than the mere act of completing and signing a consent form. Given that the majority of my readers will be unfamiliar with the process, I provide an overview here.

The vast majority of organ donors' deaths result from head traumas that are sudden and thus unexpected, and many are violent as well. Primary causes include motor vehicle accidents (car or motorcycle collisions, or cyclists or pedestrians being struck by moving vehicles); gunshot wounds to the head (ranging from the misuse of firearms by children to intended acts of violence between teenagers or adults); suicides (involving a handgun, hanging, or carbon monoxide poisoning from car exhaust fumes); and severe brain hemorrhages (in adults and children). Whereas in the past age limits were set on donor eligibility, today virtually anyone—ranging from newborns to octogenarians—might qualify for donor status. Nevertheless, a widespread understanding within this specialized medical community is that by far the best donors are young people because they are assumed to be healthier (that is, less disease-ridden) than older adults. At work here, too, is the understanding that the deaths of children are especially tragic, and so it is most important that some goodness emerge from the horror of their sudden loss. Fifty years ago it would have been impossible to save— or salvage—brain dead patients. Once identified as potential donors, the severely brain damaged may later be disqualified for a host of reasons that can include (but are not limited to) failure to meet brain death criteria, detected infections, organ damage, or medical histories marked by certain cancers. Currently, one becomes a donor in the United States if next of kin grant consent. Even in those states where donor cards are legally defined as a form of advanced directive (a recent trend I will raise again later), procurement staff remain reluctant to take organs in direct opposition to kin. At the onset of my research, patients were automatically disqualified as donors if they were even suspected of having HIV, and later hepatitis B and C virus, infections. Advancements in immunosuppression, on the one hand, and treatments for AIDS especially, on the other, have led to a recent shift in accepting organs from such patients for transplantation in others who bear similar infections. These and other "marginal" donors now define an increasingly common source of "extended criteria" organs (Reynolds 2005) as surgeons, driven by organ scarcity anxiety, seek transplantable parts for growing numbers of patients in need. I will address the clinical and social relevance of "extended criteria" later in this chapter and again in chapter 4.

The artificial ventilator now routinely enables EMTs, as well as staff based in emergency wards and trauma centers, to administer CPR to damaged patients' bodies, place them on artificial respiratory support, and then, through the assistance of drug therapies that control pain and blood pressure, for instance, maintain such patients in relatively stable states in ICUs. Many procedures are performed on patients already pronounced dead as a prelude to acquiring consent and procuring their organs. It is at these highly liminal moments in clinical care that procurement professionals become intimately involved with patients and their kin. Although such policies are not necessarily enforced, the majority of states in this country now mandate hospitals to alert their local OPO if they have a patient whom they believe may soon be brain dead. Some states even require hospitals to report *all* deaths to the OPO so that field staff can assess all deceased patients as potential organ and/or tissue donors. Whereas a decade or so ago many OPOs were based within hospitals that specialized in transplantation, today this is the exception rather than the norm. Typically, OPOs maintain separate offices off site, working instead with a network of hospitals that may actively assist in identifying organ donors and/or perform transplant surgeries.

Once alerted to the potential demise of a particular patient, OPO field staff enter the hospital and perform a range of tasks. Sometimes one person performs all the necessary tasks; in larger OPOs the duties may be split between two people, in part because the work at either end is exhausting, especially when a case extends over the course of several days. As one OPO staff member explained, it can be an emotionally trying experience for the same individual to tend to the clinical needs of a depersonalized body while also trying to comfort a family in the throes of grief. Here I offer perhaps the most complex version of OPO hospital work, involving a pair of employees who work side by side, as typified by the style of a large, urban OPO whose staff I observed during the mid-1990s. Following this account, I will briefly describe other arrangements.

Knowing what to call OPO staff is itself problematic: many procurement professionals employ the title "transplant coordinator," but this is both confusing and misleading for several reasons. First, staff who work directly with recipients in transplant units also go by this title; second, the work of OPO staff in fact focuses specifically on *procurement* (otherwise known as "retrieval" or "harvesting") and *donation,* not on transplantation. Furthermore, OPO field duties involve both clinical and counseling roles, and so in my discussion here I use labels that reflect these responsibilities. When duties are split between two staff members, their activities typically play out as follows. The first, or what I will call the *clinical coordinator,* works directly at the bedside of a potential donor. If brain death is thought imminent, the clinical coordinator often assumes duties previously performed by hospital nursing staff, who retreat in order to care for other, more viable patients. The clinical coordinator takes regular readings of the patient's status, and he or she may even write orders on the patient's chart, providing directives for administering medications, especially vasopressors (or "pressors" for short) that control drops in blood pressure. Clinical coordinators generally have backgrounds in critical care nursing, so that many have worked previously in hospital ICUs. It can be difficult for lay visitors to distinguish clinical coordinators from in-house nurses because they frequently dress in hospital scrubs, wear no badge that identifies their employer, and may make little effort to clarify to family members for whom they actually work.

The clinical coordinator may be paired, in turn, with a *family counselor,* someone who arrives dressed in a suit or somewhat formal street clothes. The primary duty of family counselors is to provide emotional support to family members; typically they explain that they specialize in helping families cope with end-of-life issues. They also respond to a range of pragmatic concerns. For instance, when overtaxed nursing staff are too busy to help family members find meals or coffee, or a private room in which to talk or rest, the family counselor will respond to these needs. As with their clinically trained partners, their purpose (and employer) may be left unstated at least at the onset. Family counselors generally wear no identification badge (save that required by hospital security), allowing them the option of passing as hospital employees rather than proclaiming outright that they are from an OPO. Such practices are justified by OPO employees who stress the importance of establishing social bonds with kin before raising the topic of donation. A badge that declares that one works in organ retrieval would subvert their ability to breach the topic gradually with kin, and only once they have gained their trust as compassionate health workers. The fact that many OPOs have altered their names in recent years also facilitates this process. Whereas ten years ago most agencies bore composite names consisting of their state or region plus "OPO" (for instance, NWOPO or Northwest Organ Procurement Organization), many have assumed new titles that emphasize organ donation as an act that saves lives (thus, NWOPO is now LifeCenter Northwest).[10] Today only a few OPOs are based within hospitals, but ten to fifteen years ago such relationships were common, only further complicating the duties of procurement work. I can only hypothesize at this point, but drawing from my data culled from fourteen OPOs of a range of sizes, it appears that employees from smaller offices are less likely to attempt to pass as hospital staff. The question of how OPO field staff should introduce themselves to the kin of prospective donors is currently a topic of heated debate. As my descriptions reveal here, procurement strategies in the United States are, oddly, both compassionate and covert.

Successful procurement rests heavily on the shoulders of family counselors. Particularly important is their skill in engendering trust among family members, for without this their attempts at procurement will fail. In those cases where family members experience callous treatment from overextended hospital staff, the OPO family counselor provides a sympathetic ear and shoulder, allowing kin to express their sadness and rage openly and free of judgment. An important strategy employed by many OPOs today is referred to as "decoupling," where successful procurement is understood as relying on the sequential acceptance of two messages by a patient's surviving kin (DeJong et al. 1998). The first message concerns brain death criteria, and OPOs generally rely on hospital physicians—preferably neurologists—to explain this initially to patients. OPOs thus expend much time and energy running in-house educational seminars for hospital staff on the dos and don'ts of talking about brain death with patients' families. The OPO family counselor then follows up with another discussion or series of conversations about brain death, sometimes supported with visual aids but, more frequently, by employing vernacular language devoid of mystifying clinical jargon. As I will explain in greater detail later, metaphorical analogies abound. Only once kin begin to show signs of accepting brain death criteria (they start to talk about funeral arrangements, for instance) does the family counselor shift to the second message: that is, the great social value of organ and tissue donation.

Within one East Coast OPO in particular, I found that family counselors defined a well-developed area of in-house expertise. This OPO is based in a large and ethnically diverse city, and in the mid-1990s the director hired a team of counselors who represented an eclectic range of professions, religions, and ethnicities. This hiring practice was based on the premise that it would facilitate the rapid establishment of rapport with families whose backgrounds overlapped with those of individual counselors. Such an approach was nevertheless highly controversial within this OPO and beyond because of a dominant assumption in the realm of organ transfer that all patients or bodies are equal beneath the surgeon's knife (Sharp 2002b). Nevertheless, in this particular OPO, if it was known in advance that a potential donor was, say, Latina, the team's director would make every effort to assign a family counselor fluent in Spanish and, preferably, also of Latin American descent. Similarly, an Orthodox rabbi, who often agreed to be on call, would respond to requests to meet with Jewish families of a range of levels of observance; and an African American woman, who had worked previously as a Pentecostal minister within a storefront church, was regularly matched with inner-city African American and Caribbean families.

These elaborate pairings generally characterize only the nation's largest OPOs and were more typical in the 1990s than they are at present. Financial pressures (linked in large part to false hopes that donations would grow substantially each year) have forced some OPOs to scale back, rendering specialized hiring practices an unaffordable luxury today, except where linguistic barriers may prevent successful donation outcomes. Similarly, clinical coordinators and family counselors may have reverted to a single position in some OPOs. Smaller OPOs, such as those that serve primarily rural regions or midsize cities, have much smaller staffs (perhaps five to fifteen employees rather than fifty), their members shouldering all duties, including the clinical monitoring of a donor, talking to family members and providing emotional support, and sometimes even assisting with the actual procurement of the organs (a task performed elsewhere largely by transplant surgeons who arrive on site to retrieve organs for patients under their care).

Successful procurement also relies on support from a range of other, non-OPO employees. Family members may raise the topic of donation themselves, making the task of acquiring consent much easier. Many donor kin frequently report that a staff nurse (but rarely a physician) broached the topic of organ donation and, further, that it was this nurse's extraordinary level of emotional support that led them, in the end, to consent to donation.

Many OPOs now train ICU staff as well as other hospital employees, among whom clergy are especially important, to approach families about donation. Chaplains, after all, regularly tend to families faced with end-of-life decisions, and they define a significant target for OPO training sessions (UNOS 2000). Ruth Yoder, a chaplain based in a midwestern hospital, explained her approach as follows, one that echoed those used by local OPO staff during the early 1990s:

> With families, almost universally [donors] are people who were young, vibrant and healthy—they died in a car or motorcycle accident, from a gunshot or an aneurysm in the brain. So the family has a tremendous adjustment—the person was fine only a little while ago, unlike [with] terminal[ly ill patients where families have been coping for a while with death]. . . . What I show [the family] is that their breathing is exactly the rhythm of the machine. I explain that their blood isn't cold and that there is only a little color change, but that it is the machinery that is keeping them alive. The machinery is traumatic [for kin] when family members see someone like this suddenly all hooked up to these machines. . . . I [then] ask them, "Have you ever talked to so and so about organ donation? How would they want to be remembered?" That helps a lot. . . . The initial reaction is, "He/she has suffered enough." What this means is "*I've* suffered enough." Most people are very sympathetic [to donation]. Donorship helps them make sense out of the loss. With sudden death, people do want to make sense out of it. Terminal [illness] is much harder—usually family members will say, "They have suffered enough" . . . [and that's precisely] what they mean.

Procurement is far from an easy assignment: within one East Coast OPO where I conducted research over the course of a full year, of all potential donors identified, only 18 percent in 1993 and 28.5 percent in 1994 resulted in successful procurement. The reasons the remaining cases did not succeed included the failure of patients to qualify for brain death status; the inability of OPO staff to approach kin on time; obstructionist hospital staff; and medical complications (including advanced age, history of cancer, serious heart disease, or the body "crashing," as staff so often put it, before procurement could occur). Finally, within each year more than 30 percent of kin refused consent when asked.[11]

Procurement is emotionally trying work, exacerbated by hostility toward such work among some hospital staff, as reflected in the range of derogatory slang applied to OPO workers. Common labels include "ambulance chasers," "vultures," and the "death squad."[12] The ability of OPO staff to remain true to their course hinges on their great dedication to the humanitarian principles that drive organ transfer. The dominant messages they convey to potential donor families include emphasizing that donation allows some good to emerge from a terrible tragedy; that loved ones, though suddenly lost, may live on in others through organ transplantation; and that multiple organ donation especially means that donors' "gifts of life" can pull a number of people back from the brink of death, allowing them to return to normal, productive lives.[13] When I began my research on organ procurement, I was informed repeatedly that the typical burnout rate for this line of work was around eighteen months, whereas transplant coordinators who worked with patients awaiting organs often remained on the job for a decade or more (Sharp 2001). Recently, both AOPO and UNOS have begun to address the effects of what one OPO employee referred to as "sympathy burnout" among procurement field staff.

OPO staff speak specifically of the work that involves direct contact with (potential) donor families as simultaneously the most trying and rewarding of experiences. Staff put in long hours at the hospital, each assignment frequently spanning several days. Because rapport with kin is essential, OPOs are especially reluctant to switch family counselors midstream, even when they are exhausted from lack of sleep. Their primary tasks involve assisting families faced with unimagined traumas, fresh grief, and, at times, internal strife among kin on issues that may include guilt, anger at one another or even the dying patient, frustration with hospital staff, or disagreements on treatment trajectories, funeral plans, or donation. OPO work is exacerbated by the need to approach families under time-pressured circumstances—that is, a successful procurement hinges on the ability of kin to offer consent when they are still numbed by the sudden onset of grief. Donors' deaths often result from unexpected, and often heartrendingly violent, situations: a little girl has a massive aneurysm on the playground; a young boy is struck by a car on his way to school, makes his way home alone, and crawls into bed, only to fall into a coma; a sleeping teenager is shot by a friend who is playing around with his father's handgun; a fiancée has a head-on car collision and sustains a major head trauma two blocks from her lover's house; a cornered young man is shot in the head by police at the end of an hour-long car chase; a college student home for the holidays, recently rejected by a lover, shuts himself in the garage and turns on the car engine soon after his parents have left for a Christmas party; an elderly gentleman collapses in the street from a massive stroke during his lunch break and is rushed to the hospital by EMTs. These sorts of stories are all too familiar to procurement coordinators.

At times individual counselors are accepted by kin as a source of support and guidance; at others, and especially in the case of male counselors, they might even be physically assaulted by family members who want no part of a stranger speaking to them of death. As all counselors underscore, they are often deeply moved by their encounters with donor families, whom they view as an inherently unique group of people who have made horribly difficult decisions at terrible moments in their lives. At times the catharsis of these sudden and unexpected encounters generates a level of closeness that may extend for weeks, months, or longer. All counselors who have been on the job for a few years can speak of donor kin who contact them personally when grief strikes anew. When a donation has gone well, donor kin, too, speak of compassionate counselors whom they remember with great fondness.

In part to relieve field staff of the burden, as well as to provide sustained aftercare for donor kin, by the late 1990s a number of OPOs began to hire grief counselors. Today these specialists typically direct a subsection of their OPO, offering a range of aftercare programs and more intimate forms of counseling. Prior to 1998, however, aftercare was limited to annual commemorative events, generally staged by OPOs or sometimes by regional hospitals. As Chaplain Yoder explained in 1992, at that time donor families had to fit into a particular niche by joining a six-week support group for widows and widowers, or another for parents who had lost a child. Among the most impressive shifts in OPO work is the growing understanding that donor kin, by virtue of their unusual end-of-life decisions, experience grief in specialized ways (Maloney and Wolfelt 2001). (This reality defines a key focus for the following two chapters.)

A Special Kind of Death

Sorting through the literature on brain death is a complex affair, given that the manner in which brain death has been defined or described varies, especially if traced from the 1960s through the early 2000s. Early on, for instance, brain death was regularly referred to as "irreversible coma," as phrased by the Harvard Ad Hoc Committee (HMS and Beecher 1968). Today it is generally contrasted with, rather than equated with, coma and vegetative states, although such references linger.[14] The refinement of brain death's definition stems from more recent advances in neurology, a burgeoning specialty that now relies routinely on sophisticated forms of imaging technology to diagnose and treat brain traumas (Gean 1994). I will begin, then, with a technical description offered by Eelco Wijdicks, a neurointensivist and recognized specialist on brain death criteria. As he explains, "'Brain death' is the vernacular expression for irreversible loss of brain function. Brain death is declared when brainstem reflexes, motor responses, and respiratory drive are absent in a normothermic, nondrugged comatose patient with a known irreversible massive brain lesion and no contributing metabolic derangements" (2002: 1). Embedded within Wijdick's statement is the understanding that brain death is detected through the systematic application of diagnostic procedures (Wijdicks 2001). (I will return to this issue later.) Among the more confusing aspects of brain death for the clinically uninitiated is precisely how much or what part of the brain is in fact irreversibly damaged. During fifteen years of field research I have received a range of answers to the question, What is brain death? when speaking with OPO educational and clinical staff, as well as internists, transplant surgeons, and neurologists. OPO staff typically underscore what it is not: brain death is neither a coma nor a vegetative state. OPO staff are especially averse to these terms (even when either condition is described as "irreversible") because they evoke within the lay public images of injury followed by spontaneous recovery. Other interviewees (especially those who are clinically trained) sometimes describe brain death as "full" or "total" brain failure.[15] Neurologists whom I interviewed in 2004 preferred to speak of brain stem failure (cf. Hill 1999; Matta 2000; P. Young and Matta 2000). As Dr. Needler, who regularly diagnoses brain death in patients, explained, "During my clinical training I learned what any physician learns—we learn about the hierarchical organization of the brain—if the brain stem has ceased to function, then the upper brain's capabilities will fail, too. This is why we speak of [the] brain stem in reference to brain death." Another neurologist, Dr. Valentine, underscored that the damage sustained from this form of head trauma is irreversible and, further, that the brain may begin to "liquefy" or "grow necrotic" even as procurement staff are in the process of assessing a donor's status. All that is left is perhaps some residual spinal activity, nothing more.

Diagnosis by a physician is a relatively straightforward procedure that requires few specialized tools, but from a lay perspective brain death is a truly confounding medical category. Oddly, too, whereas several professional organizations—such as the American Academy of Neurology and the American Academy of Pediatrics—have published diagnostic guidelines, brain death criteria have yet to be standardized either within this country or internationally (AAP 1987; Gelb and Robertson 1990; J. Lynch and Eldadah 1992; University of North Dakota 1998; Wijdicks 1995a). Within the United States specifically, mandated diagnostic criteria vary from one state to another, among OPOs, and even among hospitals located within the same city. Dr. Lazarre, a neurointensivist who described himself as one who has "diagnosed literally hundreds of brain dead patients," stressed that "brain death is a clinical diagnosis. You don't need special tools or tests to do it. It only takes me about four minutes—it's very quick. It is not difficult for me [to recognize]—diagnosis is not [a] difficult [task]."

Regardless of protocols, in the end, the purpose of diagnostic criteria is to confirm the absence of brain activity. The systematic assessment is generally conducted by a neurologist, although any trained physician is capable of the task. (Sometimes, though rarely, a nurse may assume this duty.) In-house protocols almost always require that the assessment be administered twice and by two separate physicians, although the period of time between the two varies significantly from one institution to another. Dr. Lazarre, who proudly stated that he had "streamlined" his unit's protocol, put it thus:

DR. LAZARRE: I . . . got rid of the observation period.

L. S.: But don't two separate doctors still evaluate the patient?

DR. LAZARRE: You still need two different doctors. Some places they [conduct separate observations] six, twelve, twenty-four hours apart. I got rid of this. You don't need it. I can do the [tests] two minutes apart with two people [and that's all it takes]. If you really understand brain death—[after all] you can't become *un*-brain-dead. [He then describes the function of the hypothalamus.] You will [then] have cardiac death. We [might be able to] keep you alive for two to three days. There are those who write [about] people who can be brain dead for two to three months— but the body [falls apart eventually]. I find it hard to believe [that maintaining someone this long] is realistic or happens [very often at all].

Drawing from the literature and my field interviews, I offer the following review of brain death assessment in *adult* patients.[16] First, the patients must be deeply comatose and artificially ventilated, their CAT scan and spinal fluid tests generating abnormal results. Before proceeding with diagnostic tests for brain death, the physician must also know the origin of injury, so that he or she can exclude other causes that can mimic brain death. These include hypothermia, endocrine crisis, severe acid-base abnormalities, intoxication, the presence of barbiturates and other sedatives (self- or hospital-administered), as well as neuromuscular blocking agents.

Once these are ruled out as probable causes, the physician tests systemically for brain stem activity in response to excessive noxious stimuli. The physician exerts pressure on the nail beds of the hands and feet and on the sternum (located in the upper central region of the chest). Throughout such tests the physician watches for such reflexes as eye opening, facial grimaces, head movements, and reflex movements of the limbs. The purpose of these tests is to make certain that the patient's condition results not merely from a damaged cerebral cortex but specifically from brain stem failure. For instance, the pupils can be any shape, but they should exhibit no response to bright light. There should be no evidence of normal eye closure as the corneas are stroked, or eye movements when the head is moved briskly or when the interior of each ear is flushed with cold water. Also, brain dead patients do not gag or cough in response to a throat swab or tongue blade, or when the physician wiggles the ventilator tube within the trachea. A range of more sophisticated (and technologically mediated) diagnostics, referred to as "confirmatory tests," might then be applied. (Although required in Europe, they do not define a mandatory component of U.S. protocols.) They include cerebral angiography, electroencephalogram, transcranial doppler, and other brain imaging techniques.

In the United States the single required confirmatory technique is the apnea test, whose purpose is to document that the patient is incapable of breathing spontaneously when disconnected from the ventilator. (This ability is marked by such responses as coughing or gasping.) As recently as the mid-1990s, the apnea test was considered highly controversial within those OPOs where I conducted research. A widespread fear was that cessation of ventilation could induce cardiac arrest or other forms of trauma, circumstances that threatened the viability of organs for later transplantation (Wijdicks 1995b). The apnea test has since evolved into a normative practice, in part because of a range of more recent techniques designed to prepare and stabilize the patient before and during the procedure. Common precautions include using a warming blanket to increase the core temperature of the body and administering vasopressors to counteract low blood pressure, as well as other medications to control fluid levels. Prior to the test patients are also typically oxygenated; once the patient is disconnected from the ventilator, the physician must document blood gas levels (paying particular attention to carbon dioxide [CO_2] readings) for several minutes. Depending on the hospital, the apnea test may last anywhere from three to eight minutes. As Dr. Lazarre explained, "This is the biggest stimulus to the brain [to start breathing]. You look, watching with your own eyes for no breathing movements. In the end you . . . document that there's evidence that the blood is [saturated] with CO_2 and not oxygen. . . . you draw arterial blood and then document the CO_2 [level this way]." In some instances the apnea test is repeated, although staff whom I interviewed (drawn from OPOs of a range of sizes) all reported that this was strictly optional in locations where they worked.

Today the administration of diagnostic tests defines a ritualized form of witnessing for patients' kin in some hospitals. As a neurologist, Dr. Needler prefers to have family members present when she tests for brain death because this helps her to explain more clearly what is wrong with the patient. A troublesome element here is that brain dead patients sometimes manifest what clinicians refer to as a "Lazarus sign": that is, their bodies may move as a result of residual spinal activity. Wijdicks stresses that such movements frequently occur following an apnea test, and he thus offers these cautionary words: "It should tell you that the family members should never be present during this procedure [because] it might be very difficult to discuss organ donation after this occurs" (University of North Dakota 1998). Nevertheless, some OPOs have taken the radical step of encouraging the kin of prospective donors to be present during the apnea test. Dora Tuckerman, who directs her OPO's donor family aftercare program, underscored the power of this form of clinical witnessing:

> This is a very [important part of understanding] brain death because they [that is, ventilated donors] don't look dead. I ask our people [in the field] to ask if [donor kin] want to see the apnea test. They have a right to this! Otherwise, you're asking them to take on faith that this breathing thing is dead. Docs—I wish, please tell them to say *dead*. . . . I know one donor mom who was told she couldn't be there for the apnea test—she snuck in [anyway] and she was so glad she did. Then she believed [her son] was dead.

Variability and Trust

As reflected in Dr. Lazarre's statement, brain death criteria are more streamlined in emergency rooms, ICUs, and trauma centers when their directors enthusiastically support organ donation. The presence of large transplant centers in such cities as Pittsburgh, Cleveland, San Francisco, Dallas, New York City, and Rochester, Minnesota, for instance, as well as long-standing and large-scale OPO operations, also inevitably shapes brain death protocols. Individual OPOs frequently assist smaller hospitals in forging in-house policies for brain death declaration; at the very least they initiate the declaration process by observing individual patients and assessing their medical status. Based on their readings, OPO staff may then request that proper neurological tests be performed. The varying level of engagement and willingness on the part of hospital staff to work with OPOs ultimately shapes the time lag between the two physicians' assessments, as well as the urgency with which additional confirmatory tests might be applied.

The manner in which OPO counselors approach families is driven in part by a widespread paternalistic assumption that kin do not want, nor do they need, to know the specific details of brain failure (or, for that matter, organ procurement). Such knowledge is understood as too difficult to comprehend, too traumatic, or too cruel to describe to kin in the throes of grief. Also, too much knowledge might threaten the opportunity to acquire consent. As noted earlier, OPO coordinators generally prefer that a neurologist speak first to the family, but he or she should then withdraw so that a counselor can work directly with kin. Dr. Lazarre, who is highly supportive of organ donation, put it thus: "[They say], 'your job is to [try to] save the patient and diagnose brain death and ours is [to talk about] donation.' But they have this really patronizing attitude—they're afraid we're going to fuck up [the process]. But it's like the eight-hundred-pound gorilla—look, the family knows—they're already thinking about donation—and it helps them to see some good come out of the tragedy [of the death] and so, I say, I just want to let them know that I support this, that I support organ donation."

OPO family counselors regularly stress how important it is for them to follow the neurologist's presentation with their own, one devoid of obscure clinical jargon. OPO counselors rely heavily on a rich array of metaphors to communicate the severity and irreversible quality of brain death to surviving kin. This range of variability in brain death protocols may account in part for the paucity of print material made available to donor kin by OPO family counselors. It may spring as well from the assumption that counselors must gauge the education level of kin on a case-by-case basis, choosing their language accordingly.[17] Instead, reading materials—if they exist at all—tend to focus on two other, albeit related, themes. The first involves advice on how to cope with a sudden and inexplicable death. The second focuses on pragmatic concerns. For instance, will donation cost family members anything? Will procurement surgery disfigure the body and thus affect desired funeral arrangements? Do any religions prohibit organ donation? Even if donation is said to be anonymous, will recipients try to establish contact? Are brain death and coma the same thing?[18] The answer supplied to each of these questions is a resounding no.

The Clinical Art of Procurement

While kin struggle to cope with the potential death of a loved one, the clinical coordinator evaluates the patient's status by drawing blood, extracting lymph node samples, and monitoring life signs to determine blood and tissue type, assessing, too, the patient's general health and thus his or her viability as an organ donor. In some regions of the United States, OPO staff may actually initiate such procedures before brain death has been declared, and even, in some instances, before kin have arrived at the hospital. The clinical coordinator rapidly assumes responsibility for the care of an imminently brain dead patient, administering blood pressure and perhaps other medications to try to prevent the patient from "crashing" before brain death can be declared or organs procured. The clinical coordinator also orders diagnostic tests to determine the following: Does the patient test positive for various strains of hepatitis or HIV/AIDS? Does he or she have self-administered tattoos or track marks from drug use that would indicate a higher chance of exposure to such infections? How well do the vital organs appear to be functioning?

Once in communication with next of kin, the coordinator pursues other data in order to amass a more detailed health history. For instance, has the patient ever been diagnosed with or treated for cancer? If so, what kind, and how long ago? Did he or she smoke or drink heavily? What of the patient's sexual history? Has he or she ever been incarcerated? Ten years ago these complications would have rendered most patients unsuitable as donors. In response to the growing sense of urgency over organ scarcity, however, these are now treated as *cautionary* signs by most OPOs. As a coordinator from a midwestern OPO explained in a videotaped 1998 hospital training session, exclusionary criteria had shrunk dramatically in response to the demands of transplant surgeons: "We've changed our criteria in the last year; [there's] no [upper] age [limit, for example,] . . . as more and more people are added to the list and more and more people are dying every day, because of the lack of organs, the transplant surgeons are getting more and more aggressive and more and more liberal with the criteria they will accept. . . . [For us today the] only contraindication is HIV/AIDS. . . . [We] will still assess those with sepsis, [hepatitis B and C], [and] cancer . . . for instance" (University of North Dakota 1998).

Staff based in other OPOs report a similar trend in recent years. As Liza White, a clinical coordinator with eight years of experience, explained in 1994, at times she felt she had to be the guardian for potential recipients; as she put it, "some of our [region's] surgeons are so desperate [for organs] they'll take anything short of road kill."[19] This shift toward "more aggressive" and "liberal" criteria is a recent one. For example, in 1995 I watched an exasperated family counselor seek advice from his supervisor when he learned that a local cardiac team wanted to accept a heart even though the donor tested positive for hepatitis B. As he later explained to me, "This case is a clear rule out, but [they] still want the heart. . . . I keep telling [my boss] to tell them *no!* Otherwise it will come back to haunt you. If you say yes, it's nothing but *greed.* This sort of thing makes [our office] look really bad."

In the end, the supervisor's judgment call prevailed, and the patient failed to qualify as a donor. Yet nearly a decade later, placements such as these have become routine within this and other OPOs. The cautious, selective use of donors with cancer, for instance, has recently been endorsed by UNOS (Buell et al. 2003; Kauffman, McBride, and Delmonico 2000), as have those infected with HIV and strains of hepatitis, provided their organs are transferred to patients with similar infections.

In response to a question about shifting boundaries for exclusionary criteria, Dr. Salvador, a liver surgeon, offered this explanation in 2004:

> With [transplant candidates whose liver failure is already attributable to] hepatitis C, we know that there is an 80 to 100 percent chance that the patient will have hepatitis C [again] within one year post transplant [and so] we ask ahead of time if [we might transplant in them a liver, say,] . . . from a donor [infected] with hepatitis C. Now, when the donor has [benign] tumors, [we might use his liver, but we have] talk[ed] to the [transplant] patient ahead of time [to acquire advanced informed consent]. We tell them that it can lower their chance of survival if they wait [for an organ] without such risks attached. [We tell them,] "You might have to wait much longer—too long—if you say no to tumors, or hepatitis C"; but if [they are] willing to take this [sort of organ,] they might get a liver sooner.

Such transplant recipients are thus faced with a lethal trade-off between severe disability or death from organ failure, and the long-term consequences of infections stemming from flesh acquired from anonymous, diseased organ donors. Acquiring informed consent from patients at the outset of joining a unit's in-house waiting list may not necessitate asking patients later if they are willing to accept a specific organ known to be infected with a particular pathogen; more often this judgment call is made by the transplant surgeon at the time of procurement or surgical implantation.[20] The problems associated with diseased organs only compound the already known dangers associated with long-term ingestion of potent immunosuppressants and steroids. Nevertheless, current perceptions of the ever-increasing scarcity of organs inhibit surgeons from protecting their dying patients from a range of subsequent posttransplant infections; after all, a transplanted organ bears the promise of extending the patient's life for years.

If all goes well—that is, if brain death has been declared and the donor can be maintained in a physiologically stable state, kin have consented to donation, the OPO has determined that the organs and tissues are viable for transplant, UNOS has successfully placed the organs, and surgical teams can arrive in time—the donor then proceeds to the operating room for procure-

ment surgery. AOPO provides a helpful—though somewhat sanitized—
summary of what its authors term "the donation process." I quote it at
length here because this statement represents the public face of procurement as communicated to donor kin:

> Once all suitable organs have been accepted by transplant programs,
> the surgical teams travel to the hospital to perform the organ recovery
> procedure. The ventilator continues to provide oxygen to the donor's
> bloodstream, which in turn allows the heart to keep beating and the
> blood to circulate. The organ recovery surgery is performed in the same
> fashion as any other operation, in the operating room, under sterile
> conditions, using standard surgical instruments and techniques. The
> operation may take from one to four hours, or longer, depending on
> which organs are recovered for transplantation. The organs are flushed
> with cold preservation solution, which lower[s] their temperature and
> ensure[s] safe preservation until the time of transplantation. Blood
> samples and lymph nodes are also removed for tissue typing to ensure
> compatibility between the donor and the recipients. When the organs
> have been removed from the body, the ventilator is turned off. The sur-
> gical incisions are closed and the donor's body is prepared for transfer
> to the morgue. Throughout this process, the donor's body is treated
> with respect and dignity.[21]

Although this statement from AOPO is certainly informative, it fails
to mention a number of procedures essential to procurement work. As one
physician put it, "Surgery is messy business." OPO staff know this all too
well, and thus they filter or sanitize their descriptions of procurement surgery out of fear that too many details will undermine their ability to acquire
consent for donation from kin. Some readers may be offended by some of
the information that follows. I provide such details not for their shock value
but to underscore the complexity of procurement work. As I will show
through a careful consideration of excluded details, a key aspect of organ
procurement involves the ability to depersonalize donors.

How, then, does actual procurement work differ from AOPO's description of the "donation procedure"? First, it remains unstated who, beyond
surgeons, is involved in the procurement of organs. Sometimes OPO staff
bear this responsibility, especially if they work for smaller offices involved
nearly exclusively in kidney and tissue procurement. Today, however, many
transplant surgeons (especially when hearts, lungs, and livers are concerned)
insist that they or, at the very least, another surgeon from their unit be
present for and conduct the actual surgical removal of parts destined for their
own patients. Thus, the timing of procurement hinges on the ability of surgical teams to coordinate their arrivals so that they can work side by side.

In addition, among the more intriguing aspects of procurement is that even though organ donors have been declared dead, they are regularly anesthetized at the onset of surgery. As several interviewees explained, this is done for two reasons: first, anesthesia relaxes the body by dampening residual spinal cord reflexes; second, it helps bolster surgical personnel psychologically in case they worry that the patient can still experience pain. Furthermore, during procurement, unlike normal surgical procedures, organs are removed, not repaired; also, because time is of the essence (and the patient is understood to be dead), the physical opening of the body and techniques for organ excision more closely approximate an autopsy or, in the acerbic words of one non–clinically trained witness, an "evisceration."

One transplant surgeon, when asked whether procurement was in fact so different from regular surgery, responded as follows:

DR. SALVADOR: It's *totally* different. Look, the abdomen gets completely excavated. [After all,] we're not allowed to put artificial material back into the abdomen when we're done [to fill it up again and] give it shape.

L. S.: [So, then it's] no different from an autopsy?

DR. SALVADOR: Oh, no, it's *completely* different. But the patients are already deformed—many were in auto accidents and the face is damaged—they don't look like themselves at all. And the family knows that. But it is totally different. If you do [regular] surgery on a patient who is alive you try to think about how the patient will look afterwards, you try to [minimize] the scars [for instance].

As Dr. Salvador went on to explain, the incision made is much larger than in regular thoracic or abdominal surgery, designed here to expose the torso's full interior so that the surgeons can investigate the body for tumors or other abnormalities (cf. Hogle 1999, esp. chap. 9).[22] Again, unlike standard surgeries, the donor's body is fully flushed of all its blood and then perfused with solutions designed to eliminate the danger of subsequent blood clotting in recipients, to stave off sepsis, and to keep the organs "alive" at the cellular level. Although a patient enters surgery on a ventilator and is administered anesthesia at the onset, once perfusion begins these earlier technological interventions are no longer necessary. Also, although not mentioned in AOPO's summary supplied earlier, among the most important surgical moments is when cross-clamping occurs—that is, when blood flow to and from the heart is clamped and stopped, at which point the ventilator is no longer of any use. In other words, it is not "when the organs have been removed from the body" that "the ventilator is turned off," but, instead, just prior to organ excision. I have found, though, that most OPO staff are unaware of this fact unless they regularly assist in the operating room and assume technical roles during surgery.

Clearly, the surgical extraction of organs is a complex process (Gelb and Robertson 1990; Hogle 1999; Levinson and Copeland 1987), and here I focus only on those few details significant to the specific concerns that drive this chapter. Following perfusion, and while the organs are still intact, the torso's interior is covered with ice, again to preserve organ integrity. In cases involving a multiple organ donor, thoracic and abdominal surgeons may work side by side, later handing the donor's body over to the kidney team.[23] The last step involves various forms of tissue procurement, which may occur either in the operating room or later in the pathologist's lab or the morgue. The last person to leave surgery bears the responsibility of closing up the donor's torso. This might be a member of a kidney or tissue team; in other instances hospital or OPO surgical staff assume this task. The remains of the donor's body may require additional repair work in preparation for the mortician: eye caps will cover the scars of cornea removal, and dowels will be slipped in to replace the long bones of the arms and legs.

Procurement Aesthetics

Although OPO staff vehemently deny that the donor body experiences any form of mutilation, they nevertheless take precautions to shield donor kin from the details that surgeons themselves know to be true. In recent years OPOs have also begun to work closely with local funeral directors, sometimes even hiring a full-time liaison as a mortuary consultant. Field interviews with morticians in New York City, conducted by research assistant Sarah Muir in 1997, revealed that, technically speaking, the services necessary for preparing an organ or tissue donor are no different than those for an autopsy, and thus they pose no unusual aesthetic challenges. A significant concern voiced by OPO personnel is that donor families must not incur extra charges for, say, an open-casket funeral simply because the loved one was an organ donor. Furthermore, mortuary employees must refrain from offering graphic descriptions of the body's condition following procurement.

Some surgeons pride themselves on ensuring that a donor's body is handled with dignity. As Dr. Salvador explained:

> I try to take into account [the donor's background]. If I know, for instance, that the donor was Catholic and female, I know the family will probably want to put a cross on her right here [tapping his own upper sternum]. [With such a donor] I try [to do a] Y[-shaped] incision

[on her upper chest instead of cutting straight up] so we can preserve the shape of the chest. This is what is referred to as "the aesthetics of the donor"—there's a lot written on this. If this person was nice enough to donate their organs—and this family doesn't want to see the body disfigured, don't I owe it to them [to take such care?] But not all [surgeons] do this. . . . We [on our team, we] try to preserve the body—aesthetics [matter].

In those rare instances where members of the surgical team actually know donors or their kin, they will make heroic efforts to ensure that bodies are handled in a dignified way. One OPO staff member reported an extraordinary case involving a nurse who had assisted at countless procurement surgeries. When she suffered fatal injuries in a car accident on her way home from work late one night, her kin consented readily to donation. When it was time for her to enter the operating room, this nurse's colleagues insisted that they alone perform the surgical procurement of her organs. Staff interviewed from two additional OPOs similarly reported that either they themselves or their colleagues assumed full responsibility for the preoperative care and oversaw the actual procurement of organs from a colleague's child. As one interviewee explained, the task was both horrific and cathartic for all involved precisely because everyone wanted to be certain that the donor was handled lovingly and solely by those who knew either the child or the mother.

Other Ways to Die

The demand for transplantable organs has increased rapidly over the last ten years, the waiting list shifting from just under 38,000 in 1994 to more than 88,000 in mid-2005. This trend stems from a number of interrelated factors: improved surgical techniques, the burgeoning of transplantation as an attractive medical specialty, and an expansion in the number of transplant units located in cities throughout this country. In contrast, the cadaveric donor pool has only grown incrementally, from 5,099 in 1994 to 7,150 by the end of 2004.[24] Even if, ideally, all brain dead patients could become multiple organ donors (the full count ranging from seven to nine organs per patient, depending on how one counts), it would still be impossible to meet the nation's ever-growing demand.[25] According to UNOS in 2004, "On average, 110 people are added to the nation's waiting list each day—one every thirteen minutes," and "on average, sixteen patients die every day while awaiting an organ" (UNOS 2004b). In response, OPOs and transplant units engage in a constant quest to identify new organ sources. These include relying on living donors for kidneys and lungs (whereby they offer one of a pair) or livers (transected livers will regenerate), domino procedures, and experimental research focusing on artificial (mechanical) organ replacement, organ cell seeding followed by tissue regeneration, and transpecies transplantation (the latter defines the focus of chapter 4).[26] As noted earlier, the lifting of restrictions has already expanded the donor pool. Yet another strategy involves expanding allowable causes for donors' deaths.

One of the most significant shifts to occur in recent years involves procuring organs from patients who die not from brain death but instead from medically assisted forms of cardiac arrest. As noted briefly in the introduction, such donors are variously referred to as "non-heartbeating cadavers" or "non-heartbeating donors" (NHBDs), or the process itself as "donation after cardiac death" (DCD) or following "asystolic" death (UNOS 2004a; DuBois 1999; Fung 2000; Institute of Medicine 1997; Mandell et al. 2004). These are patients who never qualify for brain dead status. Instead, clinical staff have determined these individuals will suffer cardiac arrest, at which time they will not be resuscitated. When under such circumstances kin grant consent to organ donation, they and OPO staff inevitably become involved in a death watch of sorts. Cardiac arrest may occur spontaneously or when a patient is removed from the ventilator, in either the ICU or the operating room. When the heart stops beating, all pause briefly so that kin may have a final moment with the patient; then the patient (now donor) is rushed off to surgery, or else kin are ushered out of the operating room so that procurement work can begin (Greenberg 2003; Roach 2003: 167–95). Just as brain death protocols vary among hospitals, so, too, do those for NHBD or DCD. For example, the amount of time (or what is generally referred to as "the count") allotted between cardiac arrest and the surgical opening of the donor may range from as little as three minutes in state-of-the-art transplant centers to eight minutes in smaller and more cautious hospitals.

Such circumstances require an advanced directive from the patient (as stated in a living will, for instance) or from close kin who agree to a "do not resuscitate" order in anticipation of cardiac arrest. The actual procedures involved are, at the very least, murky. In some quarters they represent a blatant defiance of the credo that medicine must do no harm (Agich 1999; Fox 1993; Lynn 1993; Veatch 1997). Prior to surgery (and, thus, cardiac death), such patients have already endured a range of invasive procedures designed specifically to assess their viability as donors and even prepare them for organ procurement. As one OPO staff member explained, such procedures can be hard on field staff, for whom the excision of lymph nodes from the groin area for medical testing is especially troubling precisely because the often comatose patient is still alive and thus can conceivably experience pain. Such patients are regularly administered medications to control their blood pressure. In addition, as one perfusionist attested, some teams who work in "high crime areas"—where patients are likely to be people of color and poor—may even initiate organ preservation techniques before family consent has been obtained. Critics underscore that such procedures defy rules of informed consent, favoring procurement needs over very basic forms of patient care and perhaps even endangering the patient's life. Renée Fox, a sociologist who has conducted research in the realm of organ transfer since its onset in the 1950s, has gone so far as to describe the DCD protocol as "an ignoble form of cannibalism" (1993: 231). As she explained during a PBS Online Forum:

> This [protocol] consists of a set of procedures for obtaining organs from patients on life support who have suffered a brain injury and lack a neck pulse, with presumably no chance for recovery, but who are not brain-dead. This protocol entails administering high doses or [sic] two drugs to the patient-donor—the anticoagulant heparin and the antihypertensive phentolamine mesylate (Regitine)—in order to prevent blood clotting and widen blood vessels so that the organs procured will be optimally viable for transplant. I am not a physician, but as I understand it, these medications provide no benefit or comfort to the patient who is the prospective donor, and there is the possibility that they may mask the continuing activity of the patient's neck pulse. In the case of Regitine, there is the danger that through its secondary effects, it may induce or hasten the patient's death. (Fox, DeVita, and Ritchie 1998)[27]

Transplant surgeon Dr. Salvador expressed his reluctance in obtaining organs from such patients:

DR. SALVADOR: I have a really hard time with this. . . . Actually there is a reason why [there is the category] of the non-heartbeating [donor], how it came about. Initially this was [tried] in Spain. They actually have an organized system for this kind of donation. [In Spain] it's for people who have an acute heart disorder—they suffer heart failure in the street and then they bring them to the OR. The Spanish system . . . [is] a very well organized system. The other system [like what happens here in the United States is very different]: [here] you have a family who wants to donate but only if it's cardiac arrest. This part gets more tricky. Here they bring the patient to the OR and they stop all support— the vent[ilator] and hemodynamic [support] and then, hmm [pause] . . .

L. S.: You sit and wait?

DR. SALVADOR: Right. And when the heart stops you harvest the
organs. . . . In this case you can't harvest the heart,
I think. I don't like [to harvest organs from these]
patients, but others [here on my team] don't mind.

As liver surgeon Thomas Starzl wrote, "Acceptance of brain death in 1968
was a boon to transplantation" (Starzl 1992: 150); so too, he could later argue for DCD, for by 2003 some OPOs had embraced this protocol with gusto.
Whereas in the 1990s the testing of such protocols in Pittsburgh and Cleveland was hotly contested in the transplant literature (Agich 1999; DeVita
1993; Lynn 1993; Weisbard 1993), today DCD is experiencing rapid rou-
tinization.[28] By 2003, DCD had become a standardized procedure within five
of the eight OPOs where I conducted on-site interviews. As an employee
in one of the nation's smaller OPOs explained, for three years running her
staff had obtained organs from only three DCD donors per year, but by 2003
the number had increased to thirty.

The use of DCDs or NHBDs is hardly new. As Starzl's memoir (1992:
chap. 14) reveals, cardiac death was the precursor to organ procurement in
the early days of experimental transplant surgery in this country. The practice dropped out of fashion as CPR techniques became standardized, alongside advanced knowledge on how to medicate patients in such a way that
they could be sustained on ventilators even when brain dead. The significance
of the DCD *revival*, then, is that it marks a breakdown in contemporary ethical codes of medical behavior. The desperate search for new sources of transplantable organs has thus *re*introduced procedures that now threaten the
humanity of dying patients, adding to their discomfort and suffering and
even, potentially, accelerating their deaths.

Donation Denial

Such are the circumstances of successful procurement. Those kin who refuse to consent to donation are inevitably viewed as uninformed, superstitious, or overly conservative in their religious views, woefully uneducated, or confused by the belief that only cardiac death is a legitimate
marker of a patient's final demise. As a result, public outreach programs—
in the form of public service announcements, health fairs, and talks staged
in schools, hospitals, businesses, and places of worship—are viewed by
OPO personnel as powerful panaceas to any form of lay resistance to organ donation.

A tension that has long characterized OPO work is that staff view non-consenting kin as obstructionist, and they regularly vent their anger and frustration over failed procurement attempts during in-house staff meetings (Sharp 2001). Unfortunately, the world of organ procurement is, in some regions of the United States, fiercely competitive. For instance, some OPO directors may go so far as to attempt to impose monthly quotas on their field staff. In reality, of course, it is impossible to predict the number of gunshot head wounds, auto accidents, strokes, or suicides that will occur in any given month in an OPO's catchment area. As a result, a field team may sense that it remains inescapably in debt, so to speak, to UNOS, to whom their administration submits annual predictions that then determine their funding level for the year.

Institutionalized anxiety over organ scarcity has led some OPOs to push for national policies that approximate "presumed consent," an approach that has proved highly successful in several European countries (BBC 1999). Under presumed consent, patients who die while hospitalized are assumed to approve of organ donation unless they have officially registered their opposition with a state agency. By 2003–4, a number of OPOs had successfully lobbied within their states for new legislation that has since transformed a signed donor card on a driver's license from being mere evidence of a potential donor's desire into a mandated advanced directive (like a living will). Previously, the decision to donate lay with surviving kin to determine; under new legislation, OPO staff can conceivably override the protests of kin and procure organs without their consent. Sabrina Bowers, a staff member from an OPO based in a western state, described this new policy as "'feel good legislation' [because] no one ever votes against this sort of thing." As she explained, it would be unlawful if her staff did not act on this "directive" as designated by the patient. When framed by this new legislation, even supportive hospital personnel become new sources of frustration for such OPO reformers. As Sabrina elaborated, a doctor who counsels a family that the decision to donate is "an option" is in fact acting in direct opposition to the new law.[29]

Rather than viewing those who say no to donation as uninformed or obstructionist, I offer an alternative reading. Although such acts certainly defy the ideological premises of organ transfer, they may also be interpreted as highly creative—albeit subversive—understandings of death as a complex biosocial process. As described in the following section, even kin who understand brain death criteria and who have consented to donation may still voice the opinion in private that the donor's death occurred during procurement surgery. Even more surprisingly, an array of involved and well-informed professionals embrace this sentiment, too.

RECONSTRUCTING DONOR HISTORIES

Seeing and Believing: Professionalized
Strategies for Depersonalizing Donors

The merging of legal criteria with transplant ideology has indeed transformed brain death into a clinical reality, such that the public face of organ
donation proclaims it unequivocally as a great social good. Nevertheless, the
daily practices of organ transfer uncover a more complex set of relationships and meanings. All involved parties openly acknowledge one thing:
whereas brain death is a legitimate or "real" form of death, brain dead donors
still appear, feel, and may even behave as if they are alive. As a result, brain
death criteria evoke the disturbing sense that seeing is *not* believing: these
criteria demand that clinical knowledge override what our senses tell us.
Brain dead patients seem to breathe, but cannot think; we can touch and hold
their warm hands, but they do not respond; and they may move, but only
as a result of residual spinal cord reflexes and not because they sense that
we are there beside them.

This strange, liminal nature of the brain dead patient was expressed suc-
cinctly by Dora Tuckerman, an OPO grief counselor. Dora raised the issue
spontaneously during an interview, asking me, "Have you ever been there?"
to which I gave a puzzled look. She clarified: "Have you ever . . . [seen an
organ donor]?" I gave her a brief overview of an experience I had had while
observing two of her colleagues in the field. She then said, "I have—once.
[The donor] was on the vent[ilator] for ten days. [The sister] had been there
for many, many days [and she was exhausted]. We had a problem getting
him declared—[although] she believed he was dead. Then she called me up
[and said,] 'I don't want him to be alone—can you go?' I'd never gone [be-
fore], and when I saw—you know, they don't look any different from someone who's sleeping."

As Dora's response indicates, understanding brain death as true death is
in many ways an intellectual exercise, one dictated by the premises of transplant ideology. It can nevertheless be extraordinarily difficult for the observer to conceive of such patients simultaneously as mere bodies and thus
as *completely* dead. Among the most shattering experiences is witnessing
reflex movements from residual spinal activity. During one case where I was
an observer in 1995, an ICU nurse attempted to flee the room after a designated donor appeared to shrug in response to a question she had posed
about his status. The OPO clinical coordinator coaxed her into staying and
then calmed her down (and me as well) by explaining that this was merely
a "Lazarus response" caused by a still active spinal cord. Both mortuary lit-

erature and fiction are rife with dramatic accounts of corpses that appear to respond to external stimuli (Proulx 1993; Roach 2003: 98–103; see also Hogle 1999: 65; Wetzel et al. 1985).[30] In the words of Dr. Valentine, a neurologist, however, this is no different from "the chicken that runs around the barnyard after its head has been cut off."

Nevertheless, even highly experienced clinicians can be unnerved by movement in brain dead patients. The surgeon Dr. Salvador reported that such responses led him to delay procurement surgery in at least one instance. As he explained, "I had [a] pediatric—a baby [who] moved on the [operating] table. [The baby] had complex spinal movements. I [called] for a reevaluation [of brain death] and [we] waited five more hours for the reevaluation [before proceeding with] the harvesting." The fact that guidelines for pediatric donors are far more conservative than for adults accounts in part for the extra caution taken by a range of involved professionals. These guidelines stem from the knowledge that infants and children recuperate differently than adults in response to severe brain trauma (Ashwal 2001; Gean 1994; Otte et al. 1989; Sarti 1999). Health professionals regularly make unusually heroic attempts to save children's lives. As OPO staff member Sabrina Bowers explained, in her city's local trauma center, brain death assessments for adults occur six hours apart, but "we wait twelve hours for children because we want to be very careful with them." Field supervisors in some OPOs thus concur with Wijdicks (University of North Dakota 1998), advising their staff to keep kin away from the donor as much as possible to minimize the risk of their exposure to spontaneous movements from the dead.

The process of depersonalization is standard to medical care in this country, in which the most dramatic levels of professional detachment frequently arise in (especially non-hospice) contexts where clinicians must care for the dying (Nuland 1993; Rothman 1991). In hospital settings, brain dead patients clearly define a highly troublesome category, for they are viewed simultaneously as patients, as unconscious (albeit terribly damaged) human beings, and as still-warm dead bodies that move. On a very basic level, the semantics of organ transfer alone quickly set up layer upon layer of medical double binds for the researcher. Simply knowing, for one, how to refer to this liminal category of nonperson may be difficult. Such labels as "cadaver," "corpse," and "neomort" deeply offend surviving kin, who always refer to their loved ones by name. In contrast, procurement staff walk a tightrope between respecting the emotional fragility of kin and remaining true to the ideological premises that drive their work. Acceptance of brain death criteria requires at the very least a great leap of faith, given that seeing is not believing. Even more subtle shifts in faith are at work, too, rendered visible when transplant ideology clashes with private musings over the mystery of death. As we shall see, such shifts are reflected in professional behaviors and turns of phrase. At such moments as these, death emerges as a remarkably complex biosocial process.

Metaphors of Death

Within ICU settings family coordinators rely heavily on metaphorical thinking as a tool for talking with kin about death. Such an approach enables them to skirt the more technical aspects (and details) of the clinical management of brain dead patients. Dora Tuckerman, for instance, offered this example: "One of the . . . coordinators [here likes to say,] 'It's like you have a complex form of farm machinery and the driver falls off.' That's what the brain is," a description that is used widely by others within the same OPO. On two other occasions research participants from separate OPOs described brain death as "a house where there's nobody home." More basic explanations involve defining brain death in reference to what it is not: the patient is "not like someone who is asleep—they will never wake up," or through technical analogies, likening a hemorrhaging brain to a leaky hose or a broken and irreparable container.

Clinicians, too, may revert to metaphorical thinking. Among the more elaborate and poetic descriptions was the following, provided by the neurologist Dr. Lazarre:

> L. S.: Are you concerned with the mind or the brain when you talk about brain death?
>
> DR. LAZARRE: The brain. I'm like a plumber . . . I think about both. [But] with brain death you lost your mind a long time ago. [Look, you can] think [about this as being] just like a fully decorated house. Consciousness is [a world of] color in the [fully decorated] house. [In a] vegetative state you just have the scaffolding up. There's still some residual structure of a brain [there]. [But] with brain death [pause] everything is reduced to dust.

Metaphors similarly abound in the visual imagery used to illustrate informational pamphlets, among which the most prominent involves vegetation, or what I have referred to elsewhere as the "greening" of the donor body (Sharp 2001), a topic I will discuss in greater detail in the final section of this chapter. A pamphlet circulated nationally in the mid-1990s, one intended for use by hospital chaplains, bore an image of three aspen trees clustered before an open field void of other life-forms, with stately mountains in the distance. Imagery such as this now defines a widespread, powerful genre of representation that ultimately clouds or denies the clinical reality of hospital death and organ procurement; the stand of aspens, for instance, evokes instead a sense of serenity. Also notable are attempts to grapple with death ultimately as an unknowable category. How might we describe a rose's perfume to someone who has always lacked the sense of smell? Similarly, can the clinically trained describe a necrotic brain to a family member with no understanding of neurology? The power of the metaphor lies simultaneously in its ability to obscure the dark realm of brain failure while also rendering the intangible somehow knowable. While the family counselor walks a fine line between comforting kin and nudging them toward consent, such metaphors also inevitably facilitate a smoother transition toward the depersonalization of the patient, who may then be thought of with greater ease as occupying the newly established status of organ donor. This process is especially evident in the work conducted by OPO clinical coordinators, who oversee the actual medical care of donors.

Other Forms of Semantic Policing

In their professional efforts to dehumanize the brain dead, procurement specialists must be masters of technological euphemisms. For instance, in any other context a ventilator is typically referred to as "life support," yet this phrase is never used in procurement circles. Holly Franz and her colleagues emphasize the importance of employing what Ruth Richardson (1996) refers to as "semantic massage" when OPO staff address the kin of potential donors:

> *Choose words carefully when talking with the family about the patient's condition.* After brain death is declared, the healthcare team must declare with certainty that the patient is dead. It must be stated explicitly that brain death is not coma, that the patient will not recover, and that [although] the heart is still beating and the body is warm—the person is dead. This information must be stated simply, without obscure medical terms, acronyms, or other jargon that serve to confuse most families. The care given to the brain-dead patient should never be referred to as "life support." Better terms are "artificial" or "mechanical support." (Franz et al. 1997: 19; italics in original)

As Jacquelyn Slomka (1995) has argued, the phrase "life support" can prove detrimental to humane end-of-life care. As she explains, nurturing is pivotal to much of the work performed by health professionals, especially nurses. Among the most difficult aspects surrounding the termination of care involves hydration "therapy," which is administered through "feeding" tubes. When labeled and imagined as such, nurses may find it truly difficult to cease administering such basic forms of care to patients who lie at the brink of death. As a result, their patients may suffer more because they are not allowed to die. In response, Slomka (not unlike Franz et al.) advocates the development of more neutral terminology that shies away from references to care, therapy, and life-sustaining treatments.

OPOs are well aware of these dilemmas. Field staff are instructed to take an active part in dehumanizing brain dead individuals in a manner that goes beyond mere shifts in labeling of patients. Again, I quote from Franz et al., who offer guidance on proper decorum when in the presence of hospitalized organ donors. Shifts in language and behavior are intended to assist kin, hospital staff, and OPO workers in shaping their perceptions of donors: *"Avoid talking to the patient once brain death has been declared.* It is common for nurses and other staff to talk to patients who are unresponsive, which may continue even after brain death has been declared. Members of the healthcare team may need to remind one another to be more conscious of this habit so that their message to the family about the patient's death is not undermined" (Franz et al. 1997: 20; italics in the original).

As such instructions reveal, the ideology of organ transfer insists that ventilated brain-dead patients are already dead, and the policing of semantics and associated behaviors is critical to successful OPO outcomes. A final form of dehumanization is evident in the style of clinical care administered to prospective donors. Because the greatest urgency rests with the ability of OPO staff to preserve the integrity of transplantable organs, they must focus their efforts on protecting organ viability by stabilizing the physiological status of bodies maintained on artificial support systems. In Linda Hogle's words, this "cyborgic technology" reassigns a patient to the liminal status of "living cadaver" (1995b: 204, 206–7; see also Lock 2002, 2003). It is for such reasons that hospital nursing staff readily shift their attention to other patients whom they feel they can still heal. From their perspective, it is truly odd that such intensive care is applied to patients who have been pronounced dead. Among the more troubling aspects of brain death is that it clouds widely accepted views on how we do—or should—die, a fact that is clearly borne out by a case I witnessed in which a patient literally died twice.

The Patient Who Couldn't Die

Mr. Faustman was a forty-nine-year-old Euro-American man who collapsed midday on the sidewalk as a result of a massive stroke, and after a passerby called 911, he was taken by ambulance to a nearby hospital. For the first twenty hours of his hospitalization he remained alone because it took some time to identify and track down his kin. Relying on information found in his wallet, police eventually paid a visit to his apartment, where he lived alone. With the landlord's assistance, the police acquired the names of two adult daughters, both of whom flew in immediately to be at their father's bedside. Within a few hours of their arrival, Willie Otis, the OPO family counselor, sat down with the two sisters and explained, "Your father has had a massive bleed to the head—the hospital has done everything it can to try and save him, but there's just not anything else we can do." Willie added that Mr. Faustman was about to be declared brain dead because "much of the brain has been destroyed." The consent process was rocky: although one daughter readily gave consent, the other was highly suspicious of Willie and began to scream, "You're not going to take his organs!" Willie then asked the nurses to find a room where they could talk privately; in the end, the daughter granted consent as a means to support her sister. Soon afterward their mother (who was in the midst of divorce proceedings with Mr. Faustman) arrived from another distant city. She, too, gave her consent, as did a third daughter who was unable to be there.

Procurement is too complex an affair to proceed smoothly on a regular basis with no glitches, and this case was no exception. A few hours later a doctor from the unit approached Willie and said, "Boy, they've had a bad day, haven't they? It doesn't get much worse than this. I really feel sorry for them. A fuck of a bad day." Willie then turned to me and said, "There's always another story." Within Mr. Faustman's apartment the two daughters had found evidence that their father was gay, something their mother already knew. As Willie explained to me, "Look, this is [Metropolis]—if he's gay, the lover will show up." Indeed, within a few hours of the wife's arrival, this is precisely what happened. At this point Willie confided to the attending physician, "I don't want this gay information broadcasted." He and his supervisor back at the home office decided together to withhold information from UNOS on Mr. Faustman's sexual history until serology tests came back for HIV and various strains of hepatitis. According to Willie's partner, the clinical coordinator Kathy Green, Mr. Faustman did in fact test negative for HIV but positive for hepatitis B. Although by evening the daughters and their mother had already retreated to a local hotel to await word that the procurement surgery was over, and various local transplant teams stood poised and ready to come and begin harvesting his organs, in the end Mr. Faustman was deemed too high-risk a case to qualify as an organ donor. As a result, he never entered surgery.

Early the next morning Gabriel Evers, another clinical coordinator, arrived to relieve Willie and Kathy, both of whom had been at work in the hospital for the last two days. Gabriel's primary assignment was to assist hospital staff in disconnecting Mr. Faustman from the ventilator. As Gabriel later explained, however:

> It became a feud [over] who wanted to do what . . . and then [the hospital staff] got really confused about pulling the plug. One of the doctors said we should just keep him on oxygen but [that will keep the] heart going! This doc [then] wanted to declare the death upon *disconnecting him.* He wanted to *throw out the death certificate* [declaring brain death] *and do it again!* I said, *You can't do that! HE'S DEAD!* So I had to tell him what to do. I said, Get the family in here to say their good-byes and then get them out of here and disconnect him. . . . Most hospitals won't just take someone off the life support. But you know, a patient like this can go for six weeks just on the respirator—because as long as the heart is still getting oxygen, it can keep on beating. The heart can keep going—they can potentially die six weeks later. . . . [Eventually] they took him off the respirator—they stopped giving him oxygen. By then, I'd left—my work was over. . . . In the end, they did [reissue the death certificate].

I was curious to see how Mr. Faustman's demise was officially reported by his family, and so I searched the local paper that week for his obituary. As I recorded in my field notes, Mr. Faustman was found on the street and hospitalized on May 20, and he was declared brain dead on the evening of May 21. His obituary, however, recorded that he had died "suddenly on May 23," this date coinciding with the time he was disconnected from "life support" by the hospital physician. In the end, Mr. Faustman indeed died twice.

Personhood and the Brain Death Conundrum

The case of Mr. Faustman reconfirms arguments put forth by Margaret Lock (2002) that organ donors are a category of the twice dead. I would like to expand this argument by exploring how this specific account uncovers the manner in which shifting or competing explanatory frameworks are also at work. We might consider Mr. Faustman's case, for instance, as offering unquestionable evidence of severe cognitive disjunction. Even more compelling is how transplant ideology so readily confounds the ability to view death as an intricate social process. In contrast, Mr. Faustman's case insists on such an alternative reading.

Medicolegal guidelines dictate that death is something we can map out, track, and declare; in turn, the act of declaring death is time-bound, and thus death inevitably must occur only at a very particular, recordable moment. End-of-life hospital work and procurement activities both rely heavily on this model: in caring for organ donors, specialists in each domain must embrace brain death as absolute death. Pat Fisher, who works for an East Coast OPO, expressed this idea in blunt terms: "The donor is dead—not sort of dead, not kind of dead, but dead. D-E-A-D dead. This kind of hedging is destructive to donor families . . . and the work we do in my office." During such horribly mixed-up moments as Mr. Faustman's demise, death nevertheless emerges as both a social process and a social drama. Mr. Faustman's death, after all, involved a host of end-of-life events marked by a full range of physiological breakdowns. First, when found, he was unconscious and alone. Once he was hospitalized, staff were able to stabilize him, although he never revived as a cognitive being. As his brain deteriorated, his body nevertheless continued to function, albeit through the assistance of mechanized support. Following the removal of the ventilator, his heart quickly failed, and he turned cold and gray. Throughout this process professionals and surviving kin withdrew their support at various moments, depending on which stages they considered to be the most significant markers of his death. Nurses were among the first to withdraw, clearing the way for OPO staff; Mr. Faustman's kin retreated to a hotel only once they believed he was bound for surgery; an attending physician, however, still viewed Mr. Faustman as a living patient when he failed to qualify as a donor. OPO staff left the hospital only when procurement became impossible, although they regarded Mr. Faustman as dead much earlier than all other participants.

Significantly, parties involved in or who witness donor management do not necessarily embrace brain death as evidence of true death even if they are supportive of organ donation. Research conducted by Franz et al. (1997) vividly illustrates this. Drawing on result from a survey involving 172 families from three OPOs, where respondents consisted of 102 kin who had consented to donation and another 62 who had not, these authors found that a significant proportion on both sides had not fully understood brain death criteria (cf. Siminoff et al. 2001 for a similar discussion). A full 20 percent believed that brain dead individuals could recover; 28 percent equated brain death with coma; and 12 percent assumed the heart had already ceased to function. An additional 6 to 9 percent answered "I don't know" to each of these questions. Statements generated from interviews offered evidence for why this was so. For example, when asked whether brain death is the same as a coma, a forty-seven-year-old man, whose wife had been a donor, responded as follows: "They are dead. Well, they're not dead. . . . It depends on how you look at this." A thirty-two-year-old wife who denied consent explained: "I think a little of both. . . . My emotions are telling me that [his brain is dead], but the rest of him is still alive until I do what I have to do."

Finally, a donor's thirty-year-old daughter put it as follows: "She was breath-ing. Her heart was going. . . . They're telling you that she's dead, but she's still there" (Franz et al. 1997: 17–18).

My own interviews with donor kin generated similar responses. As one father explained of his teenage daughter, "As far as I'm concerned, she died on the operating table." In response to these sorts of answers, though, Franz et al. reach this limited conclusion: "The difficulty many laypeople have in understanding the concept of brain death cannot be underestimated [sic]" (1997: 17). The policing of language and gesture, as outlined earlier, defines the main component of the solutions Franz et al. offer in response. In do-ing so, however, these authors overlook the possibility that kin regularly consent to donation although they may not accept brain death criteria as evidence of true or absolute death. An important question that must be an-swered is, What leads some to consent to organ donation even when this is so?

One possibility is that OPO counselors are especially persuasive or even coercive at moments when kin are already destabilized by the shock of a sudden death. Those working for the nation's largest OPOs do in fact speak regularly of developing ever more "aggressive" tactics for acquiring con-sent. Yet my data support an alternative and more subtle reading. For one, I assert that those who say no to donation will probably always do so, re-gardless of the educational messages they receive, or the "aggressive" tac-tics they might endure. Nevertheless, a widespread belief among OPO staff is that most kin say no specifically because they are unaware of the official stance of their respective religious faiths. For this reason much effort has focused on culling succinct (and, thus, superficial) statements from clerics of all stripes to illustrate that there is a near-universal acceptance of organ donation (for example, see DCIDS 2004). The nonreligious in turn may be labeled as "superstitious" or "uneducated." My own data reveal, however, that informants' visceral reactions to what happens to the body at the time of death play a large role in determining consent outcomes, whether or not they are religious. Those who say no to donation understand death as a time of suffering, and this is a process that persists when the brain has failed, as the body itself breaks down and, even, at times, after the body has turned cold and gray. For such reasons these kin feel strongly that the patient—or body—must remain undisturbed and intact if death is to be peaceful. Cer-tain faiths and cultures may even view discussions of death, or of the dead themselves, as threatening to this process.[31] As such, the activities of OPO staff emerge as dangerous work because of the volatile emotional responses they evoke in kin who hold different beliefs about the *process* of death.

On the other hand, kin who consent to donation are frequently capable of embracing competing models of death simultaneously (although they generally refrain from voicing contradictory beliefs within earshot of OPO staff). Two models are particularly relevant here. The first relies on clinical definitions of death, whereas the second focuses on more intimate understandings of the selfhood of the beloved. Kin consent to donation when they understand that the social being they know and love is irretrievably lost to them. Their desire to perform a great act of kindness by helping strangers in need bolsters their commitment. Nevertheless, many kin regularly accept as well that the inner self, soul, or spirit finally dies (or departs) only once the body itself fails entirely. In cases of brain death, this occurs during procurement surgery; for DCD, it coincides with the cessation of the heartbeat. Such understandings are key to organ transfer's success, although ironically they run contrary to organ transfer's ideological assumptions about death.

Donor kin are not alone in embracing a model of the multiple death, or, when understood in its more sophisticated form, of death as an intricate social process mediated only in part by medicolegal interventions (and definitions). Procurement professionals may express similar ideas: at times this is reflected in the rhetoric of persuasion, at others, such beliefs are voiced explicitly during private interviews. For instance, among the most effective messages offered by OPO counselors is that donors can live on in others, granting new or "second" lives to transplant recipients who, in turn, frequently describe their own surgeries as cathartic "rebirths." These same professionals also privately acknowledge the tenuous quality of brain death. During staff meetings at one OPO, employees regularly distinguished brain death from cardiac death by describing individual donors as moving from the state of being "kind of" or "sort of" dead in the ICU to being "dead dead" following procurement surgery (Sharp 2001; cf. Hogle 1995a). Such donors are, in Lock's words, "good-as-dead" (Lock 2003; cf. Greenberg 2003; Siminoff 2004).

Hospital-based physicians, too, readily speak of the dissonance that prevails between official rhetoric and private beliefs (Youngner et al. 1989; Youngner, Arnold, and DeVita 1999). For example, I had the following exchange with Dr. Lazarre:

> L. S.: When you talk about brain death, are you thinking about a brain dead patient or a brain that's dead? Also, is it possible to say that someone can die twice—first brain death and then cardiac death?

DR. LAZARRE: Sure—I can keep the rest of your body alive. The rest of your body is alive artificially. Does this mean you die twice? The way you should die [is that] dead is dead. Brain death should mean that you're dead. But in [this state within the United States]—it's very conservative [politically here]. . . . You're only dead by brain death if you want to be. Only if your family doesn't accept it for religious [definitions of] death.

Another neurologist put it thus:

DR. NEEDLER: It [brain death] is synonymous with death, which we're taught to say [to families] in the ICU [but] I'm not really convinced of that [although it's no way to live]. . . . [To me] the person is irrevocably gone—we don't even expect them to do even what a baby can do. I try to convey to the family that I'm not horrified by this—I wish to see them grow, but they're not going to grow.

In these senses, then, the biological breakdown of the brain and body undermines the social functioning of the person valued for his or her sentient qualities. These and related sentiments are not unusual: Lock herself reports that "among the thirty-two intensivists (specialists who work in ICUs) whom I interviewed between 1995 and 1997, not one believes that brain death signals the end of biological life," although they embrace the understanding that the brain is irreversibly damaged and that this will eventually lead to "complete biological death" (Lock 2003: 171–72). An internist whom I interviewed, and who works closely with transplant recipients, offered yet another point of view. Rather than describing organ donors as dying twice, she stressed that "we need to view death as a process that we undergo gradually over time." When taken together, these views offered by donor kin, OPO staff, and physicians provide a more gradual and thus subtle model of donor death, albeit one that runs contrary to the official rhetoric of organ transfer. When death is framed exclusively as a biological process, typically the brain dead donor moves from head trauma, to mechanical ventilation, to brain death declaration, to anesthetized surgery, to the physiological death of the body during procurement, culminating much later in final decomposition at the cellular level. Such is the specifically medicolegal trajectory of brain death.

If we in turn trace the demise of the social person and the self, death emerges as a different sort of *social* process. We can depart from this world in various ways, depending on individual readings of what defines the key aspects of our selves. At times such readings are linked to biological processes, such as aging. As Dr. Needler said of vegetative and brain dead patients, "They're like a baby again. There's some humanity [there] but [there's] not really a developed mind." An even more stringent approach is reflected in the opinions of OPO staff, who understand that the self dissipates with coma and is irrevocably extinguished when the brain fails. As a result, such donors should no longer be treated as if they are full-fledged human beings, as evident in the range of semantic policing described earlier in this chapter.

Some kin, however, understand the social process of death in ways that ultimately defy a clinical model of death. A brain dead state (not unlike coma) renders it impossible for kin to detect traces of the person locked within. Kin nevertheless continue to respond to a brain dead person with the understanding that he or she might somehow still be there in small part. They willingly caress and speak to such patients up until the moment they are taken to surgery. The ability of kin to maintain a sense of connection is facilitated by the fact that brain dead patients do not appear dead. Thus, the unresponsive donor retains some essence of a unique life. Donor kin frequently understand the donor's private self (or, for some, the soul) as departing only during or by the end of procurement surgery—that is, only once the body has become an empty shell.

At work here is a subtle distinction between the *social person* as cognizant (and communicative) human being and the far more *private, hidden self*. With brain death, I argue, kin are far more likely to accept that the social person is no longer there (and, thus, has died) because evidence of the behaviors and responses they associate with social behavior is gone. Put another way, the social person dies as the brain fails, and it is for this reason that kin ultimately consent to donation. As for the unique, private self, kin frequently feel that this lives on in the body and persists until the donor is ultimately and truly a cadaver. Sadly, the official ideology of organ transfer denies the legitimacy of these sentiments and associated subtle distinctions. In the realm of organ procurement there is no room for such existential possibilities.

With these sentiments in mind, I argue for a radical shift in frames of reference so that we might recognize the wider range in which death is culturally constructed. Unfortunately, when involved parties question the reductionistic quality of ideological premises driving organ transfer, they are quickly silenced because they are perceived of as challenging the legitimacy of brain death criteria. For instance, procurement professionals view questioning within their own ranks as a sign of weak faith or work-related fatigue. Similarly, when donor kin state that a loved one died during procurement surgery and not in the ICU, OPO staff insist that kin have misunderstood the definition of brain death (or may assume that they themselves failed in their mission to communicate what this term means). But what if we read such statements as evidence of an acceptance of the inevitability of death, albeit under circumstances radically different from those promoted in the messages delivered by OPO counselors? I regularly encounter donor kin who embrace organ donation as among the most important decisions they have ever made in their lives, yet these same people may still question or challenge the assertion that brain death is true death or, even more important to them, that it is a natural way to die. When the father of a teenage donor states, "She died on the operating table," he does not mean that OPO staff orchestrated her death but, rather, that the essence of his daughter departed when her organs were procured and her body ultimately failed.

Anesthetizing the Dead

One of the most peculiar aspects of procurement involves the manner in which organ donors are surgically managed. As noted, although organ donors already have been declared brain dead, they are nevertheless anesthetized at least during the first portion of procurement surgery (Gelb and Robertson 1990; Levinson and Copeland 1987). This practice is rarely discussed, and it is not even necessarily understood by closely involved parties. When I posed questions about why dead patients need to be anesthetized, I was informed by three OPO staff members, two neurologists, and two internists (both of whom work closely with prospective transplant recipients) that I must be misinformed. The subsequent musings of one neurologist exemplified the responses I received from two other physicians. As Dr. Valentine responded, "I suppose it might be used in order to suppress residual spinal activity?" Dr. Lazarre put it thus: "You need to ask an anesthesiologist that one. As far as I know they don't need anesthesia. The only reasons might be that the spinal cord may still be perfused and alive, and capable of triggering vasomotor reflexes (i.e., unstable blood pressure) in response to painful stimuli such as cracking the chest open or cutting the abdomen open."

Procurement surgery is indeed complex and can generate a host of complications that require immediate response from the anesthesiologist (Gelb and Robertson 1990: esp. 809–11; Levinson and Copeland 1987). Dr. Salvador, who regularly retrieves organs from donors, offered this explanation:

> The [donor] patient is brain dead, [and] you have an anesthesiologist, but it's not really for anesthesia. They are there to oxygenate the patients [and] monitor the hemodynamic [status—that is, blood pressure;

for this] they may administer pressors—you see, the longer you
are brain dead . . . the greater the requirement is for pressor support
[in anticipation of drops in blood pressure]. [Anesthesiologists] also
give drugs to paralyze the patient to relax the abdomen more for us
[to make our work easier]. . . . But [once] the blood has been removed
[by the perfusionist] the anesthesiologist is no longer necessary.

Yet another transplant surgeon, Dr. Paluchi, explained the need for
anesthesia as follows in a note: "The donor is brain dead, i.e., dead, so that
anesthesia per se is not needed. We do need to give muscle relaxation [*sic*]
as there are spinal reflexes which lead to stomach muscle contractions while
operating. Anesthesia is also needed to[o] or at a least a nurse, so that the
blood pressure can be regulated and drugs [such as] insulin can be given."
Clearly, then, anesthesia plays a pragmatic role here, serving to relax the
body so that the donor will not move and potentially jeopardize the delicate work of removing still vital organs.

There is, however, another purpose at work. As Adrian Gelb and Kerri
Robertson write, neuromuscular reflexes "may range from muscle twitch-
ing to complex movements of the limbs and trunk. For the unsuspecting in
the operating room, this can be most disconcerting and staff may require
frequent reassurance that the donor is indeed dead" (1990: 809). The neurologist Dr. Needler similarly underscored this fact:

L. S.: I understand that brain dead donors are anesthetized—

DR. NEEDLER: Yeah, I know: Why, if they're dead?

L. S.: Exactly.

DR. NEEDLER: They are dead. My understanding is that the anesthesia
[is used] to relieve the people who work in organ procurement. . . . Although I think it's very rare, [I think
they're thinking,] "What if they've been given the
wrong information that the person is brain dead but
[they're actually in another state]?" This would be
horrible—they would feel they were assisting in an
evil cause. It is a way to avoid [participating] in the evil
cause [of being responsible for harming someone]. If
they know they are anesthetized [then they know] the
patient didn't experience [any pain].

L. S.: This may sound naive, but if someone is brain dead
from brain stem failure, could they still experience
pain?

DR. NEEDLER: [No.] Pain is a cortical phenomenon. [She offers
a detailed description of cases where patients

have experienced extreme upper brain trauma but
show no responses to intractable pain.] If the brain
stem isn't functioning you can't have upper brain
function.

Linda Hogle, who has conducted field research on this subject in both the
United States and Germany, confirms that anesthesia does, in fact, help quell
anxieties among surgical staff. As she explains, although donor bodies may
be handled as passive objects (laid out, for instance, on a gurney or operating table, with both the body and the face covered with a surgical drape),
they nevertheless exert a "type of agency" because "the body responds" to
a range of stimuli during surgery. In addition to the need to monitor hemodynamic systems, "more disconcerting are reactions not considered to
be characteristics of dead bodies. Spinal reflexes may cause the body to move,
as if the body is reacting to the incisions. Blood pressure and respiratory
changes have been reported at the moment of incision and during the procedure. Neither reaction is supposed to happen in 'dead' bodies, even brain-
dead ones, and neither the chemical agents nor the physical actions being
carried out explain such reactions in the reported cases" (Hogle 1999: 164–
65, citing Emmrich 1994; Wetzel et al. 1985).

Hogle's interviews with operating room staff in Germany uncovered
specific concerns over the limited application of anesthetics:

Since no deep-pain control is used, individuals who are unsure or
unconvinced about the implications of brain death are concerned that
the person may be able to sense pain even if he is incapable of expressing it. Therefore, he may be dying an agonizing death, according to
detractors. Neurologists insist that pain response is no longer possible
in brain death. Not using additional anesthesia is another way of cog-
nitively placing the body closer to the state of being an organic mass
as opposed to a patient in an indeterminate state of animation . . . both
opinions about pain response are theoretical because they are impossible
to test.

As Hogle concludes, both the body and the surgical staff "flinch" in response to this paired "invasion of bodily boundaries" and the "invasion of
the boundary between life and death" (1999: 165).

In recent years, these sorts of concerns have driven heated debates
among anesthetists (anesthesiologists) based specifically in the United Kingdom. The related literature proves especially helpful, given that the authors
are the very specialists who are most intimately involved in the minute-
to-minute surgical management of organ donors. Key questions focus on

whether brain dead and/or DCD donors require anesthesia; whether necessary procedures should even be referred to as anesthesia; and whether either brain dead or DCD donors are in fact fully dead. As David Hill, an anesthetist, asserts, "The greatest misconception is that the donor will be dead in any ordinary sense of the word. Most people equate death with what [another author] calls 'asystolic' donation, not the warm, pink, pulsating, breathing (albeit by machine), reactive state that we call brainstem death. It may come as a considerable shock to know that the donor will always need to be paralyzed for the surgery, and may or may not have anaesthesia" (Hill 1999, citing Pallis and Harley 1996: 46). Hill's statement is rooted in the assumption that organ donors are best imagined as liminally dead patients rather than as full-fledged cadavers.

The quandaries associated with this position are addressed in detail by P. J. Young and B. F. Matta, both of whom specialize in neurosurgical critical care. Specifically, they question the recommendations appearing in a 1999 pamphlet on organ donor procurement surgery, as published by the Intensive Society of the United Kingdom. More specifically, they object to the general statement that "brainstem dead patients do not require analgesia or sedation." Echoing earlier arguments by clinicians I interviewed, they assert that anesthesia quells the doubts of surgical staff, and rightly so, given the lack of confirmatory tests to show without a doubt that the donor experiences no pain. They also insist that death is best viewed not as a discrete event but as a process:

> Firstly, under few circumstances do we allow operative surgery with muscle relaxation and without analgesia or anaesthesia, leading to a psychological compulsion to provide anaesthesia. Second, the hypertension and tachycardia that accompanies the donation operation can be distressing for operating theatre personnel to witness and for this reason alone one should always administer anaesthesia or agents to control these reflexes. [A shift in blood pressure] . . . could be considered to represent an organism in distress and probably occurs at a spinal level, although we are unaware of EEG studies during organ collection to confirm this. Third, death is not an event but a process and our limited understanding of the process should demand caution before assuming that anaesthesia is not required. (P. Young and Matta 2000: 105)

J. Wace and M. Kai offer a more contentious response, identifying in particular the "transplant lobby" as undermining necessary anesthesia requirements for donors. Further, they challenge the assertion that DCD and brain dead donors are truly dead. Speaking of events that transpired at a conference of Medical Royal Colleges, Wace and Kai express the following concerns:

> This conference was intended to facilitate beating heart organ donation but only concluded that the state of brain stem death was a state of unsurvivable coma and, quite rightly, stopped short of equating it to death itself.
>
> Many anaesthetists clearly have been very uneasy about the transplant lobby's rather rash assumption that organ donors do not require anaesthesia. Many anaesthetists do administer an anaesthetic to these patients, with good reason, as set out [by Young and Matta]. The problem the transplant lobby have with giving donors an anaesthetic is the perceived additional difficulty in telling the donor's relatives that the donor is not dead but in an unsurvivable coma.
>
> It is time all anaesthetists realised that to not administer an anaesthetic to a donor (who is not by any definition dead) is to commit an act of possibly barbarous dishonesty. Whatever the effect on donor numbers, one cannot condone such action. (2000: 590)

In this sense, then, organ donors exist in an unusual state of nonbeing, but not full death. B. Poulton and M. Garfield, however, react "with dismay" to these assertions. They argue instead that in administering anesthesia one ultimately grants consciousness (or life) to a patient who should already be treated as dead. Unlike the other authors cited here, then, Poulton and Garfield refute the necessity of anesthetizing donors. Key to their argument (or what Wace and Kai equate with the "transplant lobby") is the assertion that, even if we view death as a process, the practice of anesthetizing donors undermines messages communicated to surviving kin:

> Appropriate concentrations of volatile anesthetics could only *produce* unconsciousness if the individual was conscious to begin with. . . . Consciousness in the absence of brainstem reflexes is a theoretical possibility, but if this was known to be the case in a particular individual, we believe that few of us would be comfortable in informing relatives that their loved one had "died." Death is clearly a process but many would argue that the persistence of consciousness, more than the function of any organ system, defines human life. Death may well be inevitable for individuals meeting the brainstem criteria, but to render a conscious mind unconscious for the purpose of organ harvest could well be considered as an act of euthanasia. (Poulton and Garfield 2000: 695; italics in the original; see also Turner 2000)

As these heated debates make clear, regardless of the stance asserted by organ transfer ideology, the uncertainty of death still haunts some neurointensivists and anesthesiologists who, in the United Kingdom at least, willingly voice their concerns. The positions asserted by these clinical specialists are fed at times by what they witness during surgery; at others, they more closely approximate the position of procurement professionals, whose work must insist that a being for whom there is no hope of revived consciousness is already fully dead.

Clearly, the inability to grasp fully the minute details of the process of death underlies this troublesome debate. The lack of universal criteria, paired with diagnostic limitations, proves particularly irksome. As Matta explains, "Defining a moment at which death occurs within the dying process is necessary but arbitrary, and differs across societies. A brain might be defined as dead in the United Kingdom, yet the same brain would not be dead in Europe and vice-versa. . . . While there is no evidence to suggest consciousness persists in these patients (with obvious reasons), the absence of a direct measurement of this makes it only a belief that has not, and perhaps cannot be, confirmed" (2000: 695–96). In the face of uncertainty, those medical specialists most intimately involved in managing the ultimate demise of organ donors frequently insist that these patients be handled as if they were still alive. Critics, though, view such approaches as unethical because they are tantamount to acknowledging that surgical teams practice euthanasia. At the heart of this conundrum is the fact that one can never be certain if organ donors retain the ability to sense the world around them.

Just as surgeons themselves should care, in Dr. Salvador's words, about the "aesthetics" of the donor body, the art of anesthesia is likewise guided by aesthetic principles in response to a troubling set of existential quandaries.[32] Given that the majority of American OPO field staff never enter the operating theater, they can embrace with greater ease the understanding that brain death is an absolute state of nonexistence. As such, they accept the premise that an organ donor can experience no further trauma during surgery. Those who have more intimate experience with the actual "procurement," "retrieval," or "harvesting" of organs, however, come face-to-face with the open-ended and unknowable qualities of donors' deaths. This then leads them to ponder the likelihood of physical pain as well as the point at which one can sense the ultimate demise of the patient. The actions of those specifically in charge of the surgical management of organ procurement are driven in part by a "what if" approach, such that they administer anesthesia as a means to stave off persistent doubts while also preserving the dignity of patients whose bodies house parts coveted by transplant surgeons.

BODY ECONOMIES

> If I wind up brain-dead with usable parts, someone's going to use
> them, squeamishness be damned.
>
> M. ROACH, *Stiff* (2003: 291–92)

As reflected in the previous discussion, the ideological premises of organ
transfer overshadow a host of contradictions, particularly about how we must
perceive of, talk about, and manage patients who are sustained artificially
in half-dead states. Responses expose the fact that potential donors (and
donor bodies) are valued in radically different ways by assorted parties. OPO
staff, for instance, insist that the technology of ICU patient care creates the
illusion that brain dead donors are still alive. Yet donor kin who grant consent may silently question this assertion, sensing instead that a damaged
brain may rob the beloved of their humanity but not necessarily their
essence or life force. All participants nevertheless agree that organ transfer
is of great social worth because it grants life to others who are at the brink
of death. Through the act of consent, goodness can spring from horrific
tragedy and grief. As we shall see, however, such principles define only a
fraction of the value assigned to organ donors and their transplantable parts.

Body Counts

As my earlier discussions make clear, brain dead patients experience a transformation in value, shifting in status from that of human being to a repository of harvestable organs. Organs, too, are similarly transformed. Once removed from the original bodies that housed them, organs shift to being prized
commodities (Sharp 2000b) that must be handled with great care. Because it
is illegal to buy and sell organs in the United States, their worth is clouded
by the language of an unusual gift economy. Donated organs have long been
described as "gifts of life," for which donor kin receive no monetary compensation, nor even reciprocal favors from OPOs, transplant teams, or organ
recipients (or their insurance companies). Within the framework of the gift
economy, donor kin also assume an elevated social status: alongside organ
donors, they are frequently described, for example, as transplant's "unsung
heroes" and "stars." Regardless of the fact that transplant medicine is unquestionably among the most lucrative of medical professions, the rhetoric
of organ transfer glosses over this reality. As James Frick, a perfusionist and
surgical technician who advocates compensation, asserted during an informal discussion, "Look, we're *all* sustained by this industry—whether through
surgery or even through [your] research—let's stop kidding ourselves, we
all profit from it, [so] shouldn't donor families get something, too?" Donor

kin are nevertheless expected to give willingly and selflessly to anonymous strangers. As critics assert, paying donor kin for their acts of kindness would debase the Samaritan act so intrinsic to organ donation, defile the sanctity of donors' deaths, and potentially drive the economically disenfranchised to place dying kin (or themselves) at risk when lured by promises of economic gain.

The medical worth of the donor body itself is reflected in a numerical language employed by a range of staff from assorted professional organizations. For instance, those who work for OPOs regularly speak of the "seven-organ donor" or even "nine-organ donor" as the quintessential success case. Currently the body's value is similarly quantified by UNOS and other organizations. A popular statement is that one body may generate fifty or more reusable parts, a figure that has climbed steadily over the last few decades as clinical medicine finds ever-expanding ways to reuse the human body (Fehar, Naddaff, and Tazi 1989; Flye 1995; Hogshire 1992; Kimbrell 1993; Machado 1998; Murray 1987). Monthly and annual tallies are also maintained by UNOS and individual OPOs as a means to track how many organs are procured and transplanted. Individual transplant units maintain their own body counts: at public forums and conferences, surgeons and their staff will inevitably cite the number of surgeries they have performed within a week, month, or year. Finally, even organ recipients are subjected to quantification, falling into a given unit's numbered hierarchy of transplants. For example, they regularly identify themselves as "the third lung" or "heart number twenty-five" from their respective hospitals. Lower numbers accrue greater value: in one hospital I watched staff over the course of four years repeatedly go to extraordinary lengths to extend the life of a recipient who held the esteemed status of "heart number one," a patient who, in turn, always signs his name on personal notes and greeting cards followed by "#1." It is worth noting, too, that an unwavering agenda within all involved organizations is the constant drive to increase their numbers of acquired organs.

Scarcity, Recycling, and Renewal

Scarcity breeds anxiety, which in the realm of organ transfer is reflected in a language that contrasts successful organ reclamation with the tragedies of lost opportunities. Evelyn Brown, a nurse whom I met in the Midwest and who was married to a lung recipient, put it thus as long ago as 1992: "I don't know too much about it, but I know there is a shortage of organs. I hadn't really thought much about it before all of this, but now it seems to me it's a shame to waste all of those organs when there are people who need them." Evelyn's words reflect an ongoing concern that OPOs consistently fail to capture all the nation's eligible donors. Beneath this sentiment is the understanding that once patients shed their personhood and revert to donor status, redefining them as vessels harboring reusable parts is intrinsically unproblematic and a natural aspect of this process.

Public outreach programs today are driven by a heightened sense of scarcity anxiety, where promotional slogans are designed to encourage people to offer their bodies willingly to meet transplant's needs. As noted in the introduction to this book, a range of genres abounds in these messages; among the most popular is a "greening" of the donor body, a strategy that draws heavily on nature imagery (Sharp 2001). Promotional campaigns, T-shirts, campaign buttons, posters, and bumper stickers all bear messages underscoring that organ transfer is a regenerative process, as one might encounter in nature. Associated imagery assumes several forms.

One dominant approach draws directly on references to recycling. Just as the ecology movement perceives bottles, cans, and plastic containers as renewable resources, within the realm of organ transfer, human body parts can be reused to replenish dying patients. Two of the most established slogans are "Recycle Yourself" (often displayed against a triangular recycling emblem) and the complementary celestial version, "Don't Take Your Organs to Heaven—Heaven Knows We Need Them Here."[33] Yet another approach transforms the donor body into an astonishing array of greenery. As noted earlier, an artist's rendering of an isolated stand of aspen trees graced the cover of one organization's pamphlet on brain death. In a range of other contexts, images designed to underscore the social worth of organ donation are similarly devoid of people, illustrated instead with pictures of trees, leaves, or flowers. Some images go so far as to offer visual puns. Consider, for instance, a change of address card issued by UNOS that featured the image of a repotted, flowering plant to illustrate the message, "We've Been Transplanted" (figure 1). Grafted tree branches and leaves appear on transplant and donation-related literature, too, offering an only slightly veiled reference to the surgical "grafting" of organs to recipients' bodies. In still other contexts, the shapes of various flora may appear reminiscent of particular organs. As I detail elsewhere, strange-shaped clouds can resemble livers and pancreases, or leaves may be clustered in such a way as to form a heart or to suggest a pair of lungs or kidneys (see Sharp 2001, figures 1–4).

The butterfly, too, has recently achieved iconic status. This image was first adopted by the National Donor Family Council, a grassroots organization that lobbies for the needs of donor families. For several years a pink butterfly has served as its logo, gracing its letterhead, newsletter, and other print materials. NDFC members also regularly sport butterfly pins at organ transfer events. The image of the butterfly is now popular among OPOs across

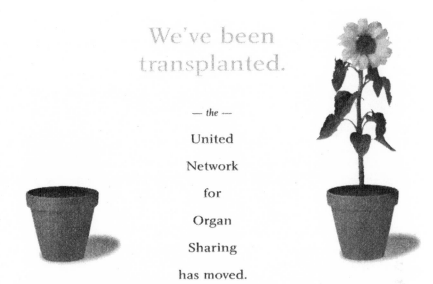

We've been
transplanted.

— the —

United

Network

for

Organ

Sharing

has moved.

Figure 1.   Moving announcement issued by the United Network for Organ Sharing in December 2002. Design by Kevin Smolen. Image used by permission of UNOS.

the nation as a symbol of the spirit of organ donors, of hope, or of the ever-repetitive circle of life and thus, again, renewal. As I will detail in the next chapter, even UNOS has adopted this symbol: in a newly established memorial on its corporate grounds, one may now stroll past a butterfly garden.

Through this ecology of the body, plant and other associated imagery draws on established traditions that recognize nature's regenerative properties (Bloch and Parry 1982). Such imagery, then, bolsters a public image of organ transfer as a life-giving force. The frequent playfulness of associated slogans and images underscores the great social worth of organ donation while successfully obscuring references to a darker reality: that is, that organ transfer relies heavily on the inevitability of tragic deaths. The power of recycling imagery lies in its ability to focus our attention on the idea that death can beget life as part of a larger circular process of natural regeneration.

The Politics of Waste and Social Redemption

Of concern, though, too, are anxieties over wastefulness. Whereas a body placed in a grave could conceivably replenish the soil, in the realm of organ transfer such an action is understood as a terrible waste of precious goods that could serve a far better purpose by rejuvenating the bodies of sickly human beings. The failure of some kin, then, to grant consent is frequently interpreted by OPO staff, surgeons, and involved lay parties as yet another example of wasteful consumerism in a throwaway society. Furthermore, whereas organ donors assume an elevated social position, procurement professionals may quickly relegate failed cases to the status of medical waste or refuse. Among the most virulent language employed by OPO staff is that reserved for those bodies that in the end are unable to generate transplantable parts.

This method of devaluing a failed donor is exemplified by the language employed by the clinical coordinator Gabriel Evers when he described in retrospect the case of Mr. Faustman. As noted earlier, Gabriel was called in to relieve two exhausted coworkers; contact transplant units and tell them that there were in fact no organs available from this disqualified donor; and assist ICU staff in removing Mr. Faustman from the ventilator over the objections of an attending physician. A day later, when I asked him how it all ended, Gabriel offered this assessment:

> It got ruled out fifteen minutes before packing the donor to go to the OR. [But] this donor was crappy from the get-go. The [medical and social] history said so! [He had a] history of hypertension . . . [and] the kidneys were shitty! And then there was the boyfriend who didn't even know he'd collapsed on the street. . . . [Later I was the one who had] to call [the kidney surgeon], and he starts yelling at me over the phone, saying, "What the hell are you giving me these shitty kidneys for?" . . . The donor was garbage from the get-go!

As Gabriel's words illustrate, the politics of social redemption define an ever-shifting ground in the realm of organ transfer. In this account, Mr. Faustman moved from being a potential source of valuable organs to little more than medical refuse. His kidneys were "shitty," and his body (and its associated history) "crappy" and "garbage from the get-go." As such language makes clear, in the end the blame or fault rests with the donor himself as his parts in essence move from "treasure" to "trash."[34] Such views have their counterparts among donor kin.

Organ donation, when it succeeds, grants surviving kin the hope that they may assist others in need. As a result, some kin opt for donation even when they know that a member of their own community will object. Donor kin often recount stories of neighbors, coworkers, and distant kin who express astonishment or disgust when they learn of the decision to donate organs, especially when the donor was a child. Some of the more strident criticisms they endure focus on their willingness to have the body cut open so its parts can be removed. Instances in which kin decide in favor of donation over widespread cultural objects become cherished stories among OPO workers. For example, Octavia Zamora, an OPO worker from the Southwest, recounted during an interview in 2003 the story of one of the few Native American donors her organization could claim in more than ten years of personal experience. In this case, the mother explained her decision to offer her son's organs as an extension of giving as practiced within her own culture, even though it defied established mortuary customs. In other instances, when kin are angered by a death, they may decide to donate because they perceive this act as redeeming the donor socially or spiritually. (Such decisions thus emerge as potentially punitive, too.) This is precisely what happened in one case I tracked in 1995. The donor, who was a teenager and a member of a notorious street gang, was shot in the head by a rival. As his mother explained to an OPO family counselor, "My son did nothing to help anybody when he was alive, but I'm going to make damn sure he does something now that he's dead!" To allow such a son to slip through the cracks would in essence only reconfirm that his life had been a wasted one.

Alternative Strategies for Recovering the Dead

As the language of needless waste underscores, the ever-growing shortage of transplantable human organs emerges as a terrible—though not inevitable—national tragedy. Yet another strategy used by UNOS and the nations' OPOs to alert the public to transplant's needs is the practice of supplying regular body counts of patients who have died while awaiting transplants. As indicated in the introduction, no publication on organ transfer is complete unless it supplies such figures. This approach serves as a powerful reminder that, as human bodies go to waste, others suffer or, worse yet, also waste away and die. For this reason, according to transplant ideology, the nation's lay public should willingly and without hesitation offer themselves in death to others so desperately in need.

In response to the chronic shortage in body parts, alternative solutions are gaining support, a trend that has become especially pronounced since 2000. Proposals now under serious consideration range from altering current donor protocols to instituting legislative reforms; each, too, has its own base of constituents. Those who work in clinical settings are more likely to advocate the need to streamline even further the criteria for the determination of death (Agich 1999; DuBois 1999; Fung 2000; Greenberg 2003; Lock 2003). To paraphrase a suggestion offered during an interview with neurologist Dr. Needler, for example, why not expand the donor pool to include vegetative and comatose patients? Given that the brain injuries sustained by such patients can compromise their chances at full recovery, perhaps we should seek permission from kin to remove them, too, from ventilators so that we might make use of their vital organs. In turn, many others—frequently from outside OPOs—enthusiastically support proposals that OPOs be permitted to offer donor families a range of financial incentives as rewards or as compensation for consenting to donation (AMA 2003; Arnold et al. 2002; Bailey 1990; Blumstein 1993; Goldberg 2003). Many OPO staff, in turn, advocate that the United States should follow the lead of European nations and institute presumed consent laws so that all dead patients could potentially be relegated to donor status automatically and without the consent of kin (AMA 1994; C. Cohen 1992; Michelsen 1991). New advanced directive laws, as outlined previously, in fact offer a version of this very strategy. All advocates assume that public outreach and education programs have failed to convince enough people to designate their willingness to be organ donors, and thus more aggressive strategies are in order.

These proposals define three key trajectories: widen the definition of death, entice donor families with financial rewards, or override the rights of next of kin to make end-of-life decisions and instead coerce donation out of the nation's general population. In my interviews I have found that the strongest proponents of such proposals have great difficulty imagining the slippery slope of these tactics. Yet one need only turn to several decades of writing in bioethics or the long-term fascination with organ banks in science fiction to realize the inherent dangers of such proposals.[35] The more pronounced criticisms identify the dangers of preying on the poor and socially disenfranchised whose kin might find financial compensation too enticing to resist; the gradual instatement of euthanasia as a means to acquire organs from a widening pool of patients who are not yet dead; the deliberate withdrawal of medical care from sickly patients who are considered of far greater value when dead; the need to rank dying patients in terms of their social worth, such that those who are less valued are allowed to die so that their parts can sustain others of greater value; and the erosion of medical professions more generally, as doctors, nurses, and others become specialists in orchestrating death rather than saving lives. When framed by the ideological premise that organs are growing increasingly scarce, current anxieties over this national tragedy sadly overshadow an already shaky ethical code that guides organ retrieval.

CONCLUSION

Within this chapter I have sought to provide a comprehensive portrait of the intricacies of organ procurement, as well as its associated ideological dilemmas. I realize that some portions of this chapter may have alarmed certain readers, leading them to question the legitimacy of organ transfer. Do procurement specialists and transplant surgeons ultimately orchestrate patients' deaths? Does corporate greed drive the desire for transplantable human organs? Do the clinical practices of organ transfer offer evidence of widespread medical failure? I am quick to answer that such reactions are far too simplistic (not to mention evidence of knee-jerk paranoia). Instead, it is the highly unusual circumstances of organ transfer that ultimately enable this discussion to occur at all. The value of these unsettling questions lies, then, in their ability to expose the peculiar and contradictory array of practices shaping transplant medicine in America.

I argue that the assertion that brain death is "true death" is a consequence of embracing organ transfer as an act of great social worth. After all, if the purpose of organ transfer is to save lives, it makes little sense for physicians to orchestrate the deaths of donors merely to acquire organs for other patients. Nevertheless, we would do well to acknowledge publicly that brain dead organ donors experience (or, perhaps better put, undergo) death in stages, the process itself carefully mitigated by conflicting cultural and medical understandings of what it means to die. As the person fades away, the body follows soon after.

Organ donation hinges on the sort of logic outlined in this chapter: its medicolegal success and social acceptance ultimately insist that we be reduced to our mind-brains. Or, put another way, organ harvesting is driven by the assertion that when the mind-brain no longer functions, we cease to be ourselves, to be full-fledged human beings and, thus, truly alive. Furthermore, the harvesting of transplantable organs and the legitimacy of cadaveric organ donation rest on a pairing of lay trust with medical knowledge of brain death as a knowable category, as an absolute and unquestionable state of nonexistence, as something easily detectible in medical and social terms. This chapter has sought to explore the pitfalls of brain death criteria when viewed through medical, emotional, and social lenses. As such, it indicates a need to move beyond the assertion that the brain dead are merely living cadavers or neomorts.

When kin decide to give to others in need, they do so because they understand the social worth assigned to the donor body. Unquestionably, the "gifts of life" reaped from a donor save a wide assortment of dying patients and may radically improve the quality of life of many others. A kidney transplant removes a middle-aged mother from dialysis, skin grafts facilitate the healing of a firefighter who was badly burned on the job, a replaced patella allows a karate instructor to walk—and work—again, and a new heart allows an infant to leave the ICU and go home to her parents. As such idealized scenarios assert, donation allows great good to arise from terrible, unimagined tragedies, so that donor kin may at least cling to this small comfort for the remainder of their own lives. As described in detail in the following chapter, "gifts of life" enable donors to live on in the bodies of others. As such, organ transfer offers truly unique ways to experience life and death in America.

2   Memory Work

Public and Private Representations of Suffering,
Loss, and Redemption

Not a day goes by when I don't think about my donor. He's my
guardian angel—and that's why I always wear this [angel] pin
in his honor.

Female heart recipient ten years after her transplant

Nothing is worse than burying a child. Nothing.

From a conversation involving a pair of mothers

On a busy street corner in Richmond, Virginia, stands a memorial complex
erected to an unusual category of the dead. The National Donor Memorial
occupies the grounds of the new corporate headquarters of the United Network for Organ Sharing and spans approximately ten thousand square feet
of outdoor space.[1] With one end wedged into a corner near the UNOS lobby
entrance, its second arm banks the corporate parking lot, shadowed by the
building's multistory garage and, in turn, by the medical examiner's office
across the street. The cost for the memorial is an estimated $1.2 million,
built with monies solicited from UNOS staff, transplant surgeons, national
organ procurement organizations, pharmaceutical companies, and local Richmond establishments. The memorial consists of a gateway, the Wall of Tears,
and three outdoor "rooms"—the Water Garden, the Butterfly Lawn, and the
Memorial Grove (figure 2)—each of which is organized around one of three
themes: hope, renewal, and transformation. The design grew out of committee discussions that involved UNOS staff, donor kin from diverse parts
of the country, an architect, and a facilitator who helped translate donor kin
sentiments into ideas that made architectural sense. The National Donor
Memorial occupies two levels of contemplative outdoor space, complemented
by a set of indoor computer terminals where visitors may consult personal
online tributes that describe aspects of individual donors' lives.

Four hundred miles away, a donor mother, Sandy O'Neill, has decorated
her house to honor her four children. Numerous tables and shelves are covered with family photos, and the refrigerator and kitchen cabinets are plastered with their colorful paintings and writings. Yet another set of artwork

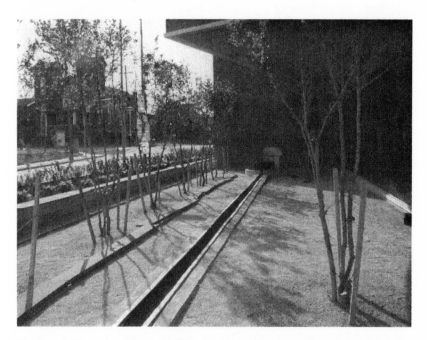

Figure 2.   Upper fountain and holly garden, also known as the Memorial Grove
(signifying Transformation), at the National Donor Memorial, Richmond, Virginia.
The lobby of UNOS headquarters is to the right; within are computer terminals
where visitors may view online tributes to donors. Photo by Lesley Sharp, spring
2004, courtesy of the United Network for Organ Sharing.

graces an entire hallway, extending as far as the ceiling's boundary. One child
nevertheless eclipses the other three, for Sandy has built a veritable shrine
in Joshua's honor. Just inside her front doorway hangs a beautiful quilt of
vibrant yellows, reds, and oranges, pieced together by machine and then in-
tricately hand-quilted. When Joshua died, Sandy could not bear to discard
his favorite clothes, and so she appliquéd them onto this quilt, which is emblazoned with images cut from two of his favorite T-shirts, a full pajama set,
a pair of bright yellow swimming trunks, and a karate jacket complete with
ketchup stains. Each of the quilt's four corners bears a photo of Joshua printed
on fabric, including one taken when he was baby, and two others at ages two
and five years. In one, Joshua looks straight out at us as he blows out the
candles on a birthday cake. The fourth photo, placed in the upper right-hand
corner, was taken when Joshua was barely seven, only a few months before
he died from a rare blood disorder and, with his parents' consent, became a
multiple organ donor.

Martha Berman, who lives about two hundred miles away from Sandy,

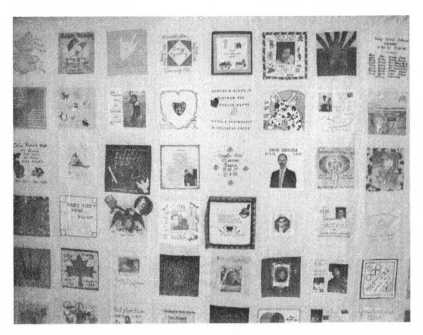

Figure 3. A portion of the Patches of Love Quilt from the National Donor Family Council, on display in the lobby of UNOS headquarters, Richmond, Virginia. Image of the National Donor Family Quilt used with permission of the National Kidney Foundation (www.donorfamily.org). Photo by Lesley Sharp, spring 2004.

is a quilter, too. For several years now Martha has directed the Patches of Love Quilt for the National Donor Family Council in New York City. Like Sandy, Martha is also a donor mother, and she is dedicated to helping surviving donor kin express their grief publicly and unhindered by the obstructionist policies of OPOs and transplant units. Today the Patches of Love Quilt consists of more than twenty panels made from fifteen hundred squares submitted from diverse regions of the country by the kin, friends, and other loved ones of organ donors (figure 3).[2] Clearly modeled after the AIDS Quilt, the Patches of Love project played a major role in subverting the ideological assumption that organ donors should remain anonymous and, thus, unnamed. Martha imposes no restrictions on the content of quilt squares: submitted pieces regularly display the full names, birth and death dates, and photos of individual organ donors. Many of these squares also bear precious mementos, ranging from police badges, athletic letters, and Girl Scout pins, to tiny stuffed animals, swatches from baby blankets, bits and pieces of children's toys, and adults' trinkets and work-related objects. Some squares clearly display or hint at the cause of the donor's death: a motorcycle, automobile, or bicycle, a surfboard, a fishing boat, a pistol, a hang-man's noose. Each square is also carefully cataloged, because Martha requests that submissions be accompanied by personal statements, letters, or essays that say something about the donor or the meaning of the square. Sections of the Patches of Love Quilt now regularly tour the nation's transplant events; the quilt is always on display at the biannual Transplant Games, and hospital units, OPOs, and UNOS frequently hang one or several panels in their lobbies.

Within recent years, individual OPOs and, in at least one case, even a tis-sue bank, have begun to commemorate the lives of their respective donors. Brandon Whittaker, who lives in the Southwest, can attest to the power of this movement. Now in his late fifties, he has always been an avid quilter, having learned the art as a child by assisting his mother, two aunts, and a grandmother, all of whom participated regularly in quilting bees in their small town in the Central Valley of California. Brandon, who is a liver trans-plant recipient, sees quilting as a way to give back to the anonymous fam-ilies that helped to save his and other recipients' lives. Brandon regularly volunteers at his local OPO, helping out at health fairs and heading the office's speakers bureau. He also coordinates several quilting bees by work-ing with local fabric stores, bringing donor kin together with established quil-ters, and providing a social setting where bereaved kin can work alongside others as they stitch together commemorative squares.

Meanwhile, in public parks and corporate parking lots, saplings have begun to mature, defining permanent donor gardens scattered across the nation's landscape. Plantings range from modest efforts, consisting of one or two trees set on the grounds of a hospital, to a project as elaborate as the National Donor Memorial in Richmond. On the outskirts of Indianapolis, for instance, in the city's largest park, stands a grove of trees, some of which are fifteen years old. These trees have been planted individually to com-memorate, in anonymous fashion, donors from whom transplantable parts were procured each year. A host of participants—including adults and chil-dren, recipients and donor kin, and transplant professionals—assemble to give thanks and then take turns with a shovel to cover the exposed roots of that year's tree. Another even more elaborate donor garden can be found in the center of the parking lot for LifeNet, a nonprofit tissue and organ pro-curement firm based in the South. Consisting of several small trees, flow-ering shrubs, a small circular walkway, and two benches, this tiny oasis beck-ons one to pause for a brief repose (figure 4). A recent addition includes several Gift of Life rose bushes, a new hybrid named specifically in honor of organ donation. As various plaques make clear, the garden honors, first,

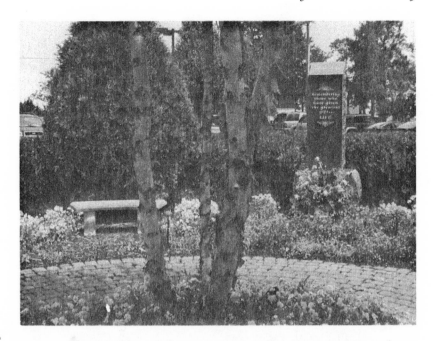

Figure 4.   Donor garden at LifeNet, an organ procurement organization and tissue bank in Virginia Beach, Virginia. The stone tablet reads, "Remembering those who have given the greatest gift . . . LIFE." Photo by Lesley Sharp, spring 2004. Used with permission of LifeNet.

an anonymous community of organ and tissue donors whose bodies were handled specifically by LifeNet, and, second, the firm's charismatic founder. When he died a few years ago, he became a donor himself, his parts procured by his own staff. At yet another corner of the parking lot stands a lone tree; a plaque buried deep within a low-lying holly bush proclaims that it honors a young man, the tree placed here by his mother as one of many ways to ensure that her son's name will remain known to others long after his death.

As these memorial efforts attest, the paired processes of remembering and forgetting shape a complex set of contradictions central to the ideological assumptions and everyday actions that characterize organ transfer in America (cf. Huyssen 1994; Sturken 1997). Over the past fifteen years I have witnessed radical shifts in the ways that cadaveric organ donors are described and, ultimately, imagined in the transplant arena. Among the most significant shifts is the recent challenge mounted by numerous donor kin against the assumption that the anonymity of donors is crucial to organ transfer's success. Many OPO and transplant professionals have long insisted that exposing donors' places of origin, names, and, at times, causes of death will undermine public trust in donation and thus threaten already fragile attempts to increase awareness and commitment to being organ donors when we die. Yet another prevailing argument is that anonymity protects both donor kin and transplant recipients. For one, anonymity offers privacy, allowing donor kin to grieve alone and free from intrusive strangers. In turn, it prevents recipients from identifying psychologically with their donors (a development considered pathological by transplant clinicians), protecting them, too, from encounters that might exacerbate the guilt expressed by many recipients that someone had to die so that they could live. When faced with subversive acts mounted by both donor kin and recipients, a number of OPOs (and, to a lesser extent, transplant units) have begun to reshape policies that once guarded donor anonymity. Such actions spring from witnessing firsthand the consequences of encounters whose uplifting results have quelled certain fears. Whereas donor kin have begun to insist on the right to tell their stories publicly, many recipients also defy transplant ideology by asserting that some essence of another person dwells within them or watches over their lives.

As I will illustrate throughout this chapter, among the most potent aspects of organ transfer is the power of storytelling. Personal narratives assist recipients and donor kin alike in reordering their lives following either a transplant or a funeral, making sense of a miraculous recovery or a donor's sudden, horrific end, and ultimately memorializing wondrous or tragic events. Both recipients and donor kin learn how to speak of and represent within a range of public forums their joys, fears, losses, and sorrows. Such actions involve mastering particular scripts and associated turns of phrase, and, in turn, responding appropriately to an array of memorial forms mounted by professional organizations. An argument that frames this chapter is that the private sentiments voiced by those most intimately involved in this medical realm frequently contradict the public face of organ transfer. Furthermore, it is during those instances when the sense of either loss or grief is likely to surface that this contradiction is most readily apparent and, therefore, problematic.

I begin with the recipient experience by exploring the hidden costs of posttransplant survival. Daily trials may range from the financial to the emotional, but the sense that one's renewed life hinges on the death of an anonymous stranger often proves to be an especially difficult burden to bear. As I will show, the inability to reciprocate the "gift of life" inevitably shapes a range of public memorial projects mounted by professional organizations: first, as a means to honor donors; second, to offer recipients a public forum in which to acknowledge their donors' sacrifices; and, third, as tools for managing the private grief of both recipients and donor kin. I offer several key examples of sanctioned memorials and then turn to donor kin, whose sometimes private and now, increasingly, collective public projects challenge, and thus subvert, bureaucratized memorials.

The paired forces of loss and grief shape the range of memory projects within the realm of organ transfer. To borrow from Dominick LaCapra (1999), a historian who writes of collective loss and trauma, recipients and donor kin might well be understood together as being "haunted by the past." An inherent irony is that memorial projects, when mounted by professional organizations, offer an inadequate response to private forms of longing. Shaped by the ideological premises so central to organ transfer, such projects ultimately silence and thus deny the legitimacy of grief. As with other groups who struggle against the force of "endless melancholy" or "impossible mourning," organ recipients and donor kin likewise "face [their own] particular losses in distinct ways, and those losses cannot be adequately addressed when they are enveloped in an overly generalized discourse of absence" (698).

All donor memorial projects—whether in the form of a public narrative, a structure built of wood and stone, or a handcrafted object, such as a quilt—are driven by desires for recovery and redemption. Although sadness and longing permeate memorial work, the grief associated with organ transfer has its magical moments. This sense of the magical is expressed vividly in personal stories. At the end of this chapter I offer accounts of spectral encounters with deceased donors, events frequently dismissed as ludicrous and illogical by professionals, yet cherished by both recipients and donor kin as an intimate form of postmortem memory work.

RECIPIENT SUFFERING AND RENEWAL

Memory work is a deeply embedded social process within the transplant arena, where one must learn how to express very private forms of pain and suffering in ways that are simultaneously translatable and tolerable in public spheres. Prior to transplantation, a recipient may have suffered from long-term chronic illness, including months, or even years, of dialysis while awaiting a kidney match; or perhaps a year of hospitalization for a progressive and life-threatening form of heart failure; or acute and irreparable liver damage from, say, acetaminophen poisoning, where the only possibilities for the future are immediate transplantation or sudden death.

Patients of all sorts quickly learn that within American society others grow weary of tales of ongoing or chronic suffering, which are often interpreted as malingering behavior and signs of emotional weakness (Murphy 1987). The bald-faced fact is that all transplant recipients, no matter how well they seem, remain dependent on their drug regimens to stay alive. In essence, a transplant marks the beginning of yet another sort of chronic condition that can extend to the end of one's life. Recipients must consume massive quantities of immunosuppressants, steroids, and a host of other counteractive agents to stave off the dangers associated with being in a constant state of graft rejection. They risk an onslaught of infections, where even a common cold might evolve into pneumonia and land them in the hospital. Although some recipients return to relatively normal lives following their surgeries—measured most clearly by the stability of a marriage, full-time employment, and the ability to exercise vigorously—many more never fully recover, instead struggling to qualify continuously for disability and Medicaid support when faced with mounting monthly bills and the exorbitant costs of prescription drugs. These problems may be compounded by social isolation and depression.

Many also struggle with what one recipient referred to in an interview as "donor guilt": during formal transplant events, recipients are reminded constantly that their well-being springs from the lost lives of others, and some find this burden overwhelming. As Renée Fox and Judith Swazey (1992) have so poignantly argued, this "tyranny of the gift" weighs heavily on the minds and hearts of many recipients, who struggle to make sense of this imbalance. Some recipients find comfort in expressing their thanks anonymously or personally, either by attending events where they might encounter donor kin or by writing anonymous letters to their donor's family; visiting prospective recipients who live full-time in the hospital; or volunteering as public speakers who promote organ donation as an important social cause. Regardless of the venue, transplant recipients soon learn that even close friends quickly grow intolerant of repeated, drawn-out accounts of their physical, psychic, and economic ills. Many recipients feel, too, that they are not entitled to speak of ongoing forms of suffering because their surgeries have saved (or, certainly, extended) their lives. They thus learn to remain silent on such matters, recounting their private and more troubling experiences only to the most cherished of intimates, or to others who now face similar predicaments.

The complexity of these constraints is only exacerbated by the exoticism that the uninformed or inexperienced assign to the reality that a dead person's parts can be placed in another, living person. The painful effects of passing remarks are evident in the following excerpt from a support group discussion I recorded in 1994. It involved Angela, a Euro-American liver recipient in her fifties; Zeb, a Euro-American heart recipient who is in his early sixties; and Pete, an African American man, also in his early sixties, who is a kidney recipient.

ANGELA: People sometimes ask me, do you still live the same way with a part from someone else?

ZEB: I was at this party one night and there was this fellow there, I don't know what his problem was, he had, well, you know, had a bit too much [to drink]. He kept saying to me, "How can you get up and look yourself in the mirror every morning and live with yourself? The man who gave you that heart had to die." [Pause] It was one of the most terrible things that has ever happened to me. That man was crazy. So I just said to [the host,] I have to go home, and I left the party.

PETE: Someone pulled the plug on them so we could live, that's what some people think. I say a prayer every night to give thanks.

ANGELA: Well it still bothers me.

ZEB: Really? Why? I don't think about it a bit. There's nothing wrong with it.

ANGELA: Well, I do. It still bothers me. It's true—someone had to die so that I could live.

Recipients such as Angela, Zeb, and Pete slowly find their way into support groups, meetings that are often organized by their transplant units, where they can speak in relatively uninhibited terms about posttransplant suffering. The most poignant moments inevitably occur, however, when the professional who coordinates such a group momentarily steps out of the room and the recipients are left alone with one another.

Some recipients opt to enter a far more public arena, speaking to crowds of the uninitiated, working beside transplant professionals, other recipients, and perhaps a handful of donor kin to spread the word on organ donation as a life-affirming mission. The realm of organ transfer is rife with public events that depend heavily on the firsthand, moving accounts that only organ recipients can provide. Their efforts range from providing solace to patients still on the waiting list to running information sessions offered at health fairs, school assemblies, business luncheons, hospital workshops, transplant celebratory events, and donor memorials. Within such public arenas, recipients develop specialized ways to tell their personal stories, their words and actions bound by taboos placed on emotional outbursts, graphic accounts of suffering or death, and the strict time limits necessary for the smooth operation of professional conferences. The most successful public speakers master a specialized narrative style for describing their life-altering experiences for initiates and strangers alike. Also, the language they employ frequently bears references to religious conversion and salvation.

Speaking of Recovery and Rebirth

"I would like to deliver my testimonial!" A burly Euro-American man with salt-and-pepper hair has just bounded from his chair and seized a microphone. It is 1997, and I am sitting in the audience of a conference plenary session organized by a local chapter of the Transplant Recipients International Organization. The status shared by a majority of the audience is clearly marked by the tiny green ribbons they wear pinned to their shirts: this is the symbolic color of TRIO, which designates that the bearer is an organ recipient. The speaker is a man I have known since 1991 whom I have already interviewed on two separate occasions. A panel of experts has just outlined a rather ordinary list of problems associated with long-term organ graft survival, skirting such volatile topics as depression and financial hardship. Standing microphones have been placed in each corner of the room so that participants may ask questions or deliver their comments. The speaker continues, relying on a narrative form familiar to anyone who regularly attends public transplant events.

"My name is Dale Sabrinski," he says, "and I'm sixty-three years old. I just recently celebrated my rebirthday—nine years ago, during the wee hours of May 14, I received the miraculous gift of a heart, a heart that saved my life." The audience applauds enthusiastically, and a man from the back row yells out a loud whoop. Nine years is an impressive span of time to have survived a heart transplant, and the fact that Dale has celebrated yet another rebirthday in recent months gives us all the more reason to celebrate. One of the panelists pulls a microphone toward her and says warmly, "That's fantastic." A few more seconds pass before it is quiet enough for Dale to continue.

"I was very ill—my doctor told me I didn't have much longer to live and that I needed a transplant—if this didn't happen soon, I was going to drop dead one day while walking down the street." He briefly details the causes of his illness, then continues, "I waited eight months—it was a killer." He chuckles, as we do, too, at his dark joke. "I carried that beeper around with me everywhere I went—even when I was in the shower! I didn't want to miss the call [from my surgeon saying they'd found a heart]. The call finally came on the afternoon of May 13, 1988. My doc said, 'Dale, it looks like we've got a heart for you. Do you think you can get over here?' 'Heck, yeah!' I said, and then he warned me, 'Now, Dale, no driving over the speed limit!' But, you know, I used to be a professional race car driver, so I couldn't help it—I drove as fast as I could!" Many of us are laughing hard at this point. After a brief pause, Dale continues: "I'll never forget that day! I was afraid I would get my transplant on the thirteenth—I couldn't help but wonder, what are the chances of getting a new heart on Friday the thirteenth? But it took time for the heart to arrive and for them to prep me [for surgery]. That's why my rebirthday is the fourteenth."

Dale then assumes a somber tone. "If it weren't for a very generous and loving family I've never met, I wouldn't be alive today." At this point his voice is shaking, and he covers his face for a moment with his left hand; he then removes his glasses and begins to wipe them with a handkerchief he has clumsily removed from his pocket. "I am alive today only because of a young twenty-year-old man who died very suddenly one fateful day." He pauses again, struggling to compose himself. "Every day I think of him— I can *hear* his heart beating inside my chest whenever I lie down to sleep at night. I am sorry I could never know him—it's only because of him that I can speak of this to you today. Otherwise *I'd* be the one who is dead in the ground."

Dale's tone shifts once again. "I think there's nothing more important than the message we can spread about organ donation. We have to do everything we can to make sure that others can have this same gift—this miracle, this gift of life. I cherish every day I have now. I look back on the craziness of my life--fast cars and all that! I love the sport! But now I live a quieter life. I thank my donor every day for the life he has given me. We've got to do everything we can to help other people understand what a gift organ donation is, and how important an act it is." The audience applauds as Dale sits down. Two chairs away sits a man about the same age as Dale, and he extends his arm in a handshake. A woman in the row behind Dale leans forward and says quietly, "Congratulations. My son's now out three years with a liver transplant and he's doing great."

Dale Sabrinski, in delivering his testimonial, relies on a narrative form that pervades the world of organ transfer. Those readers familiar with the format of twelve-step programs, especially those that characterize Alcoholics Anonymous (AA), will recognize the form, from which the organ recipient's testimonial is unquestionably derived (Eastland, Herndon, and Barr 1999; Griffin 1990; Jensen 2000).[3] Within an AA support group one typically states, "Hello, my name is _____, I'm _____ years old, and I'm an alcoholic." In their own support groups, organ recipients follow a similar format, one slightly more detailed than the self-introduction Dale provides in this conference setting. In his home state he would typically introduce himself thus: "My name is Dale Sabrinski, I'm sixty-three years old, I'm heart number seventeen from Urban Hospital, and I just celebrated my ninth rebirthday on May 14 of this year." The AA member follows his or her self-introduction with a highly stylized narrative that details the woes of alcohol abuse and, if the speaker has been able to overcome his or her addiction, an account of how this extraordinarily difficult challenge was met. There is the underlying assumption, too, that alcoholism is a permanent aspect of one's identity, and one thus draws support, first, from a higher power (a deity or other force greater than oneself) and, second, from one's peers at support group meetings. The ultimate goal is to muster the courage and strength to avoid alcohol in the future.

An organ recipient's use of a similar narrative approach is especially intriguing, given that transplantation bears little if any resemblance to alcohol addiction or other forms of substance abuse. For instance, recipients never speak of being addicted to their medications (instead, their lives depend on them). In addition, I have yet to encounter a transplant recipient who suffers from self-blame for his or her predicament, a characteristic so central to the alcoholic identity in AA. Typically recipients explain that they required a transplant because of a congenital heart condition; they come from a family with a history of kidney failure or diabetes; their lungs or liver failed because of exposure to unknown toxins; or they contracted hepatitis C through a blood transfusion. In essence, then, the cause of illness lies beyond the patient's control. In those cases where blame might be possible (as a result of poor eating habits, lack of exercise, smoking, or heavy drinking), such vices are part of the past only, a view reinforced by the fact that surgeons and transplant coordinators regularly insist on proof of reformed behaviors prior to placing such patients on their units' waiting lists. Unlike the ideology that drives AA, rarely within the clinical and public realms of organ transfer does anyone dwell on a recipient's past sins (although members of non-transplant support groups might very well do so).

Recipients are similar to AA members, however, in two respects. First, just as in AA, one assumes "Once an alcoholic, always an alcoholic," recipients of lifesaving organs (that is, the lungs, heart, and liver) often proclaim, "Once a recipient, always a recipient." Second, members within each camp consider themselves to be survivors. Whereas AA members speak of themselves as surviving the life-threatening aspects of alcohol, in the words of one interviewee, organ recipients have "beat the devil" by surviving chronic or acute organ failure and then strenuous yet lifesaving surgeries.

Both must work diligently to maintain the body in a healthy state, avoiding activities that would compromise their sobriety or transplanted organ and, thus, their lives.

Among transplant recipients, the theme of survival is often paired, in turn, with that of salvation (as it is in AA). The recipient's testimonial bears strong religious—and, more particularly, Christian—overtones. One must not assume, however, that individuals who rely on the testimonial form are practicing Christians, and Dale Sabrinski is a case in point. Although he grew up in the Bible Belt, he is not a religious man, nor did he attend church as a boy. In addition, it is important to realize that organizers of transplant events work hard to instill an inclusive, ecumenical tone. Nevertheless, the dominant narrative form adopted by public speakers such as Dale resonates strongly with testimonials delivered in Pentecostal churches across the United States. Not unlike organ recipients, reformed Christians speak regularly and in moving terms of their wayward ways and their subsequent salvation or renewed sense of faith, an awakening that generally follows a life-altering experience. The retelling of one's personal experiences serves as a means to teach others of salvation, a process that is central to the evangelical mission.

We might conceive of organ recipients, then, as an unusual category of clinical evangelicals who promote the goodness of organ donation by way of personal example. This does not mean that Pentecostalism has taken hold of organ transfer in this country, or that one must be Christian to take part in this unusual community of believers, although the long-standing involvement of chaplains, Protestant pastors, and, more recently, Catholic priests in promoting organ donation has certainly helped to shape the use of rhetoric so rich in Christian overtones.[4] More important, recipients rely on a Christian-derived genre of public speaking that enables them to describe in persuasive terms their personal suffering, transformation, and renewal. Through the testimonial they spread the word, so to speak, on transplant's miraculous outcomes and the importance of "donating life" as an ultimate form of charity. This narrative form proves highly effective in such key venues as school assemblies, church services, health fairs, and formal transplant celebrations.

This language of suffering and salvation extends beyond the personal narratives delivered by recipients. Recall, for instance, the themes around which the National Donor Memorial at the UNOS headquarters is organized: visitors are urged to imagine organ donation itself as a "journey" of "hope, renewal, and transformation." Transplantation is also regularly described as a medical "miracle" in such diverse settings as media accounts, professional publications, and public addresses delivered by chaplains and surgeons. Recipients themselves are understood as having been spared from death or further suffering through a "rebirth" made possible by the implantation of a new organ. These themes permeate the messages offered to donor kin as well: organ donation ultimately involves the sacrificial act of giving of oneself, as exemplified by the Good Samaritan. In some instances (such as an annual donor commemorative service in New York City that always coincides with Easter and is staged in the Catholic Cathedral of St. Patrick), the donor body is likened to that of Christ, who offered himself as a form of salvation to others. Regardless of the context, within the realm of organ transfer it is understood by a full range of parties that death begets life.

As is evident in Dale's testimonial, the recipient's life is transformed by this extraordinary surgical experience. Not only does the body heal in impressive ways following a successful surgery, but many recipients, like Dale, also speak of reforming their lives following their transplants, explaining that the gifts they have received are too precious to waste. This transformation is even proceeded by a "calling" of sorts: whereas the reformed Christian has responded to a calling from God, recipients always speak of receiving "the call" from their transplant unit informing them that an organ is available.[5] The sense of transformation is not simply about reform, though; recipients regularly describe their surgeries as a form of "rebirth." Transplantation necessitates a death of sorts, especially when the heart or lungs are involved. After all, patients who receive these organs have actually been dead on the operating table, lacking an essential organ for a period of time. They are sewn up and revived only once the new organ has been sutured in place and appears to be functioning well. Recipients know all too well that their surgeries have saved or extended their lives, when others they know have died waiting for an organ match or from postoperative complications. They then forever after celebrate the day of their surgery as a day of rebirth, one as significant as the one on which they were first born. Recipients also regularly describe their donors as angelic creatures, personifying this anonymous source of renewed life as a guardian angel, and many recipients wear a tiny gold angel pin or pendant as a reminder of this special relationship.

The testimonial ultimately emphasizes themes of survival and renewal, not suffering. A properly delivered recipient testimonial does not dwell on posttransplant complications, whether mundane or life-threatening. If a speaker strays too far from this prescribed format, inevitably someone in charge will make gentle efforts to bring the presentation to a close, or follow with an uplifting message of hope. Also, only the healthiest (and most upbeat) speakers are invited to give public addresses. Tales of surgical complications, life-threatening infections, the adverse effects of medications, economic hardships, or divorce are most certainly not part of the official, public face of organ transplantation in America.

The Secret Realities of Posttransplant Life

I am sitting in a small-town diner with Dale Sabrinski, an encounter that predates by five years the TRIO plenary session just described. I have asked Dale if he could tell me the story of his heart transplant. Just as recipients' public testimonials follow a prescribed format, so, too, does yet another set of personal or private histories offered during one-on-one interviews, or around the table of a support group meeting. Methodologically speaking, this type of interview can seem highly unstructured because in some cases it required posing only one rather than, say, ten preselected questions over the course of two hours or so. This is because recipients learn quickly how to talk effectively about the more private aspects of their lives, too. Many make special attempts to construct a coherent chronology of key phases, moving from sickness and near-death experiences, to the clinical evaluation that determined their eligibility for local and national waiting lists, "the call" for surgery and postsurgical recovery, and the return to daily life.

As I have learned to expect, Dale tells me first, in great detail, of his illness: the circumstances leading to his diagnosis, how the illness progressed over the course of several years, the series of heart attacks he endured, his cardiologist's decision to refer him to a transplant surgeon in the state's capital city, the intensive battery of physical and psychological tests that ultimately determined that he would be a viable candidate and compliant patient, and then the torturous period of waiting before receiving "the call" from his surgeon. Transplant recipients generally spend little time describing their postsurgical recuperation, unless this was particularly traumatic and fraught with catastrophic complications. Of greater importance to a recipient at this juncture of the story is how the surgery has radically transformed his or her life. Dale begins his account of the postsurgical phase of his life as follows:

> DALE: You know, when you come out of surgery, you're high as a kite. It's those steroids—you feel like a million bucks. Never mind that it can hurt like hell to laugh or sneeze—they've essentially cracked your chest open like a lobster or a Thanksgiving turkey. But you're really high—you feel great! I know for weeks afterwards when I got home I drove my wife and daughter nuts. My wife said I wouldn't quit talking, and it was always the same thing—how great it was to be alive, what a miracle it was. I was

ready to set up my own road show and go out and talk everywhere about it. I do this now, you know—I'm a member of the
Lions Club and I have made organ donation one of our main
priorities. Lions is already involved with eye banks around the
country. And I head up a little support group [for recipients]
in my hometown because all of our hospitals are far away—
we meet on the first Wednesday for lunch in the back room at
[my favorite local restaurant]. But those steroids, you know, I
soon learned they bounce you up and down. I soon found I was
getting really depressed—I'd cry over anything. It was weird—
I'm not the kind of guy to do this, and here I was doing it all
over the place. Sobbing like a kid, for Christ's sake! Some of
my friends were worried about me, but Julia [the transplant
coordinator] assured me it's just the steroids. But even now
when I think of my donor, you know, it's hard to not get upset.

L. S.: Do you know anything about your donor, or do you want to
know?

DALE: Funny you should ask—I was just thinking about that when I
was sitting here waiting for you. It's funny how these things
happen. [Pause] I never thought I'd know—they tell you in the
hospital all the time that this thing is anonymous. Before [my
transplant] I wasn't always sure that's the way I wanted it to
be, but so be it. And you accept it. But you know I did find out
about my donor, but not the way you'd think. I haven't written
or anything like that, like some folks I've met do. It was this
nosy neighbor of mine. You see, she likes to read the obituaries
every morning over her morning cup of coffee, and when she
heard I'd had a transplant on May 14, she put two and two
together. She came over to our house and pointed to a story in
the local paper. Seems my donor lived not two counties over.
He hung himself one night at home and his family found him
there. [At this point we both stop to catch our breath.]

L. S.: I'm so sorry to hear this. It wasn't her business—what a
busybody!

DALE: Yeah, she should have kept her mouth shut. But now I know,
and that's it. I know others sometimes think about writing to
their donor families, but I can't bring myself to do this. Too
many ghosts in the closet, you know.

L. S.: How, then, do you think about your heart, given, well, its origins?

DALE: You know, Doctor Novell, that's my surgeon, he's always saying
to me, "Look, that heart of yours, it's just a pump. It's a complex
machine that nature made. A beautiful, complex machine, nothing more. We take it out of someone else who's used it as long as

they can, and then, if they've taken good care of it, well, then, we can reuse it and give it to you." That's what I've got, this hardy pump that beats inside my chest. It's a different rhythm from my old shaky ticker, that's for sure, but it's just a pump. . . . Did I tell you I used to be a race car driver? [I nod in the affirmative, and then we both laugh, because he remembers that I'm now living in Indianapolis, a town that hosts one of the most famous annual races in the world. He then continues:] You see such beautiful machinery in that business. Beautiful stuff—so elegant in design, so perfect. And that's what I've got, a really spectacular, beautiful machine pumping away inside of me.

L. S.: And what about your life after your transplant? How has it been, living with a new heart?

DALE: Look, I am really grateful to be alive, and I'm lucky I got a heart in such great condition, and a young one at that. But, you know, there's a lot of things they don't tell you—or maybe you just don't hear them right because you're so damned sick. But it's hard. I'm lucky, I don't get sick very often. But [there's a lady] in my support group, she's the first heart they ever transplanted in her hospital, she's going on ten years out now! But, man, is she sick. She has horrible osteoporosis, for one. She can hardly *move*, she's so brittle, and every little bump hurts like hell. She's always having cancer scares, and early on had some sort but I don't know what, she won't talk about it much. Every time you turn around these days she's in the hospital, and now she's waiting for a retransplant. I've been lucky—I've only manifested serious graft rejection twice, and both times I was out of the hospital by the end of the week.

But the hardest part for me has been forced and premature retirement. I hate this. I'm as fit as a fiddle—I exercise, I'm not near as sick as I was before I had the transplant, but two weeks after my surgery they called me up and terminated me. Two weeks, for Christ's sake! That's not what they call it, of course— first it was sick leave, then disability, and then they let me go, saying my division was experiencing cutbacks. . . .

L. S.: Why do you think this happened?

DALE: You ask why? Well, I'll tell you why—they're afraid to have me around. I'm too expensive, for one—I'd bankrupt their health care plan in six months with all the drugs I have to take every day. It's a small company, and I take twenty-one pills every day. What scares me is how I'll pay for all of this another few years down the road . . . if I'm still alive, that is. Never mind trying to support my family.

L. S.: How has your wife reacted to all of this?

DALE: [Pause] Well, she's off in Texas right now. [Pause] And when will she be back? Hell, I don't know. Bought a one-way ticket, she did. She's now living with our daughter down there.

Hidden Costs

Dale's private account offers a radical counterpoint to the public testimonial he delivered during the TRIO plenary session. In a sense, Dale is among the fortunate: he is relatively fit physically and, as he explains during this interview, had experienced only two subsequent hospitalizations. Furthermore, he remains active socially, providing a driving force in his Lions Club chapter and coordinating a support group for other recipients. From a purely clinical point of view his is a glowing success story. Yet many recipients, like Dale, suffer terrible hardships, physical and otherwise. This private reality became all too clear to me during an encounter at the 1992 Transplant Games in Los Angeles, when the older sister of an adult kidney recipient leaned over to me in the bleachers and asked, "Are you a transplant victim—I mean, athlete—too?"

Among the most devastating effects of a transplant is the inability to return to or find work. This widespread experience runs contrary to what transplant professionals repeatedly tell candidates before their surgeries: that their lives will be transformed and, like many others out there, they can rejoin the nation's workforce. Many recipients are embittered by the harsh reality that they cannot find work, even within the realm of organ transfer. Brenda King, a forty-one-year-old African American woman from a mid-Atlantic state who had received a kidney-pancreas transplant six years earlier, put it thus in 1997:

No one wants to hire a recipient—we're too risky. We scare them. They think we're sick all the time and they don't want that. They get all upset about worker productivity. What if we're out for a day or two—who will replace us? It's no matter at all that quote *healthy* people skip out of work all the time, saying they're sick when they're really on vacation. It burns me up. And then there's the Transplant Cartel—they'd much prefer that we *volunteer* our work. Why pay us for our time when they can get us for free? We're easily exploitable because we're desperate for contact, and we feel we should help promote transplants because transplants changed or saved our lives. . . . But we're not supposed to talk about any of that. We're expected to be eternally grateful for everything they've done for us. So when they ask me to come address a group somewhere, I keep my mouth shut about this. I reiterate the story I know they need me to tell.

The veracity of Brenda's reflections is echoed in another man's, offered during the same TRIO session where Dale delivered his testimonial. Marty Ford is a Euro-American liver recipient in his midfifties who hails from the East Coast. As he explained to the crowd:

> I'm out two-and-a-half years with a new liver, and I just got a job that starts next week. [Before this] I went to the head of my local OPO and told him I'm a recipient and a social worker. I figured they could really use my skills. The director, he's a really nice guy, said, "We have a tradition of not hiring recipients." They're more than happy to have us volunteer, but they sure as hell don't want to have to pay us for our work! . . . [Another thing I want to know, too, is this:] Why hold [this] TRIO [meeting] here in this [expensive] hotel when so many of us are unemployed and on fixed incomes, wondering how we're going to pay for the cost of our medications?

In response to his question, the panelists offered no direct answer, save one, who stated flatly, "If you think about it, the medications aren't really that expensive. After all, you're still alive."

Alive, certainly. But numerous recipients I have encountered report bouts of serious depression, with justifiable causes extending beyond the emotive effects of high doses of steroids and other medications. Many, like Dale, face not only forced early retirement or unemployment but failed marriages and relationships, their partners ultimately fatigued after caring long term for a chronically ill person. Some never find love at all because potential partners are wary of a mate with such an extraordinary, chronic condition as an organ transplant. Contrary to the panelist's banal response, the cost of medications is no small affair. I have met two kidney recipients who stopped taking their medications so they could return to dialysis because the cost of posttransplant survival was prohibitively expensive. Sadly, neither knew that at that time they may well have qualified for long-term or even lifetime financial support for their immunosuppressants as sufferers of end-stage renal disease (ESRD) if disabled, elderly, or holders of particular Medicare plans. Such coverage stems in part from the understanding that kidney transplants have proved far more cost-effective than long-term dialysis.

Recipients of other organs are not so fortunate, however. If they are unemployed adults, they must either cobble together insurance support through a range of federal programs (none of which provide the same sort of long-term support as with kidneys) or remain dependent on a spouse whose health plan offers near or full coverage for astronomically expensive transplant medications and recurrent and costly treatments and hospitalizations.[6] Such circumstances may very well test the stability of a marriage, where the recipient is economically dependent on the employed spouse for survival. Middle-aged men in particular speak of the demeaning effects of this reality: although their transplants have extended their lives, they can no longer fulfill the social expectations associated with being the male head of a household, relying instead on their wives to support the family. Female recipients speak in turn of double forms of job discrimination, because they are women who are also permanently disabled. As Brenda King phrased it, being a woman of color is the third or "final nail in the coffin of despair."

I became acutely aware of the financial insecurities of organ transfer in 1992, when, following Dale's urging, I went to interview a Euro-American heart recipient named Margie Walker, who was a month away from her tenth rebirthday. Spunky and petite, Margie was forty-six at the time of our interview, although she appeared so frail that I had assumed she was closer to sixty. I had driven for two hours to meet with her in her rural midwestern home, where I arrived fifteen minutes early for our appointment. Resting on the porch of her tiny house was a box for milk delivery and a can full of cigarette butts; the front door was wide open, and for a few minutes, no one responded to my knocks and calls of hello. Eventually Margie's husband, Arnold, appeared from the side yard and led me inside.

Margie has never worked, whereas her husband, Arnold, has been a mechanic at a local garage for the last twenty years. Arnold also runs a small lawn care and snowplowing service, a second, part-time business he established eight years ago to help pay for Margie's medications and other exorbitant medical costs. While Arnold and I waited for Margie to appear, he entertained me with stories from his early days as a college baseball star and his short stint as a fireman. He was hilarious, in part because, as I wrote in my field notebook, every other word out of his mouth seemed to be punctuated with "goddamn-bastard-to-hell." Fifteen minutes later Margie emerged from the back of the house wearing an oversized T-shirt that read "I'm Not Perfect But Parts of Me Are Excellent" and holding in her right hand a ceramic coffee mug with the word *Sandimune* (a trade name for cyclosporine) printed on it. She looked as though she had been crying. After asking if she needed anything, Arnold turned to me and exclaimed, "Look at her! I called those damn bastards at the hospital and told them, 'You have a woman sitting here crying and saying, "I might as well be dead!"' ... I haven't gotten a bill since, and that was [seven months ago] this year. I talked to my lawyer and he said, 'If you don't get a bill, don't worry.' At that hospital, they think I don't know crap." I asked Arnold what then happened with Margie's bills, to which he responded: "Hell if I know, honey! And I don't care. As long as I'm not getting the bill, I don't give a God damn who's paying for it!"

At the time, Arnold was already paying seventeen hundred dollars per month for their health insurance, plus an additional three hundred dollars for other costs whose purpose he did not specify. Such expenses are not unusual for transplant recipients, who regularly report that their medications alone may amount to several thousand dollars per month. In essence, Arnold had to net twenty-four thousand dollars per annum simply to cover their health costs, and his income was certainly not much more than this.

I knew several staff members from Margie's transplant unit. A month later I approached Sara Klein, a social worker, and asked her how they handled cases when patients were unable to pay their bills. Sara, who guessed immediately that I was referring to Margie, offered this explanation:

> Margie's a special case—Dr. Mento has known her a very long time, and he's very, very fond of her. We know that Arnold's [fireman's] pension can't begin to cover all of her expenses, and recent shifts in his two coverage plans [are] really putting a lot of financial stress on that household. His boss dropped health care altogether as an option for its employees, and the other [extra coverage he has] is so basic it hardly makes a dent. We spent a full staff meeting talking about what are we going to do, and then Dr. Mento decided that the best thing to do was to fit Margie into one of his research projects so that his grants could cover her medical costs. We called Arnold and just told him to send us any bills he'd gotten. . . . Our motto here is "humane care". . . . I went to a convention recently and I was shocked to learn that we seem to be the only hospital doing this sort of thing. We can't keep doing this— Margie is an exceptional case.

Indeed, I have yet to meet another recipient with access to so extraordinary a safety net. The most desperate participate in what I have referred to elsewhere as the underground economy of transplant survival, whereby recipients who have adequate coverage may engage in clandestine schemes to aid others in dire straits (Sharp 1999). When a physician shifts a patient to a new immunosuppressant, for example, rather than discarding any unused pills from a former prescription, the patient might then deliver them to a local contact person. In one network I learned of in the mid-1990s, a blind recipient served as the key contact because he could claim he could not see who dropped off packages of medications on his doorstep. In two other instances, social workers explained that they coordinated these efforts within their transplant units, keeping track of an altogether different sort of waiting list, where they recorded who might be short of what medication at any given time. Such operations are ultimately illegal because they involve dispersing medications without prescriptions, and thus supervising surgeons may be kept in the dark about what is happening within their own units. Also, recipients often prefer to rely on independent networks. They fear that, if found out by less sympathetic transplant professionals, they risk being labeled as noncompliant or even suicidal because, for financial reasons, they have ceased filling prescriptions at the pharmacy for the very drugs that keep them alive. A recipient's decision to cease taking his or her medications is a serious breach of medical trust because any resulting graft failure would be interpreted as the deliberate waste of a precious organ (and even a suicidal act where life-saving organs are concerned). Part of the medical contract that binds recipients to their units includes the expectation that they will take good care of themselves and their transplanted parts.

Silence as a Key to Survival

Organ recipients ultimately emerge as a compliant body of participants at least in terms of how they construct their public narratives. Most certainly, disruptive or incoherent speakers will not be chosen by their transplant units or OPOs to appear repeatedly at public events. Yet even recipients who seize the microphone, as did Dale at the TRIO conference, are generally careful to leave out the more troubling aspects of their lives. At this point I can only hypothesize as to why this is so, but I believe it springs primarily from the importance of compliance as an overarching factor that initially determines one's eligibility for transplantation. Transplant units regularly screen recipients for compliance as if it were a dominant personality trait. When doubts arise among staff about a prospective transplant candidate, they may call in a psychologist or psychiatrist to make an official determination. Of great concern to surgeons and other support staff is that recipients follow to the letter the directions they are given regarding their drug regimens and daily behaviors. In turn, recipients are ever mindful that their lives have been radically improved and even saved by organ transplantation. All recipients understand that their days are numbered and that they might one day require a retransplant. Among the most common fears expressed privately by recipients is that if transplant professionals perceive them as troublesome, controversial, and, thus, even socially noncompliant, they risk not qualifying for a second transplant if and when their initial graft fails. In Brenda King's words, recipients are always careful "to walk the line" when they speak of their experiences in public. They are thus complicit in the understanding that transplant events must be joyous celebrations, where one must not dwell on the hardships of chronic rejection, exorbitant bills, unemployment, or the failure of one's marriage.

As Dale's paired narratives reveal, transplant survival has two faces, the one public, the other intensely private. Despite the inherent contradictions within and silencing of particular messages, many transplant recipients nevertheless enjoy speaking publicly of their experiences, and it requires little effort to represent a transplant as a life-altering experience. Kidney recipients, for instance, speak of the freedom of no longer having to endure dialysis in centers where they inevitably witnessed other patients' deaths when a machine failed or was mishandled by a technician. Many thrive on a new sense of energy, too, which they contrast to the profound fatigue associated with renal failure or the listlessness that follows a dialysis session. The transformation accompanying a heart, liver, or lung transplant is even more dramatic; without a transplant such patients will eventually die, a fact made all too clear by the death tolls posted on the UNOS Web site and reiterated endlessly at all transplant events. As Dale Sabrinski likes to say, "Without this new heart I'd be a dead man."

In the public arena, organ transplantation is always represented as a radical and successful form of personal transformation, where the generous gifts from one person have offered renewed life to others. This transformation is considered so extraordinary that recipients like Dale regularly speak of their surgeries as "rebirths," and they publicly celebrate their lives twice each year: once on their birthdays, and then again on their *re*birthdays. The latter frequently involves a party where those present consume a cake baked in the shape of the transplanted organ. In addition to these relatively small-scale affairs, much larger public celebrations recognize the paradoxical value of the cadaveric donor body, which is capable of rejuvenating other salvageable yet dying patients who anxiously wait their turn on the nation's transplant lists.

HONORING THE DEAD IN SAFE, PUBLIC PLACES

As outlined earlier, participation in the public realm of organ transfer necessitates various forms of silencing. The ideological premises of organ transfer delineate a range of taboo behaviors, where accounts of intense suffering (and, thus, potential failure) are considered especially dangerous. Those recipients who wish to reach out and promote organ donation as a public good must honor strict rules of decorum that shape personalized forms of story telling. As I will illustrate, a highly particularized iconography circumscribes the boundaries of public grief in the realm of organ transfer. This is especially transparent in the public memorials that now dot the national landscape, erected specifically to honor the selfless deeds of organ donors.

The Greening of the Donor Body

National Donor Awareness Week, Spring 1993: It is 2 P.M. on a Sunday at the end of April, exactly one week after Easter. I am seated in a crowd of approximately one hundred people, of whom a fifth are children of a wide range of ages. All, save for a handful of local transplant and procurement professionals, are dressed in casual clothing. I recognize six recipients in the crowd, yet the majority here today are the kin of deceased organ donors. We have gathered on the edge of a city park, and although this is a large midwestern metropolis with an ethnically diverse population, the crowd is almost exclusively Euro-American, save for two African American women in their early fifties. We soon learn that they are the mothers of organ donors. A smartly dressed woman in her thirties is handing out programs printed on gray paper with blue ink. On the front is a drawing of a large, leafy tree reminiscent of an oak, and pinned to each program is a small blue ribbon. We have been instructed to pin these to our clothes in recognition of organ donation. A string trio has started to play a selection that makes me think more of a wedding than a funeral. This is, however, an organ donor memorial event, staged through the combined efforts of three transplant hospitals and our local OPO.

The seated part of the ceremony is brief, spanning at most thirty minutes. The first speaker is a transplant coordinator, who strives to set the tone for the event: "We are here for some sadness, but not too much, and to rejoice [in] organ and tissue donorship and transplantation. We are here to mix and chat and share stories. If you look out on the hill next to us you can see some small trees—we have created a space that is everlasting—so you can come here with your family and remember and picnic, in sorrow and in happiness."

The speakers who follow clearly have been instructed to limit their comments to five minutes each. The next speaker is the park's director, who talks briefly of the ecological value of tree planting. We then pause to hear an unidentified choral piece, followed by a third speaker, a nurse from a Catholic hospital who weeps throughout her rushed presentation, telling a fragmented story of a Catholic priest and a nun, both of whom died under her care while waiting for lung transplants. As she explains, "To be alive was to talk for them. Their particular pain was that they couldn't talk, they had no breath. This was the cruelest thing of all. Theirs was a long sense of losses, a long sense of letting go. They had no fear of death but it wasn't on their agenda to go. . . .

Too many people go to their graves with things they don't need." I am struck at this point by the incongruity of her speech. "Isn't she preaching to the choir?" I write in my field notebook. After all, this event honors those who have already consented to donation to save the lives of others.[7] My musings are interrupted by the delivery of a Protestant hymn by the chorus.

The first speaker then returns to the podium and asks the two donor mothers, who sit beside her on the stage, to stand. They are not invited, however, to say anything. Instead, the speaker returns to the subject of the environmental importance of trees; then, on cue, the two mothers step down from the platform to remove a drape from a large stone in front of a cluster of saplings alongside the edge of the tent. We are instructed to go read its plaque after this part of the ceremony has ended. A chaplain then stands and delivers a three-sentence benediction.

The audience rises, and we reassemble just outside the tent, filing solemnly past the stone marker. Children tentatively approach and touch it, whereas adults stand back nervously. Eventually small groups of people— a few couples, and then a group of three women locked arm in arm, approach and read the plaque on the stone. Several people are crying silently to themselves. Next, a man carries a small boy over, holding him out and encouraging him, too, to touch the stone.

A two-man camera crew from a local television station has appeared. A reporter is interviewing the two donor mothers, who only now are offered the opportunity to speak, albeit very briefly and in clipped form: "My daughter was seventeen years old; she was coming back from a church choir concert. There was a man who fell asleep at the wheel." Before she can say anything else, the reporter abruptly shifts the microphone to the second mother, who, in a flat tone states, "My daughter was brain dead. She saved eight people. She gave sight to two. It eases it . . . but it doesn't get rid of the pain." When I watch the local news later that evening, at both 6 and 10 P.M., the coverage of the ceremony is devoid of any sound bite derived from these two mothers' brief accounts.

As others remain clustered awkwardly about the stone, I decide to approach the woman who had handed me the program and ask her why neither donor mother had spoken. Although I do not recognize her, she knows who I am. She leads me slowly to a corner of the tent and says, "I've been fighting for this all along, but I've been told that this wasn't appropriate. [The local OPO] and the hospitals organize this. Everyone tells me it's too risky—they'll [i.e., the donor mothers will] get upset and then they'll upset the audience." I explain that this policy strikes me as odd—the year before I had attended the Transplant Games in Los Angeles, and the moment when a donor mother spoke—and wept openly—proved to be cathartic for many in the audience. The woman then hands me her business card, which indicates she specializes in grief work, and she asks me to give her a call.

Meanwhile, a recipient whom I know well has appeared with a shovel in hand. He, like several other people here today, is wearing a bright blue shirt with the slogan "Recycle Yourself" plastered across a large, pink recycling emblem. He approaches an upright sapling that has only recently been placed in a hole in the ground, its roots still exposed. He puts several small shovels full of earth around the base of this little tree. Other people soon fall behind him, taking turns doing the same. Quite a number encourage especially young children to try their hand at covering the tree's roots. This act is not unlike the practice of throwing dirt into a grave after a casket has been lowered into the ground, a ritual I will reenact approximately seven years later with my own young child in tow during the interment of his beloved paternal grandfather. For another twenty minutes or so, small clusters of people take turns posing for family snapshots in front of the stone or the sapling. Within an hour all have dispersed to their cars, the donor garden now void of human life.

I realize later that at no point in the ceremony were we told explicitly why we have planted a tree. The plaque itself, however, offers some guidance, explaining that this garden, now three years old, honors organ donors who helped save or enhance the lives of others. An implicit understanding, too, is that this memorial has been erected for an anonymous collective of local dead. They died here in this city or state, and in a sense, some essence of them might dwell here, their fleeting presence stirred by our collective memories when we visit this small stand of young trees. We have been encouraged to revisit the garden from time to time to contemplate our losses and celebrate other lives that have been saved. It is hoped, too, that those who stumble upon this modest grove while visiting the park might come to realize the value of organ donation.

The Sanctioned Iconography of Donor Deaths

As far as I can determine, the use of trees and other flora as a means to symbolize the process of organ transfer originates with TRIO. As its founders, a husband-and-wife team, explained at one TRIO conference I attended, when they sat around a table at home in the early 1980s formulating the purpose of what was to become a grassroots movement in support of recipients' needs, their young daughter thought they were speaking of *trees*. She then drew a picture that would later serve as a model for this organization's logo, an intertwined pair of leafy, green trees.[8] Regardless of such seemingly accidental circumstances, the now frequent use of plant imagery is regularly described by recipients and transplant professionals as a *natural* (and here I intend the pun, although they might not) symbol of organ transfer because trees and other greenery easily convey such themes as rejuvenation and renewal. Just as many trees shed their leaves in the fall, to sprout anew in the spring, organ donation similarly renews the lives of individuals who might otherwise die from organ failure. TRIO has even incorporated green as its symbolic color, as evidenced by the ribbons many participants wore during the 1997 plenary session. TRIO's iconography has inspired OPOs and other transplant-related organizations to employ greenery in their own promotional materials and corporate logos (Sharp 2001). Today, the individual identities of the nation's organ donors are regularly obscured through a wide assortment of flourishing plant life.

Donor gardens, like the one just described, are now scattered across the nation. They are so prominent that I frequently ask when I visit a transplant unit or OPO not *if* but *where* its garden is located. In some instances, trees are planted annually, slowly establishing a small donor grove. In others, a lone tree (sometimes accompanied by a bench to sit on for contemplation) stands in for the myriad donors whose bodies have been handled over the years by a given organization. Still other memorials consist of a range of elaborate plantings, typified by the LifeNet garden described earlier in this chapter. In those instances where it is difficult to find space in which to plant trees (as is true in Manhattan, where I live), other greenery may stand in for donors' bodies: at an annual commemorative service hosted in New York City by a local recipient group, donor kin are always given long-stem roses. These might vary in color depending on whether the donor died and became an organ and/or tissue donor, or served as a living donor from whom one of two kidneys or part of a liver was procured.

The Nation's Garden

The earliest donor gardens were modest undertakings. In contrast, the massive project that now occupies the corporate grounds of UNOS heralds the overt bureaucratization of donor memorial work.[9] The National Donor Memorial serves a range of purposes. First, it signals publicly a corporate commitment to recognizing how vital donors are to the process of organ transfer in America. Second, with a price set at more than $1 million, its construction is justified in large part as providing a potent tool for public outreach. UNOS staff envision their newly erected headquarters as a site that local school groups can tour and then learn even more from an employee's formal presentation about the value of organ donation. This justification is especially important, given that it is difficult to imagine donor kin making a potentially costly pilgrimage to this site. One can, nevertheless, visit the space online through a home or library computer, taking a virtual tour of the memorial and consulting or even authoring individual donor tributes simply by logging on to the UNOS Web page. Third, as James Young reminds us, at times, "rather than embodying memory, the monument displaces it altogether, supplanting a community's memory-work with its own material form" (1993: 5). Such is the case here, for the memorial is a masterful example of public relations work, drawing upon, and ultimately reshaping, private forms of grief for its own use in the public arena. As one of my personal tour guides reiterated throughout my visit in 2004, the success of organ donation rests on professionals' abilities to "sell" it to potential donor families and, more generally, to the public. As is true of all donor gardens, the National Donor Memorial's symbolic logic serves to raise public awareness while skirting the more disturbing details of donors' deaths. Among the most common approaches is to obscure the full identities of donors. Much to UNOS's credit, a set of Web-based tributes helps counteract this practice, although some visitors will inevitably require assistance before they can effectively use the computer terminals in the lobby.

At first glance the National Donor Memorial seems strangely mundane, and passersby may even miss it, although it rests on the corner of a busy intersection. Visitors are expected to tour the three interconnected outdoor "rooms" in a designated order, for together the rooms offer a metaphorical reading of the "emotional journey" of "the organ donation and transplantation process," where dominant themes consist of "hope, renewal, and transformation," three words that are engraved on an interior wall. The structure itself, rendered in stone, gravel, bronze, and wood, is surrounded with carefully conceived plantings of flowering bushes, evergreens, and bamboo. This landscaped space is evocative of well-established symbols and rhetorical language that now pervade the public commemorative sphere of organ transfer. Here one encounters a small grove of holly trees (an evergreen also associated with Christmas), butterfly bushes (the butterfly being a widespread symbol used by donor kin), and running water (which nurtures the garden, just as donors' parts sustain recipients).

At the memorial's entrance, one first encounters the Wall of Tears, which bears an engraved display of these words: *friend, wife, son, daughter, mother, sister, husband, brother, father.* As one UNOS employee explained, together these represent "the full range of the donor family." Water falls over these words to symbolize the "tears of sorrow and joy" of organ donation. This surface also offers the visitor a tactile experience: the architect

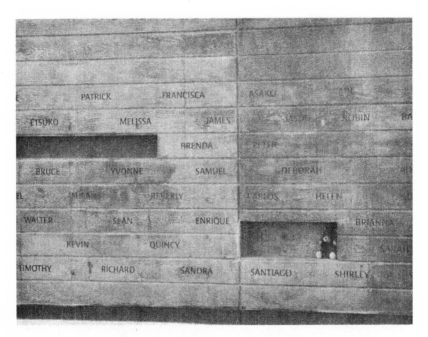

Figure 5. Names on the wall in the Water Garden, with teddy bear, at the National Donor Memorial, Richmond, Virginia. Photo by Lesley Sharp, spring 2004, courtesy of the United Network for Organ Sharing.

has mounted a small platform at the base so that water can flow over visitors' hands as they touch the wall.

An entryway to the left beckons the visitor to follow a descending path, walk under a small bridge, and then enter an oblong, enclosed area that defines the first room, the Water Garden. Upon entering this room, one is confronted with a lengthy wall upon which are engraved a wide assortment of first names, selected with care from more than six thousand donor files stored within the UNOS database (figure 5). As I learned during my visit, the names that appear here are meant to convey the "diversity of organ donation." These lines catch my eye:

Jude   Carol   Jung   Cheryl   Jose   Li

Elizabeth   Dorothy   Khalib   Berdena

Szbo   Tyon   Anthony   Joseph   Omar

Oscar   Maria   Choyta   Bruce   Yvonne   Samuel

The wall is also dotted with small niches in which visitors may place mementos. During my visit in mid-2004, two teddy bears were placed there as

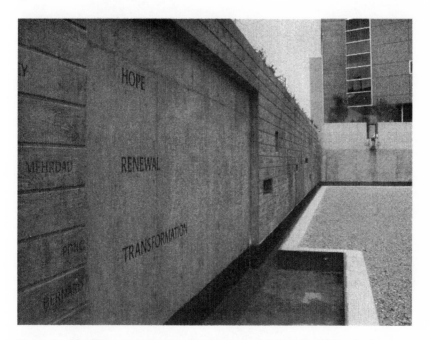

Figure 6. The Water Garden (signifying Hope) of the National Donor Memorial, Richmond, Virginia. The wall is etched with the first names of donors culled from the UNOS database. Photo by Lesley Sharp, spring 2004, courtesy of the United Network for Organ Sharing.

examples for others to follow. In the middle of the wall, three words are engraved on dark stone: HOPE, RENEWAL, and TRANSFORMATION (figure 6). The visitor is to understand, too, that this first room is intended as the site of Hope. At the far right end, set perpendicular to the wall of names, is a fountain, fed by a modest waterfall from above. The fountain itself, cast in bronze, consists of a large pair of human hands, palms turned upward to signify the act of giving.

Next, the visitor should proceed up a ramp bordered by a delicate wooden fence to a grassy area planted with shrubbery intended to attract butterflies. This is the Renewal site. After pausing here, one might wander into the UNOS lobby to consult the computer terminals by logging on to the National Donor Memorial Web site, where online tributes to individual donors are stored. At the opposite end of the lobby, set above an imposing reception desk, a shifting set of photographs of individual donors' faces are projected on an overhead screen throughout the day.[10] These are the faces of "America's heroes—organ and tissue donors." In a nearby conference room, where education sessions are held, one might also have the opportunity to view sample quilt panels on loan from the Patches of Love project. The visitor should then return to the garden outside, this time to enter the memorial's third and final outdoor "room" of Transformation (see figure 2). Here, paired rows of sapling holly trees bank a rivulet of water that cascades gently onto the sculpted hands below, in the room of Hope. This flow originates in a fountain where water falls from a small pipe, drop by drop, and into a bronze disk. These water droplets are meant once again to be reminiscent of falling tears. As each drop falls into the basin, it creates a ripple, symbolizing the far-reaching effects of organ donation. One might sit here for a moment in the shade, before a small border hedge of bamboo, to contemplate the significance of organ donation as a life-affirming gift. Just as the donor (or, more appropriately, the donor's dispersed parts) assumes an unusual journey in the realm of organ transfer, so, too, do visitors journey within this memorial site as they follow the flowing water back to its source.[11]

Sanitized Renderings of the Tragedy of Loss

As Erika Doss (2002, in progress) argues, the act of erecting monuments to the dead has evolved in recent years into a national obsession, or what she refers to as "memorial mania." Contemporary commemorative projects focus on a range of subjects: from immigrants and soldiers, to the victims of terrorist acts and cancer patients. Memorials expose a blending of collective desire and anxiety, particularly about the past, where such projects are imagined as possessing the power to heal former wrongs and shared traumas. Memorials ultimately stand as a form of witnessing, seizing upon private forms of mourning and then thrusting these into public arenas. As a result, monumental projects also inevitably serve cross-purposes, and thus they are rife with contradictions. Consider, for example, memorials erected to soldiers killed in war, or patients who die from AIDS. It is the parents, siblings, partners, friends, and other intimates who initially mourn these losses; later, public memorials transform these private losses into a national concern.

The transformative process, as illustrated here, has several consequences. First, it legitimates forms of grief that were formally expressed only in personal or individual terms. Second, it broadens the representation of grief, frequently obliterating private expressions of sorrow to capture the sentiments of those with no direct exposure to the event. One need only consider such recent projects as the Oklahoma City National Memorial (again, see Doss 2002), or current debates set in New York City over how best to honor those who died on September 11, 2001, to witness the public reworking of private grief. Memorials, as permanent structures rendered in stone, metal, and concrete, shape or guide collective memory while also ensuring its permanency (see Huyssen 1994). When built on an especially grand scale, memorials not only offer a public place to mourn but also strive to generate a profound sense of catharsis within each visitor, who, it is hoped, will sense the redemptive power of the public project.

Memory work is clearly a complex affair. Because they honor only certain categories or aspects of loss, public memorials inevitably define the limits of legitimate expression. As a result, individual expressions of suffering are silenced and, thus, erased because they are considered too upsetting or provocative for public viewing. This shift in representation is facilitated in large part by the fact that memorials, as permanent, static structures, draw on a very particularized and thus restricted set of symbols to convey meaning. They may even display words (such as *hope* and *renewal*) to direct sentiment. It is important to realize, too, that memorials are erected to honor specific categories of the dead. As a result, the processes of remembering and forgetting are inextricably intertwined in the public space of the memorial project.

Whether erected to honor soldiers, cancer patients, or organ donors, the memorial most frequently excludes the darkest or most disturbing representations of suffering and loss. Soldiers, for instance, when rendered in bronze and lifelike form, may appear injured or dead, but, even when dying, they always assume heroic postures, and their bodies are invariably whole, not blown apart by bullets, bombs, or shrapnel. Within the realm of health care, there may be a total absence of bodies of any kind; or, when patients appear in sculptured form, they are healthy and able-bodied. They are also inevitably fully clothed, and not portrayed, for instance, as vulnerable individuals in hospital gowns. The subject's individuality is lost, too, as one soldier or patient must stand in for the whole. Memorials, then, risk representing generic categories of the dead. This is precisely why the AIDS Memorial Quilt—coordinated, incidentally, by the NAMES Project Foundation—insists on proclaiming the identities of each individual who succumbed to the disease (Sturken 1997: 186–91). A key aspect of this particular memorial involves the ongoing, public reading of the full names of people honored by the quilt.

The entwined processes of remembering and forgetting are similarly evident in organ donor memorial projects, with the National Donor Memorial standing out as an impressive example. The fact that it is a garden is especially striking. Plant life is pervasive because it easily facilitates the abstract representation of life and death, excluding references to individual donors or their deaths. By focusing visitors' attention on nature imagery, the National Donor Memorial encourages them to consider the social significance of the donation process, and to think about the goodness associated with giving to strangers in need. One is to think in general terms about the processes of rejuvenation and redemption, not about private sorrows.

The memorial also standardizes, in a seemingly unproblematic way, the social ties that define who donors are to us. The selective choice of words and first names ultimately obliterates individual identities and blends them into a larger generic mix. At the entrance gate, for example, carefully selected words such as *mother, son,* and *husband* direct us to imagine donors as members of one great nuclear family. The only exceptional (yet hardly subversive) category is *friend.* There is no reference to a stepsibling, or ex-wife, or godparent, or lover. Instead, donors fall into highly conventional and unproblematic categories of sociality. A similar process occurs inside the first room. When one views the engraved wall within the Water Garden, one most certainly encounters a broad array of donor names, some of which are strikingly exotic. Nevertheless, they are first names only; as such, they, too, inevitably constitute a generic list that emphasizes the nation's diversity, but most certainly not the discrete or traceable lives that have furthered organ transfer in America.

The eclectic mix of symbolic genres similarly serves to universalize the representation of grief, where references range from Christian to Buddhist symbols, thrown together in hodgepodge fashion in an attempt to inspire a contemplative mood. As an anthropologist trained to think in culturally specific terms, I found it difficult at times to know how to respond to this space, not only because of the odd mixing of religious genres but also because the structure itself is simultaneously reminiscent of a war memorial, a mausoleum, and a suburban garden.

The world of organ transfer is in fact rife with references to war. First, as I have argued elsewhere, teams of procurement professionals may speak of their work as placing them on a "battlefield" of sorts, and they readily describe themselves as if they are at war with hospital staff or the resistant kin of potential donors. Some even speak of "dodging bullets" as they strive to bring a difficult case to a successful end. The fact that many organ donors die from gunshot wounds only further promotes the sense among OPO staff that they work in "war zones" or, at the very least, within hostile urban environments (Sharp 2001). Second, during celebratory and commemorative events, organ donors are regularly referred to as "heroes" who gave their lives to others.[12] The act of granting consent to donation is regularly celebrated, too, as the quintessential altruistic act. As the iconography of an array of donor memorials attests, cadaveric donors in particular are understood as having much in common with soldiers who sacrificed their lives for noble, patriotic causes.

Notably, soldiers and organ donors are mourned and memorialized in similar ways in the public sphere. Tree plantings have long provided a means for commemorating wartime dead, for example. Within Central Park in New York City stands an imposing grove of memorial trees. Consisting of pin and red oaks, this grove was planted long ago, as a commemorative stone explains, "To the Dead of the 307th Infantry A.E.F. / 590 Officers and Men / 1917–1919," otherwise known in some quarters as the "Lost Battalion" of World War I (figure 7). It is here, as a smaller bronze plaque states, that "They Sleep." Scattered throughout the grove are fourteen commemorative plaques, each of which has been set at the foot of an individual memorial tree. Each plaque bears a typeset roster of soldiers' full names, from as few as a dozen to more than sixty.[13] A complete assemblage of these names can be found, mounted in bronze, on the reverse of yet another central stone marker; some appear yet again on a monument erected more recently and placed to the side of the grove specifically for those who had belonged to various lodges of the Knights of Pythias. This repetitious quality of naming exposes an unending anxiety that, with time, these soldiers' names risk being lost and thus forgotten, as was the battalion itself in the Argonne Forest in October 1918.

This intense desire to name those who died in war is central to many twentieth-century projects, among which the most famous in this country is perhaps the Vietnam Veterans Memorial in Washington, D.C., sometimes referred to simply as the Vietnam Wall. This memorial's power lies in the act of naming as a means to honor this war's dead (Sturken 1997: 58–63). Today it bears more than fifty-eight thousand names etched into a wall of stone. Clearly, the National Donor Memorial draws its inspiration from the iconography of the Vietnam Veterans Memorial, which is only one hundred miles from Richmond. The central piece of the National Donor Memorial is, after all, a wall of names. Nevertheless, it fails to commemorate the very individuals it seeks to honor precisely because of the reluctance to include or even distaste for including organ donors' full names. I do not doubt that pragmatic concerns play a part: it would, after all, be expensive to add names each year as the nation's organ donor roll increases.[14] UNOS must certainly be concerned, too, that such an endeavor would require obtaining consent from donor kin before listing the names of those initially understood as anonymous. As such, the National Donor Memorial inevitably has

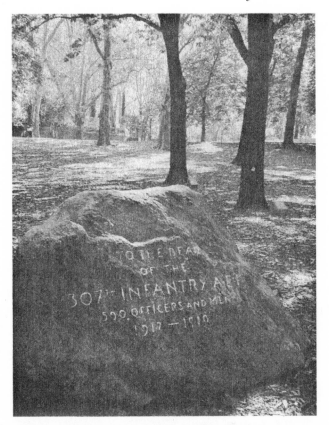

Figure 7. The 307th Memorial Grove, Central Park, New York, planted in honor of the 307th Infantry, or Lost Battalion, of World War I, the majority of whose members perished in the Argonne Forest, October 2–7, 1918. This marker is one of three stones occupying the site; the other two bear the full names of soldiers and officers. Note the smaller plaques at the foot of each tree. Each marks a "memorial tree" and, again, bears lists of full names of infantry members. Photo by Lesley Sharp, spring 2004.

much in common with other donor gardens, in that its primary purpose is to serve as a public relations tool. Its design is driven by the desire, first, to celebrate organ donation as an act of great kindness and, second, to offer evidence of transplant medicine's dedication to issues of equity. The memorial thus skirts such troublesome topics as the very real inequalities that plague access to health care (and thus eligibility for transplantation), the loneliness of hospital deaths, and the heartrending aspects of individual loss.

An occasional breach in practice nevertheless exposes the fact that even UNOS, as a corporate entity, is all too aware that surviving donor kin hunger for the display of individual donors' names. Within a special edition of the publication *UNOS Update*, one focusing solely on the groundbreaking, construction, and dedication of the memorial, donor mother Norma Garcia is pictured placing her hand over the engraved name of Jasmine (UNOS 2003a: 5, 8–9). This is the name of the thirteen-year-old daughter she herself lost, a child she will never forget.

THE PRIVATE LIVES OF DONOR KIN

On the final evening of the 1997 TRIO conference, I am seated at a circular dinner table with seven other people, five of whom are organ recipients, the other two donor kin. We are nearing the end of the festivities that define the Celebration of Life banquet; over the meal we have listened to an array of speakers and watched a life-affirming visual program about organ transfer. As servers circulate to fill our cups with coffee, the master of ceremonies returns to the podium, inviting us to come to the front of the ballroom to decorate two ficus trees, each of which is illuminated with bright white holiday lights. As he explains, these have been placed here so that we can decorate them with the "small tokens of thanks and remembrance" that we have brought with us as a means to honor our donors. Only a dozen or so people file to the front, forming a small line and then slowly transforming the trees into modest memorial sites. Although the holiday season is several months away, I cannot help but think that they look like a pair of frail Christmas trees. "I *hate* those tree ceremonies," quips Evie Leon, a donor mother of forty-six seated to my left. "I don't want a tree—I want a podium!"

Whereas recipients master narrative forms that underscore the celebratory aspects of organ transplantation, donor kin come to realize that once the initial (or official) grieving period has ended—that is, once the body has been cremated and the ashes scattered, or the coffin lowered into its grave— they are expected to shed their grief and assume their quotidian duties. In this sense, the absence of the tangible body marks the onset of a process inevitably referred to as "closure" in our highly medicalized culture, where grief is understood as a finite or time-limited experience. The dominant message donor kin receive is this: regardless of the tragedies they have faced, it is time to get on with their lives. This message may be delivered in blatantly callous terms. As donor kin frequently report, friends, neighbors, acquaintances, or coworkers might say that their problem is that they have "loved too much," insinuating, it seems, that personal weakness renders one culpable for one's own suffering (see Cowherd 2003: 22–25). Still others, though intending to offer solace, suggest that perhaps it is time to find another spouse or attempt another pregnancy, as if a dead husband or child can be replaced like a lost puppy.

A range of support systems has long been in place to assist organ recipients: all transplant units have specialized social workers on staff who help patients solve clinical, financial, and logistical problems. They also frequently run support groups for those who await or have received transplants, as well as workshops where guest speakers might describe the latest immunosuppressants or changes in Medicare coverage. Local TRIO chapters, scattered throughout the country, host everything from monthly symposia to potluck suppers and holiday galas. In contrast, throughout the first five years of my research, I was hard-pressed to find any professional who claimed specialized knowledge of how donor kin expressed or coped with grief, especially over the long term. Instead, I was cautioned repeatedly (and often bluntly) to "leave donor families alone." Such words were bolstered by the dominant assumption shared by many OPO employees that donor kin had already suffered enough, and the questions they believed an inquisitive anthropologist would pose would only reopen wounds and renew the suffering associated with sudden losses.

Although troubled by this assertion, I decided to follow orders and, for several years, to leave well enough alone. I knew through my early training in rape crisis work and, subsequently, as an anthropologist whose mother was also a clinical psychologist, that the act of speaking of past traumas can indeed have devastating psychic effects on the narrator-as-witness when guided by an inquisitive novice. As I explained recently to an exuberant yet untrained graduate student who hoped to work with the victims of war crimes, asking someone to recount traumatic experiences might very well force the interviewee to relive them. I was nevertheless troubled by the lack of data to support the assertion that it was essentially immoral to ask donor kin to describe their experiences.

Former field research in a radically different setting led me to consider other possibilities. A decade earlier, I had conducted dissertation research in Madagascar, an African island nation whose inhabitants often struck me (at least from my own Eurocentric perspective) as being obsessed with death. For example, many Malagasy spend much of their adult lives investing in tomb structures where they intend to have their bodies interred; and a multitude of women in the community where I work are in regular contact with the dead, serving either as mediums for royal spirits or as clients who seek their curative services (Sharp 1993). Such experiences have taught me that death is part of the natural flow of life (although the majority of my own kin back home still do not embrace this idea, instead shying away from discussions of burial preferences and the like). In Madagascar, children die with much greater frequency than they do in the United States, and funerals for kin of any age are public affairs, where bodies lie in state in homes for several days, and coffins are carried in broad daylight through the streets. In other parts of the island, kin periodically disinter their dead and dance with decomposing corpses that they have wrapped lovingly in hand-woven shrouds or mats (Bloch 1971). When the local king died suddenly in late 1993, I returned to northwest Madagascar to record the elaborate funeral rites. As I learned, the body of a deceased ruler requires around-the-clock care, where a caste of specialized retainers painstakingly oversees the month-long decomposition of the corpse, in the end retrieving bones and other remains as relics so crucial to royal rituals (Sharp 1997).

By the mid-1990s, then, I was perplexed by the taboos that silenced potentially rich discussions of how donor kin grieved for their own dead. A number of accidental encounters at various public donor memorial programs made me realize that at least some donor kin searched in vain for venues where they could speak openly of their experiences, either at publicly staged events or in smaller supportive settings with others who shared similar losses. I slowly learned that the concept of closure is fraught with misunderstandings of how myriad parties grieve. Furthermore, I realized that hospital deaths that culminate in organ donation radically alter the manner in which surviving kin comprehend death and, ultimately, express their suffering over the long term. Through donation, the vital parts of the loved one are literally scattered across the nation, housed in the bodies of other people who, in turn, are reborn as a result of their surgeries. The act of grieving the death of an organ donor stimulates, even among the nonreligious, profound existential thoughts on the integrity of the body, the nature of the afterlife, and sudden and very peculiar social connections to anonymous strangers.

Surviving the Donor Crisis

Donor kin never refer to their stories as testimonials. They do, however, follow seemingly scripted forms of storytelling when speaking of donors' deaths. As with organ recipients, I frequently need to ask only one question to initiate an entire interview. Collecting these stories is emotionally trying work for the ethnographer and narrator because, unlike recipients' stories, they rarely culminate in a joyful conclusion (although they may contain miracle stories, a subject I will address at the end of this chapter). Again, like organ recipients, donor kin attempt to reconstruct their histories in chronological fashion, speaking first of the donor's life and of one's personal relationship with the donor (including the conflicts). Donor kin then move to the tragic and often unexpected death of a donor, followed by an account of the donation decision. This part of the story often focuses on a series of quandaries and personal dilemmas: how they themselves struggled to accept that their loved one was dead, disagreements with other family members over donation, or run-ins with callous hospital staff. Still others speak of extraordinary acts of kindness from chaplains, nurses, and OPO professionals. Some then describe how they were affected emotionally the first time they met an organ recipient. Others now correspond with or have met the very recipients whose bodies house their particular donor's parts, an experience I will explore in detail in chapter 3.

Donor kin speak, too, of their ongoing struggles with grief. Grief, as a process, varies according to whether one has lost a spouse, a child, or a parent; donor kin are also acutely aware that not all family members cope with a tragedy in the same way. Several factors define donors' deaths as exceptional, heartrending ones. Many donors seemed fine only hours or days before they died, their lives ending suddenly and tragically: a daughter in her twenties suffers fatal head and chest wounds while driving home from her grandmother's on a stormy night; a husband in his fifties has a massive aneurysm following a rigorous yet regular exercise regimen at the gym; a teenage girl offers her boyfriend a gun and dares him to shoot her, which he does, later turning the gun on himself; a woman in her thirties is shot in the head by an estranged lover who breaks into her apartment one night; a college sophomore hangs himself in his dorm room following a heated argument on the phone with his beloved.[15] Even the most intimate of confidants may find such stories too difficult to bear, and so they distance themselves from a donor's surviving kin. Some adult kin eventually find solace by volunteering at their local OPO, hoping to offer support to others faced with similar losses. Nearly all kin describe the hurdles they repeatedly encounter as they search for public venues where they might speak, uninhibited, not only of the wonders of organ donation but of the terrible, ongoing pain associated with an inexplicable loss.[16]

The Lost Child

I first encountered Sandy O'Neill at a donor memorial event in the mid-1990s, one that is staged each year, around Christmas, by her local OPO. At the time, Sandy was pregnant with her fourth child; she was in the company of her second husband and her two daughters, one a toddler, the other a teenager. Sandy, of Irish descent and with fiery red hair, was thirty-four at the time, yet her youthful appearance made me guess her age as ten years younger, the incongruence surprising me given she has experienced more tragedy than many people endure even in half a century of life. Six months later she was honored at yet another commemorative event as Donor Mother of the Year by a local group of organ recipients. A year and a half later, at her prompting, I drove the long distance to conduct an extensive interview with her in her home.

Sandy describes herself as having been a rebellious Catholic in her youth, one who was firm in her convictions on the value of her faith, while rejecting what she saw as invasive forms of dogma, such as confession and confirmation. Although her zip code implies she comes from an affluent family, she in fact lives in a cozy and carefully landscaped community of tiny, and nearly identical, prefabricated houses. Sandy had just completed her requirements for a B.A. degree at a local state college and was scrambling to find work alongside her husband, who had lost his job of five years at a mortgage company. Among their greatest fears was that they would soon lose access to affordable medical insurance for their three living children, of whom the middle one faced potentially serious health problems.

We settled in at the table in Sandy's kitchen, and for the next four hours we talked of nothing but her son, Joshua. Throughout the interview her husband and her two older children took turns caring for and playing with the baby while listening silently to our conversation. Only once did anyone else utter a word, when Sandy asked her oldest daughter to clarify what someone had said to her when Joshua was in the hospital. Sandy, who is a skilled cook, served me a bounteous meal before the formal interview began.

As Sandy explained, Joshua had a rare blood disorder, one that is not necessarily fatal but was, nevertheless, the cause of his sudden decline and death. Her experiences thus overlap with those of myriad donor kin I have interviewed. For one, the majority of kin I encounter are parents who have lost their children. Donor kin often respond initially to a call from an emergency ward and soon find themselves beside a loved one housed in the intensive care unit as a result of an aneurysm, or a severe head injury from an auto accident or gunshot wound. Although Joshua had suffered from a chronic illness, Sandy had not expected to find herself at the bedside of a dying child.

Sandy first explained to me the nature of Joshua's illness and then provided an overview of its symptoms and the treatments Joshua had endured over the course of several years. Remaining calm throughout, she then described the shock of his death:

I wasn't with him when he was hospitalized—he had slept overnight at a friend's house and by the end wasn't feeling well at all, and so his father came and picked him up, and then took him to the hospital. My [then] husband and I weren't living together anymore, and so they had to call here several times before I got home. I rushed over, but I figured it was all going to be OK—he had been in the hospital before. My biggest worry was that he might be alone there, or that they were going to give him a transfusion or something. I didn't know he was going to die—what he had is *treatable*. But he didn't get better. He was in the hospital for six days straight. In his final days he was suffering from repeated cerebral hemorrhages, and he died in an intentionally drug-induced coma [from which he never awoke].

My experiences with the hospital were very mixed—the head doctor was *very* difficult—but the nurses helped clean him up so his sisters could come say good-bye. My [oldest] daughter walked in and found a nurse massaging Joshua's legs with lotion, and she was crying while she was doing it. . . . It meant a lot to know that someone else is there when I'm not [there to care for him]. One thing that made me crazy was they kept mistaking my [then] husband's girlfriend for me, and she'd sit there in my chair next to Joshua and wouldn't get up and let me sit there unless I put up a fight. I wanted to kill her! I had to tell my husband to get her out of there. We finally worked it out that she'd leave before I came in.

I could see he wasn't going to make it, and I'm the one who brought up donation myself. I told them I'd consent, but that I needed to see him off the ventilator, I had to see it with my own eyes first. I needed to know that Joshua couldn't breathe on his own. The pediatrician [in the ICU] was heartless—he refused to let me be there! I made such a fuss that a nurse and the coordinator from donor services had to sit him down. He finally said I could watch through a window from the nurse's station. A nurse held my hand the whole time and told me everything that was happening. I was numb with rage. But I could see Joshua couldn't breathe. When it was over, I walked out of there and I said to my [then] husband, "When all of this is over, I'm going after him. I want [that doctor] off the floor!" And that's exactly what I did— a week after Joshua died, I went straight to the hospital administration and said I wasn't going to leave until they did something about it. They put him through an institutional review and then called me back a week later to tell me he was scheduled to go through sensitivity training later that month.

. . . We went to say our good-byes together as a family, and I asked if I could have a bit of Joshua's hair. One of the nurses asked me if I'd like hand- and footprints, too, just like they'd done when he was born. So we went in together with finger paints and we put it on his hands and feet. You know, I have those from when he was really little. I wanted

to hold him when they took him off the monitor [in preparation
for taking him to the operating room] but there was so much [con-
nected to him] so I did what I could by lying near him and holding
his hand.

It was a beautiful day [on the way home from the hospital]. It
was very surreal. You know how you can have a day that's really
beautiful? I was thinking, I'm here but I'm really not here. Sometimes
even now, when I'm outside and it's that kind of day I get that same
surreal feeling. I was thinking about Joshua in the OR, and how his
life was over. I later got a call [from the procurement coordinator] who
said it had taken longer [for him to go to surgery] and my heart sank.
I thought it was over. I just started to pray for the recipients. I thought
of their excitement that everything will be OK. They called me the
next day and told me about the recipients . . . I was high on adrenalin
after that. Having a child [the same age as one of the recipients]—well,
I put myself in that mother's position. . . . [And then] exactly one
week later I went down to the [the hospital] and I went after [that ICU
pediatrician].

Much later, as I made my way to the front door, I paused one last time
to admire the magnificent quilt that Sandy has mounted in her front hallway. At this moment, as well as others during our day together, I struggled
not to cry, in contrast to Sandy's serene demeanor throughout the lengthy
interview. She turned to me and said, "You know, I love this quilt, and I'll
never take it down. But sometimes it makes me sad to look at it because I
realize there are no new memories [of Joshua]."

Private Forms of Memory Work

Sandy's painstaking effort to stitch together this quilt is but one example
of an extensive array of memorial forms generated by donor kin. Many
women, and some men, make quilts of their own, or they provide squares
to be added to corporate quilts that now hang in OPOs across the country.
More than fifteen hundred households have generated squares specifically
for the Patches of Love Quilt coordinated by Martha Berman, as described at
the opening of this chapter. Family members may also carry photo albums
that record aspects of donors' lives to conferences and commemorative
events, where both donor kin and recipients will page through them with
care, asking in delicate yet direct ways about the person pictured within.

By and large, it is mothers—and women more generally—who engage
in memorializing projects.[17] Men do, nevertheless, exhibit a range of strategies for expressing grief and loss. Fathers, for instance, may establish memorial funds or scholarships in the names of their deceased children. As grief

counselors from two separate OPOs explained to me, whereas mothers typically engage in public outreach activities and willingly accept speaking engagements, fathers prefer to work behind the scenes, assuming responsibility, for example, for the management or the financial end of things.[18]

Yet other projects offer evidence of the often intensely private—and thus overlooked—participation of men in memorial work. I became acutely aware of this during a 2004 gathering of donor kin, hosted by an East Coast OPO. An unusual number of men attended a series of workshops on managing grief, and by the end of the day several began to speak openly of their lives. As Jeremy Helder explained, soon after his fiancée died in an automobile accident, he erected a roadside shrine in her honor. He and his father worked together to build a small picket fence around it, which they have repainted together for the last three years on the anniversary of her death. They also take turns mowing the grass in and around this memorial site, and Jeremy's mother and sister assume the task of placing fresh flowers within. Another father, Paul Fenster, produced a heavy, two-volume scrapbook dedicated to his daughter, Lisa, who at age nine succumbed to a fatal brain disorder that was diagnosed only a few weeks before she died. Fearful that his memories of Lisa were fading over time, Paul sat down one evening and created a flowchart on his computer, where he began to generate entries for every memory he could recall of her. Within a short time he found he had more than fifteen hundred memories. Paul has set himself the task of writing one page or so about each of these memories, which he then prints out and stores in the scrapbooks in chronological order. On each facing page he puts an image that corresponds to that particular memory. Echoing Sandy O'Neill's anxieties, Paul's greatest fear is that one day he will reach the end of his list of memories, and the scrapbook project will come to a close.

Radicalizing the Public Face of Organ Donation

Until at least the mid-1990s, a range of public events, designed either to celebrate transplant's accomplishments or to honor organ donation, relied inevitably on the silent presence of donor kin. The period that followed marks the onset of a number of grassroots efforts that challenged the proviso of donor anonymity. One such effort was launched by a donor mother whose daughter died suddenly at age six. Under this woman's direction, the NDFC defined a new, catalytic force, ultimately transforming the public face of organ donation through its tireless efforts.[19] By 1994, the NDFC had issued the Donor Family Bill of Rights. With this document in hand, its board members agitated within their local OPOs, the National Kidney Foundation, and other relevant organizations for the right to tell their stories, express their grief openly, and publicly proclaim the full names of their dead. The Patches of Love project is but one example of the council's rebellious innovations. Clearly modeled after the AIDS Quilt, it enables donor kin to represent their dead however they please (as long as their squares fit the prescribed size). For the first time, donor kin were welcome to provide photos of donors, give donors' full names alongside the dates of their deaths (even though these correspond to recipients' transplant dates), and write essays on aspects of their lives.

Transweb, launched in 1995 by a group of Michigan-based recipients, proved to be another innovative venue. Its early efforts in this first year included mounting a virtual cemetery on the World Wide Web, one that featured tributes both to patients who had died awaiting transplants and to organ and tissue donors. Among the most striking aspects of Transweb's site was that it enabled kin to post text and photos publicly and unencumbered by the dictates of professionals (Sharp 2001).[20] The potential for contact between recipients and donor kin was rendered explicit by an early image that graced this group's Web page and promotional banners. It consists of two seemingly weightless bodies floating above the earth; one is a vibrant pinkish red, its right foot touching the earth; the other, a ghostly white, is fully airborne. Each figure's left arm is extended, reaching toward the other, and a circle of white light defines the area where they nearly touch (figure 8). In the words of Andreas Huyssen, subversive efforts such as these emerge as "countermonuments" (1994: 15). In the realm of organ transfer, they celebrate the very identities that medical professionals prefer that kin and recipients bury or forget.

As Katherine Verdery (1999: 21) reminds us, the act of retrieving the anonymous dead may prove cathartic for those who knew them intimately and who mourn their loss. Starting in the late 1990s, a handful of OPO staff began to realize the detrimental effects of donor anonymity, and some questioned policies that silenced donor kin. They started to experiment by inviting donor kin to speak at public transplant events, and by 2002 or so I found that several now proudly proclaimed during interviews that they had been "mentored" by NDFC board members. Yet another shift in OPO attitudes toward donor kin grief springs from a current, growing interest in the inspirational writings of and workshops run by Alan Wolfelt, who advocates the importance of "companioning" rather than advising or counseling those in the throes of grief (Maloney and Wolfelt 2001; Wolfelt 2002). As Wolfelt, writing with Raelynn Maloney, has helped others realize, the decision to donate organs from the bodies of dying kin may shape the trajectory of grief in exceptional ways (Maloney and Wolfelt 2001). The fact that

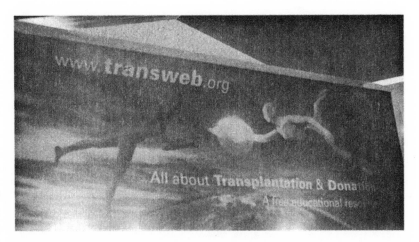

Figure 8. Early logo image for Transweb, a Web-based organization run by staff at the University of Michigan, Ann Arbor, that promotes organ and tissue donation and transplantation. The image consists of a pink figure (to the left) intercepting a pale, whitish one. Artwork by Kurt Parfitt (art director) and Matthew Quirk (designer) for www.TransWeb.org. Used with the permission of Transweb. Photo by Lesley Sharp.

NDFC's founder wrote the foreword to this volume, titled *Caring for Donor Families Before, During, and After,* bolsters its legitimacy as a guide for donor aftercare activities.

The late 1990s, then, marks the onset of OPO experimentation with institutionalized forms of donor family aftercare. At that point a few OPOs made tentative arrangements, testing the waters by hiring a part-time staff member with counseling experience. As one such counselor, James Keller, joked, "By the end of the first week my part-time assignment had turned into a full-time job," an experience echoed in interviews with staff from three other OPOs. The presence of these counselors has radically transformed the manner in which donor kin are treated in public and private arenas, as circumscribed by the activities of OPOs. Five years earlier, donor kin might have made an appearance at various pubic events, but rarely were they permitted to speak. In contrast, today some OPO grief counselors insist that donor kin have the right to speak publicly, and that no limits be set on what they say. As Dora Tuckerman explained, "When someone calls and asks if I can suggest a good speaker, I tell them [quite firmly] that you can't tell them what to say. Storytelling is part of their healing experience."

A range of OPOs now understand, too, that tangible, permanent memorials matter; some staff members may even spurn anonymous memorials, such as tree-planting ceremonies. The larger (and seemingly wealthier) OPOs invest a significant amount of energy and money in providing donor kin with small-scale and personalized memorial items. Several OPOs, for example, now hand out "memory boxes" as gifts to families just before they leave the hospital for the last time. Examples range from simple plastic picture frames that can be filled with images, poetry, and mementos; to cigar boxes covered in expensive, handmade paper; and even, in one instance, polished wooden receptacles with two recessed frames set in their lids, one for holding a photo, the other for valued objects. Nurses have long offered to snip a bit of hair for kin when patients die, and OPO staff now regularly offer to do the same, sometimes placing the lock of hair within the memory box. At least one OPO presents kin with an angel figurine (supplied by a local nonprofit grief organization concerned with lost children) if the donor was under eighteen; its field staff also offer to make a plaster cast of a donor's hand, mailing this to kin several weeks later. Such highly personalized memorials define only the first step of what might be a yearlong, comprehensive outreach program, including activities such as sending personal letters and making phone calls; sending out newsletters, pamphlets, and books; and organizing private and group support sessions.[21] Some programs are so elaborate (and well funded) that they are tailored to the highly individualized needs of each household or its members.

The Dispersal of the Body and the Consequences of Hybridity

A question I am often asked when I tell others of my research is whether organ recipients find they have changed somehow because they now house body parts from other people inside them. I have, in fact, collected a wide range of descriptions from organ recipients who clearly embrace this sense of embodied hybridity, speaking of new emotions, tastes, and desires that they interpret as being derived from their donors. Several men have told me they are gentler people or more sensitive to others' needs because a woman's heart beats inside them, and a double lung recipient once explained that he was ten years younger because his lungs came from an athlete half his age. New food preferences also abound, including unexpected cravings for, say, beer or chocolate; one recipient reported a new attraction to a wider range of colors because, as she later learned from her donor's kin, the donor was an artist who preferred a bright palette. As anyone who watches daytime television can attest, these sorts of tales provide regular fodder for off-beat talk shows in America. Their sensationalist aspects aside, such transformations stand as ghostly images of the imagined qualities of organ donors. These shifts in preference, behavior, ability, or taste provide a framework within which recipients legitimate and—often humorously—describe the deep yet confusing sense of intimacy they associate with their organs' origins. In essence, they normalize the strange transgressions associated with transplanted, hybrid bodies.

Yet another set of spectral images prevails in the narratives supplied by donor kin, so much so that I have grown to expect interviews to conclude with what I will refer to here as ghost stories. A typical scenario reads as follows: after spending several hours recording a personal story, the interview comes to a close, I shut my notebook and put it away, I express my thanks, and the interviewee and I say good-bye. It is at this point that the interviewee might say, "There's just one more thing." Sometimes I even respond, "You're going to tell me a ghost story, aren't you?" And, indeed, this is precisely what happens. As Denise Fisher, who specializes in donor family care, explained, "For recipients, it's personality traits; for donor families, its ghost stories." The next section provides an extensive, exemplary account.

Where There's Smoke, There's a Fireman

I met Cindy Hartley at the Wall of Remembrance, a temporary structure mounted by the NDFC as a place where surviving kin could place memorial stars with donors' photos, names, and other information in full view of recipients during the 1998 Transplant Games in Columbus, Ohio. I was standing there with Katie Kilroy-Marac, a graduate student who has assisted me over the years in countless ways with my research. Katie and I were discussing the array of stars that were posted on the wall. Cindy, a blond and tan woman who stood within earshot of our conversation, stepped up and offered to show us the one that she herself had mounted on the wall. Taped to a star was a photo of a fortyish, handsome, and muscular Euro-American man sporting a big, dark, loopy mustache. As Cindy explained, this was her deceased husband, Brian, a firefighter who died three years ago from a "massive bleed" while on Christmas vacation with her, their son, Teddy, and their best friends at a mountain resort close to home. Cindy and Brian had met just after Brian's divorce while they were working side by side as emergency medical technicians. They subsequently married and two years later had their son, Teddy, who was five when Brian died. Brian also had a thirteen-year-old daughter by a former marriage who lived with her mother. After talking informally for half an hour about my research project, Cindy and I decided to ride the campus shuttle bus together to a distant dining room, where we ate a horrible dinner of chicken that tasted like hot dogs. Cindy expressed a strong desire to tell her story, and we decided to move outside to escape the odor of the cafeteria and so that Cindy could take a break to smoke a cigarette. We sat there and talked for several hours until it grew dark.

Cindy, who was thirty-eight at the time of the interview, had worked for more than ten years as a paramedic. Although she thoroughly enjoyed her work, Brian's pension has proved generous enough to allow her to quit her job after his death so she could stay home and care full-time for her son. After Brian died, Cindy sold their house and moved in with her sister, with whom she is very close. As Cindy explained, she finds great comfort in this arrangement because she knows there is always someone available to watch Teddy when she herself cannot be there. These two sisters have since bought a duplex together, and although they inhabit separate quarters, they share their evening meals. Cindy possesses a remarkable ability to find the humor in many situations, even during moments of great pathos. She began her narrative thus:

CINDY: Have you ever heard of Mt. K.? It's a resort area in the Rockies. Every Christmas they have this ice sculpture contest, and we decided one year to give it a try with our best friends. We had been planning the design for months—it was great! The winners get an all-expenses-paid, weeklong vacation there for four the next year. We got there early and set to work right away, and then I went in to find the judge [who was scheduled to view our sculpture] while Brian and [the other couple, Sam and Mimi] kept an eye on the kids. Suddenly Sam came running in to find me—he said I'd better get out there right away— something had happened to Brian. He had collapsed on the ground and wouldn't get up. As soon as I got there, I knew, I could just tell—you know, I'm a paramedic, after all—I just had this feeling it was a massive bleed [i.e., cerebral hemorrhage] although it took a long time [before the doctors confirmed this]—at first they thought it was a heart attack. A couple of people called 911 while I did CPR, and when the ambulance came it turned out I knew the driver, so they let me ride along—you know, they never let you do that! It helped a lot that Brian was a fireman. He had a pulse, he was breathing about four times a minute. [To make a long story short, we first took him to a local hospital], and then he was airvaced by helicopter to [a state-of-the-art trauma center]. Sam and Mimi took all our kids home with them, and then they watched Teddy for me the next day and night [until] my sister and mom [came to get him]. It was horrible [that I couldn't be with Teddy] but it mattered a lot to know he was safe with someone I could trust.

When we got to [the trauma center] they had [already] called ahead, and the doc there knew we were both paramedics, so we were immediately on a first-name basis. They had everything ready—[in the first hospital they had done] a CAT scan [and] it showed a massive bleed . . . then they decided to fly [Brian] to [the larger hospital] that is renowned for its neurology unit. [Chuckling, she adds,] They let me ride [in the helicopter] with Brian—I felt like I was Queen for a Day! The whole time I [chanted] the words to our favorite song—[she sings:] "If you get there before I do"—to him over and over until they had put him in [the hospital] bed [in the ICU].

When they told me the injury would affect his personality— Lesley, you know, it was at that point I hoped more that he'd die than live. The man I knew had died. If God needed a brain surgeon, Dr. S. would be the one to do it [and he was there for Brian]. . . . We talked, and then they were going to take Brian in for surgery. I said [to Dr. S.], "Look, if you're doing surgery to send home a body, don't do it—don't give me a turnip!" I asked, [too], "If two to three years down the road he can't be a firefighter, don't go down that road!" Dr. S. said, "I'm glad you're saying two to three years because that means you know what we're talking about." I then said, "When do we start discussing DNR [do not resuscitate] orders?" [Brian went in for surgery but did not recover.]

I had incredible support—family [on both sides were with me constantly, and] the firefighters [from Brian's company] rented a hotel room near the hospital for me where I could stay. I was there for ten days. [One night] I went to sleep at 2:00, [then] they called me at 3 [A.M.]. He'd erupted the aneurysm. I called [Brian's first wife] and told her to get [her daughter] Maddie down there now if you want her to say good-bye to her dad. That morning they started testing for brain function. He did OK on one test, but he failed all the others miserably. The nurse then asked me about donation. I said yes! It's funny, I hadn't thought of it as something to bring up to them. The only thing they did [that I didn't like] was that the organ coordinator came in that morning [and told me] flat out that they'd pronounced him dead [fifteen minutes before] and they hadn't told me. Someone just came in and said, "Oh, he's dead." Just like that. They just hit me with this . . . I asked them to wait until Brian's best buddy could be there before filling out the papers [for the official declaration of death]. I took Brian's ring off his finger, and now [holding up her right hand] I wear it here [on my thumb]. . . . You know, and then a friend called to say we'd won the contest! But Brian never knew. There's a tree dedicated to him there [at the resort], and there's a plaque there in his honor. Every Christmas they decorate it with lights. The first year his company went up there and built an ice sculpture [of a fireman's helmet] in front of it.

. . . The decision to donate was an easy one—I made all the decisions, and to my joy no one ever objected. They were 100 percent supportive. I was sitting and talking to Maddie about donation, and I said, "We're the family in the waiting room— he's gonna die. But there are other families—think how happy they'll be." And she said, "Oh, yes, let's do it." By that point my parents were taking care of Teddy, and when I got home, he'd hug me a lot and hold on to me, but he didn't cry, but I knew he was obviously upset. He said, "Can I see Daddy before the funeral?" So we talked, and I explained, "Remember how when we moved, and we had an empty house, and there wasn't anything left of us there? Well, that's what Daddy's like—his spirit's left and there's nothing in his body any more. His body is like that empty house."[22] And he understood. . . . We had a closed casket, but there was a [private] viewing for the family beforehand. Teddy needed to see him one last time. So I took him in there. He looked at [his dad] and he said "OK," and then we left. He was OK and he understood. . . . This was a full firefighter's funeral—although there couldn't be a casket in a fire truck because he hadn't died in the line of duty. There was a mile-long procession of trucks . . . all the neighboring counties sent a truck! As we drove down the street, even a delivery guy stopped and took off his hat and saluted the procession. . . .

But I gotta tell you the story of the lime green underwear. [Cindy pauses to extinguish her second cigarette.] I once bought Brian some underwear. You know, those packages you can pick up at the store. He opened it up and said, "Lime green? Do you have any idea what the guys at the station would say if they knew I had bright green underwear?" So he never wore it. There I am going through his stuff [looking for clothes for the funeral] and everything's got holes in it. Everything! Every- thing I find has holes in it except the lime green underwear. [Both Cindy and I are laughing at this point.] So for all eternity, that's what he's wearing! [She shifts the topic again, abruptly.] You know, he used to install carpets.

L. S.: [Puzzled] You mean, Brian?

CINDY: I'm sorry. I mean Ryan—he's Brian's heart recipient. How I met Ryan. It's funny, Brian used to always have people calling

him Ryan, so he'd say, "It's Ryan with a B." I'm going to tell
you some things I haven't told anyone else. I've only told these
to my sister and my mother. Last night at one of the [meetings
for donor families] we were talking about closure and someone else said, "I hate all this talk about closure! There's never
closure!" and others there agreed. But I think I've found it
somehow, a little bit of it, anyway. I gave myself permission
to grieve and go on, to have fun while I'm doing it. I don't feel
guilty if I'm having fun. Other widows do, though, you know.
[She then lights her third and final cigarette.]

This funny thing happened at the funeral. It was this bright
sunny day, but when we got to the graveyard, it was weird—
this bank of fog moved in, and then it just stood there, stopping
just beyond the place where we were all standing by Brian's
grave. [Where I live] isn't the kind of place where you get a lot
of fog, and definitely not in the midmorning like that when the
sun is shining. But you know how they say, "Where there's
smoke, there's fire?" Well, I like to think there's a fireman there,
too. When the service was over and we turned to leave, and
they started up the engines on the trucks, then the fog just
went away!

[A short time afterward] I wanted to get the grave marker,
and I had been thinking a lot about what to put on it. He had
died just before his birthday. I didn't just want "firefighter"
and his name and rank and date of birth on it. [I wanted to
personalize it.] Another firefighter took me down [to the place
where they made the monuments]—he didn't want me there
alone. [I told them what I wanted them to put on it.] There
was a steady rain all that day. [Brian's friend] walked away
so I could be by myself. I said [to Brian under my breath],
"Honey, I'm so sorry, I gave you a tombstone for your birthday! But it's all I could give." The sky was all cloudy, and there
I was outside—it was raining steadily. And you know, I smelled
his aftershave.

. . . Now, Ryan. Ryan was fifty-six and was waiting at
death's door. They transplanted him [the second Sunday after
Christmas]. They almost [gave him a different heart instead
of Brian's]. He woke up and felt better than he ever had in his
life. He was out of the hospital in seven days. I wrote a cathartic
letter [that was sent on by my local OPO]. I said, "I want you
to know something about the man whose heart you have." I
knew only [their] first names.

I [later got a letter from his wife, Pam]—they wanted to
meet me. They wrote me a letter with their address on it, a
long letter with [Ryan's story in it—where he grew up, what

he did, why he needed a transplant]. We wrote back and forth every month. Then I moved [closer to where they live to be with my sister], and they invited me over for dinner. . . . I had all these expectations about meeting the person who had Brian's heart [but] you know, I feel like I've parted out a '54 Chevy! [This is because Brian was born in 1954 and drove a Chevrolet pickup truck.] . . . I'm not particularly brave or sacrificial. I did it for me. To make something good out of something bad. I've seen them three times now. I'm closer to his wife—she's closer to my age. I call her every once in a while. . . . I'm not here to monitor your health [I've told him]. It's a gift. It's not mine anymore.

L. S.:   Why did you decide to meet them?

CINDY: For the affirmation [that] something good had happened.

L. S.:   Can I ask what you think of the expression "the gift of life"?

CINDY: Organs are inanimate objects. It's a muscle that pumped blood in Brian. But it's not Brian. It's like I give you his shoes. When you walk in them, does Brian walk on? No! I'm playing down the emotional part—actually, I didn't send his clothes to the Goodwill—[But with his heart] I did it because it's been used and I don't need it [anymore] and someone else can use it. He was someone who saved lives. When I went to meet Ryan and [his wife] Pam I apologized; I said, "I'm sorry, I'm [a scatter-brain today] . . . I forgot to bring a photo of Brian." And Ryan said, "That's OK, I've seen him"!

[You see,] Pam had kept a diary of everything that happened [around the time of Ryan's transplant]. Without it I wouldn't have believed this. On Christmas Day he was put on the list, in less than two weeks he had the transplant. Ryan was talking night and day. Pam kept a log. He'd hallucinate every time he'd close his eyes. He kept saying he saw a big guy with dark curly hair and a mustache and a big grin. I told them, "That's Brian!" Everyone always remembers his big grin, not to mention that mustache of his! "He's just dreaming," is what the nurses would say.

The next day he felt like there was smoke under the bed. The big guy [sitting next to his bed then] said, "It's OK, I'm a fireman." Then, the next day, [the fireman] told [Ryan] he had two kids, a boy and a girl. On the fourth day, Ryan collapsed in his [hospital room]. He was unconscious. He [that is, the fireman,] said good-bye. "And I never saw him again," said Ryan. Pam called a friend [on the phone] and told her about the fireman. [After Ryan came home from the hospital] the friend came over and put a newspaper in front of him [showing him a recent obituary page from a local paper]. Ryan said, "That's him! What is this?" He was so happy!

I went to see my pastor the next day [after they told me this]. It shook me up. I said, "The Bible says we shouldn't mess with the spirit world, but I need to know what this is all about." My pastor was really cool about it, and said it really was OK [and] not to worry.

Extending the Flow of Memories beyond the Grave

Cindy's stories of her husband's ghostly presence offer the most elaborate set of postmortem memories I have collected to date from any individual interviewee. They nevertheless typify a particular subgenre of storytelling (or, perhaps more appropriately, of ending a personal narrative) employed by donor kin. OPO staff who run donor aftercare programs often provided similar tales during my meetings with them. In one instance, at the *onset* of an interview concerning in-house programs, a staff member, who is herself a donor mother, blurted out, "You want to hear about experiences with the afterlife, right?" All donor family counselors have stories about how various parties read peculiar events as evidence that donors can assert themselves beyond the grave. For example, two counselors on separate occasions described requests from transplant units whose recipients were puzzled by various events. One case involved the regular sighting of three numbers in the same sequence; in another, a patient's dreams were dominated by the color purple. The recipients hungered to know if these occurrences might be expressions of a donor's presence or preferences. Scoffing at such ideas, each OPO counselor nevertheless followed through with a promise to call the donor's kin, learning that, in the first case, this was the number on the donor's car plates; in the second, it was the donor's favorite color.

Robin Cowherd, a practicing Episcopalian who directs donor family care at LifeNet in Virginia Beach, has assembled a collection of such stories culled from accounts offered by kin he himself knows. Published under the title *Healing the Spirit*, Cowherd's modest volume consists of nine stories, six of which include "after-death communications" (ADCs). As I have described earlier, a key promotional message within the realm of organ transfer is that donors may "live on" through their recipients, a theme that is reflected in the first story of Cowherd's book, entitled "Shannon Lives On." A sudden thump from a closet led Shannon Brown's mother to an unknown box of photos and gift bag left by her daughter, who, at age twenty-three, was involved in a fatal car accident when driving home from her grandmother's. Another story tells of the disembodied voice of Jaimie Knight, a boy shot during a robbery attempt, who instructs a member of his parents' church to "watch for the yellow dog," a creature that later mounts a senior citizen van and places its head in the lap of Jaimie's grandfather. There is also Kathy Balentine's vision of and phone call from her daughter, Mia, who died in a car crash at seventeen; and Sandy Clarke's auditory and visual signs from her husband, Cres, who died from a brain aneurysm. Another mother reports regular sightings of butterflies and, later, an angel in a car, both of which she reads as communications from her son, Stephen Tayman, who died during a severe asthma attack; and little Cori Conrad has a prophetic dream about her sister Jessie Hooker, a donor who died from a cerebral aneurysm. Cowherd encourages readers to view these communications not as "frightening or unbelievable" events but, rather, as "comforting representations of life after death" (2003: x). Although Cowherd rejects the overt simplicity of the closure model, these published accounts nevertheless resonate with the sentiments expressed by Cindy, offering at least temporary solace during moments marked by intense feelings of isolation and hopelessness.

My purpose here is not to defend or refute the legitimacy of these stories—this I leave for the witnesses themselves to sort out. I do wish to note, however, that anthropology is rife with ethnographic accounts drawn from a multitude (if not perhaps a majority) of the world's cultures, where encounters with the dead are common or even typify quotidian life. My work in northwest Madagascar provides one such example, where my research interests ultimately required me to interview the dead on a regular basis. When speaking with spirit mediums of their work as indigenous healers, I found that they would inevitably reach the limits of their own knowledge and instruct me to call up their spirits to ask them more detailed questions about curative practices. History, in turn, is considered sacred knowledge in this region, and thus educated schoolteachers, elderly peasants, and royal retainers all made it clear that if I wished to reconstruct a comprehensive history of the region, I had best speak to the royal spirits, who were the guardians of the past.

As a result of such early field experiences elsewhere, I view ghost stories told by donor kin as a key component of the complex narrative structure so intrinsic to organ transfer. Because ghost stories frequently fall at the end of an interview, I conceive of them as a mystical denouement of sorts, providing one of many ways to make sense of a sudden death and tragic loss. As David Schneider, an anthropologist, once wrote, both ghosts and dead men are ideas (1980 [1965]: 2). Although Schneider's concern with the past was framed by kinship and not organ donation, his statement nevertheless provides a helpful directive for deciphering the significance of these peculiar tales. Like kinship (a topic that defines a key focus for my next chapter), ghost stories told by donor kin offer a means to pull what would otherwise be a lost or irretrievable sense of the past into the here and now. That is, they define just one aspect of a much larger project on memory work.

When understood as such, donor ghost stories may readily be understood as a genre of folklore with a wide circulation at least within the transplant arena, stories that are simultaneously emotionally troubling and cathartic. As such, they uncover the limitations of public forms of mourning in a context where—as I have illustrated here—professional management inevitably silences the pathos of individual loss. As Dominick LaCapra reminds us, mourning is framed by "the interaction between life and death." Further, as a shared and thus social process, mourning is rooted in "ways of working through the past." Whereas public donor memorials obscure personal suffering, among those who grieve "something of the past always remains, if only as a haunting presence or revenant" (LaCapra 1999: 698, 700; cf. Freud 1974).

When framed as such, donor ghost stories expose a widespread hunger for encounters with the dead; such encounters inevitably thrust the past into the present. Further, if grief is understood as a form of longing, then postmortem encounters potentially generate an unending flow of *new* memories. They thus offer fertile ground for generating new forms of intimacy with lost loved ones. By way of conclusion, I offer a few reflections on how such experiences enable donor kin to reorder their worlds by extending the life, so to speak, of a donor beyond the grave.

Building a Future with the Dead

As noted earlier, a significant anxiety articulated by both Sandy O'Neill and Paul Fenster is the unsettling finite quality of memories involving lost children. This sentiment is echoed as well by Kathy Eldon and Amy Eldon, a mother-and-daughter team who have produced *Angel Catcher*, a published journal guide for coping with the death of a loved one. The process of "journaling," as it is called, is a frequent suggestion offered by OPO staff to kin following a donor's death, and some offices distribute copies of *Angel Catcher* or other journal materials to families (Eldon and Eldon 1998; Ledoux 1993). The Eldons model this project after their own efforts to cope with the death of Dan Eldon, who was their son and brother, respectively, a young Reuters photographer who was stoned to death by a mob in Somalia at age twenty-two. As Kathy Eldon explains in her introduction, "The idea of for-getting Dan, even for an hour at a time, felt like a total betrayal of my son. Worse still, I found that my vivid memories of our life together were be-ginning to blur; his characteristic gestures and outrageous wit were not as clear as they had been; the stories I loved to tell were fading from my mem-ory. I couldn't remember incidents we had shared, moments I had always thought were indelibly etched in my mind" (Eldon and Eldon 1998).

Some donor kin indeed find comfort in journals or diaries, where they express in private form their anger, frustrations, and sorrow. Still others transform these projects into communicative devices, where their entries offer one side of a conversation with the dead. Among the most elaborate projects I have run across is one authored by a widow who writes to her de-ceased husband every evening about what happens to her each day. It is a project she looks forward to working on each night before she goes to bed.

This intense desire to capture and preserve memories is likewise illus-trated in especially poignant fashion by Paul Fenster, the father who system-atically records and stores every memory he can retrieve of his daughter. As he explained during a gathering of donor kin, the despondency he asso-ciates with the limits of his memory shook him to the very core. After his daughter Lisa died, Paul often found it impossible to sleep, and he would pace throughout the house at night for hours on end. Then he began to re-ceive what he refers to as "signs" from his daughter. As he explained, "[Other] people will tell [these sorts of stories] to me [too,] a bit sheepishly, saying 'No one is going to believe me if I tell this,' and then they tell me their stories of 'signs' and of how their [loved ones] communicate to them." Paul offered to a rapt audience brief accounts of a toy that moved and sounded on its own; the mysterious appearance of a child's Christmas present although no member of the extended family could claim they had bought it; and the sudden, fleeting utterances of a child heard by others late at night. These signs now define a new chapter of memories that Paul types up and adds to the back of an already voluminous set of fifteen hundred scrapbook entries. "According to my faith . . . I know where Lisa is, and I know that she is here with me all the time," says Paul. Donor parents like Paul in-variably speak of their lost children in the present tense and bristle when others ask if that child is in fact the one who is dead. As Paul's memory project attests, encounters from beyond the grave can ensure that the dead are always among us, defining the shape of an inexorable flow, rather than a finite set, of cherished memories. In a sense, too, they defy cultural asser-tions of the importance of closure, allowing one to pull the loved one along-side throughout the remainder of one's own life journey.

CONCLUSION

Memory work assumes an impressive array of forms in the lives of transplant recipients and donor kin. Members of both parties learn early in their careers within the realm of organ transfer to master sanctioned forms of storytelling. Each adopts guarded narrative styles that allow them to speak publicly of their transformative experiences while simultaneously promoting organ donation as a profound social act. Recipients' public testimonials, as well as the sanitized accounts of donor kin, offer but a glimpse at life, for well-crafted tales shelter audiences from the more devastating details of survival. Instead, the intimate, and often troubling, minutiae of their lives are reserved for private encounters with trusted friends and family. Professionals who orchestrate pubic events reward speakers who emphasize uplifting moments associated either with organ transplantation or with the decision to consent to donation. This patina of compliance ultimately silences accounts of the tribulations of long-term surgical survival and the open-ended nature of grief. The decision to obliterate troubling details from the public record is driven, ultimately, by professional fears that darker tales will dissuade the lay public from supporting this problematic medical realm, one already plagued by organ scarcity.

The complexities of survival are poignantly illustrated by a wealth of memorial projects that honor donors and their kin. The public face of organ transfer is dominated by a range of official events staged by transplant and procurement professionals, where donor gardens emerge as a pervasive form of expression. Rife with an iconography of renewal, these projects conceal the more intimate and troubling aspects of organ transfer. The recent assertive acts of several grassroots organizations—representing patient or donor kin needs—together define a subversive counterpart to obstructionist professionals. In recent years, these efforts have had a profound impact on reshaping official policies.

Close attention to private memorials reveals a bounty of projects that bear witness to a widespread and deep-seated longing that donors not be forgotten. On the one hand, recipients may understand donated parts as harboring some essence of their origins; on the other, surviving kin resist attempts to relegate donors to an anonymous category of the dead. Recipients honor the dead by viewing a transplanted organ not merely as a grafted part but as a lifelike entity capable of merging with a new body to form a hybrid self of sorts. Donor kin in turn refute the professional assertion that donors remain unnamed. Donor kin are especially prolific in generating an ingenious array of memorial projects, many of which defy professional decorum by proclaiming donors' identities. Still other expressive acts reveal elaborate forms of record keeping that seize upon inexplicable events that ultimately unravel the assumed absoluteness of death. When taken as a whole, memory projects challenge the secretive aspects of organ transfer in America, in the end exposing a unified desire for redemption, one shared by recipients and donor kin. As detailed in the following chapter, personal encounters define yet another form of defiance.

3   Public Encounters as Subversive Acts

In August 1998—for the first time ever—the surviving kin of organ donors arrived in large numbers to attend the Transplant Olympics, a biennial event organized by the National Kidney Foundation and held that summer at the Ohio State University in Columbus. Until that year, the Transplant Games had always been staged primarily (if not exclusively) for the benefit of organ recipients. Others in attendance included their families and friends, as well as health professionals from their respective transplant units, all of whom came to cheer them on in a host of competitive categories. This was a momentous occasion: hospital transplant staff had spent the last eight months or so rallying their members, designing team apparel, and holding fund-raisers to help pay for transportation and housing expenses. Transplant athletes now roamed the campus dressed in coordinated workout suits as well as flashy T-shirts with such names as "Team Indiana" and "Team Philadelphia" emblazoned across the front, and perhaps "Be an Organ Donor—It's the Chance of a Lifetime" or "Recycle Yourself" on the back. Frequently these outfits were further enhanced with buttons and pins bearing other slogans, and nearly all competitors wore small green ribbons signifying that they had received the "gift of life." Fresh encounters were often marked by a flurry of exchanges of small tokens of friendship, and state pins figured prominently. By the end of any given day, participants' shirts were often covered with buttons from around the country. The majority of participants were special athletes—men, women, and children of all ages who had survived organ failure and transplant surgery. Athletes were also grouped by their organs during casual conversations and in public addresses, identified as "the hearts," "the lungs," "the livers," and "the kidneys," or even complex combinations such as "kidney-pancreas" or "heart-lung." These organ-driven identities were sometimes marked clearly on more individually tailored T-shirts that bore such witty statements as "A Change of Heart" or the more ribald "I'm Living with My Daughter's Kidney."[1]

From a recipient's perspective, the Games were lively and highly inclusive, offering a place for all. One could register for events such as distance walking, golf, bowling, and badminton or compete in more strenuous events staged at the pool or track. Active participants ranged from four-year-olds who could barely hoist and toss a basketball, to those who were blind or wheelchair bound yet who expertly circumnavigated the track, to muscular Olympians whose remarkable physiques inspired awe among an admiring crowd. Some—and especially the swimmers—frequently dressed to display their impressive chest or abdominal surgical scars. Transplant athletes were housed and ate together in centralized dormitories, and they swarmed across the university's expansive grounds throughout the day. One could not help but notice this event if one were to visit this campus, where all athletic facilities were festooned with banners, posters, and tethered chains of colorful balloons.

Meanwhile, in an isolated convention center located on the campus periphery, one could encounter a hundred or so donor kin clustered separately in a high-rise hotel. Events organized specifically for them occurred almost exclusively at this location. Their participation had been made possible only after careful and persistent lobbying by the National Donor Family Council, a small advocacy group based within National Kidney Foundation headquarters in New York. Donor kin were invited to attend all the events organized for transplant athletes, but the majority of these competitions were held some distance away, necessitating that one catch a sporadically scheduled shuttle bus to reach them. Donor kin also stood apart from athletes in their appearance: unless they had accompanied a specific team as a small faction of cheerleaders, donor kin lacked the flashy, matching uniforms, wearing instead street clothes that might be decorated simply with tiny butterfly pins and salmon-colored ribbons, both of which were supplied by NDFC staff. Only a handful of events were designed to draw together donor kin and transplant recipients. Although these were held on the main campus, recipients were frequently unaware that donor kin were present in substantial numbers. These few joint events were held exclusively in a large auditorium based in the university student center, a spot that most athletes visited only when they first registered for the Games. Nevertheless, it was here that all attendees, regardless of affiliation, could walk the halls and view the Patches of Love Quilt, which by 1998 contained hundreds of squares crafted within individual donor households.

Throughout the course of the Games, donor kin and organ recipients were most likely to remain separated as isolated groups in radically different locations. They neither ate together nor, for the most part, attended the same scheduled events, be they athletic competitions, discussion groups, or instructional workshops. During the organizational phase of the Games, staff from the National Kidney Foundation had expressed great unease over the potential dangers of allowing donor kin and Olympians to mix at a time that was meant to be primarily a celebratory event for the latter. In contrast, among NDFC staff one encountered a boiling anger over what was perceived as a deliberate exclusion of their own constituency. The presence of donor kin was recognized nevertheless by all organizers as a clear landmark event, and this controversial experiment did in the end establish a trend that is now standard practice at the Transplant Games. They have since become a far more inclusive biannual celebration, one understood as being of equal importance to those who have survived organ failure and those whose decisions made transplantation possible.[2] This new trend is echoed, too, in a slowly growing acceptance of the inevitability of donor kin–organ recipient communication, a subject that defines the focus of this chapter.

BUREAUCRATIC CONSTRAINTS ON SOCIAL DESIRE

As described earlier in this book, an interlocking set of ideological premises guides both professional and lay behavior within the realm of organ transfer. Particularly relevant to this chapter are anxieties surrounding organ scarcity, rendering professionals especially reluctant to instigate new policies that could further threaten the all too fragile trust the lay pubic invests in their highly specialized medical realm. Professionals dedicatedly guard the anonymity of cadaveric organ donors and, in turn, respect the privacy of transplant recipients who, they feel, need not learn too much of their organs' origins. In a realm inevitably overshadowed by death, anonymity mandates secrecy, too. Nevertheless, as we shall see, the desire for intimate (that is, face-to-face) contact is one shared by some donor kin and transplant recipients. This chapter is an account of those who defy rules of anonymity and successfully locate one another.

I will explore an unusual form of social desire, one expressed by disparate parties now connected to one another as a result of the sudden deaths of individual patients. More specifically, I focus, first, on the taboos associated with donor kin–organ recipient communication, and the myths associated with donor kin grief that drive professionals to assume that contact is laced with danger. I then turn to the process of communication itself, its history marked by shifts from early openness to great secrecy (and, thus, subversive communicative acts), to more recent albeit carefully orchestrated encounters now overseen by professional gatekeepers. A series of detailed case studies, which dominate the central section of this chapter, exposes the motivations that compel organ recipients and their respective donors' kin to seek out one another and share details of their personal histories. A pervasive belief is that the donor body links these disparate parties to one another as blood kin. As a result, the idiom of fictive kinship generates new sentimental ties of sociality, enabled by the sharing of donor flesh. As such, this process minimizes the strangeness of the hybrid body—one composed of parts of disparate human origins—replacing it with the shared sense of intimacy. In the final section I analyze the significance of this creative strategy of fictive kinship by comparing organ transfer with other contexts, such as anonymous adoption and gestational surrogacy. As this comparative approach will reveal, ideas about blood ties shape identities and their histories, generating in turn elaborate and highly unconventional social strategies for transforming strangers into kin.

The Danger of Public Grief and Donor Kin Propriety

A dominant assumption that inevitably shapes the programs at transplant events is that donor kin define an emotionally volatile social category, and their very presence endangers the tenuous stability of the ideological premises that drive celebratory events. On the one hand, professionals consider donor kin to be valuable participants because their personal narratives supply powerful messages about the great social worth of organ transfer. Nevertheless, the complex experiences of donor kin are frequently reduced to the basic assumption that they are wracked with grief and thus obsessed with death, rendering them unpredictable in public contexts. Donor kin are frequently described as prone to spontaneous outbursts of sorrow, and thus they potentially threaten the emotional calm of transplant events. As described in the previous chapter, when invited (or, as some donor kin would say, allowed) to speak before a crowd of organ recipients, donor kin representatives are selected with great care, and their statements may even be scripted by professionals who organize these events. Those donor kin who do become actively involved as spokespersons for the transplant industry learn quickly that their narrative style and topical focus determine whether they will be invited back. In turn, organ procurement organizations may claim ownership of especially gifted (and cooperative) speakers, describing them in possessive terms as "our donor families."

Overall, dominant assumptions about the heightened emotional states of donor kin are unfounded. Such myths cloud the reality of how donor kin actually speak of their tragic losses in public. In fact, I have found that recipients are far more prone to spontaneous emotional responses than are donor kin. Male and, to a lesser extent, female recipients may weep freely and openly at support group meetings, during one-on-one interviews, and when standing before audiences of hundreds or thousands of people. Their expressive acts are naturalized in peculiar ways, for, as noted in this chapter, the outbursts of recipients (especially adult men) generally are not accredited to emotional weakness but instead are identified as an uncontrollable side effect of their medications. Thus, the causes of recipient sorrow are located beyond the individual, or, at the very least, weeping is interpreted as evidence not of suffering but of the complex, overwhelming joy recipients feel in having been granted a second chance to live, but always at the expense of the death of another.

In contrast, among donor kin, mourning and loss eventually settle in as facts of life—the reality that their lives will never be the same following the terrible and sudden death of, say, a beloved child or spouse. Contrary (or in response) to professionals' fears, donor kin rapidly learn to adopt a matter-of-fact tone when speaking publicly of their tragedies. In short, public and thus disturbing expressions of grief are rare. Instead, donor kin may hold their grief inside so well that some may even exhibit a flatness in affect as they tell—yet again—their stories of tragic loss. As many donor kin explain, in the context of their daily lives they frequently encounter a low tolerance among family, friends, and strangers for their unending sorrow. Many donor kin endure their grief privately, for an implicit cultural ideal insists that mourning is finite and, thus, when experienced properly, moves smoothly toward a sense of peace. As a result, donor kin are expected to get on with their lives and seek joy in what they have: laborers should return to work, widows should remarry, and grieving parents should have another child to replace the one they lost.

Among the most problematic issues at work here is a dominant framework derived from the writings of Elisabeth Kübler-Ross (1969, 1975, 1981), who argued that death and subsequent mourning are marked by stages of internal growth, the last of which is acceptance (often referred to elsewhere as "closure"). Procurement professionals may even promote donation as a means to speed closure, a message I have heard OPO family counselors voice on several occasions as one of the great blessings of organ transfer. My own data reveal that organ donation most certainly *transforms* the mourning process, but rather than offering closure, it may instead help extend the mourning period indefinitely (Sharp 2001). These findings are echoed in the sentiments of one OPO's grief counselor, who explained, "I think Kübler-Ross has done more damage—those five stages are for the dying, *not* the survivors! . . . There are no stages, it's . . . forever."

Three factors are at work here that render closure impossible. The first is the very nature of donors' deaths and identities. The majority of organ donors die suddenly and with no warning; as a result, surviving kin frequently express the terrible angst they experience in being robbed of the chance to say good-bye. When one is among the brain dead, there is no final conversation or an opportunity to express one's wishes or simply to squeeze a receptive parent's, spouse's, or sibling's hand.[3] The unending sense of loss is especially profound when donors' deaths result from car accidents, or from suicidal or murderous gunshot head wounds. In these contexts surviving kin always ask, could they have prevented these tragedies? Parents who outlive their children are wracked by special forms of grief because of the injustice of the death, and the belief that one should never outlive one's own offspring. Second, the impossibility of closure rests, too, in the very nature of the donor testimonial: each time donor kin publicly recount their tales, they inevitably relive aspects of their tragedies. Third and finally, the ideological underpinnings of organ transfer render closure highly problematic. If transplanted organs embody the essence of deceased donors, then organ transfer literally scatters bits and parts of selves about the country. In this sense, organ transfer simultaneously engenders, first, a special category of wandering dead (as exemplified by the ghost stories recounted in chapter 2), and, second, a peculiar type of body transgression or hybridity, involving the melding of parts from one donor to the bodies of several strangers.

Donor kin, then, occupy a terrible, liminal status in the public arena. Their narratives play an essential role in illustrating the wondrous qualities of their personal sacrifices, yet donor kin nevertheless define (albeit subtly) a category of pariah whose members must internalize their pain and grief if their presence is to be tolerated at public celebratory events. It is health professionals (including those who work in transplantation as well as procurement) who are most likely to be worried about donor kin attending transplant celebrations. In contrast, organ recipients express awe and wonderment when in the presence of donor kin. More specifically, organ recipients frequently use the term *honor* to express the sentiments they feel. It is not unusual, for instance, to hear recipients say to donor kin such things as "It's such an honor to be here with you today," "It's an honor to have met you," or "I feel so honored to have had the privilege to hear the story of your loss."

Rather than insisting on silence, when donor kin and organ recipients are together they openly voice the desire to learn the details of each other's lives, expressing deep sensitivity for one another's plights. Each also acknowledges the inability to experience the other's suffering, underscoring with deep conviction the limits of their empathy. For example, organ recipients frequently tell donor families that they cannot fully imagine what they must have gone through, but after listening they offer heartfelt thanks for having been allowed to hear the story. When donor kin and organ recipients sit together, whether it be in the bleachers at the Transplant Games or at a banquet table at a commemorative event, they inevitably ask one another, "How did you get your transplant?" and "How did your [loved one] die?" These are the sorts of direct questions that coworkers, friends, and even close family members may hesitate to ask because they fear the consequences of direct probing: they do not wish to be nosy, or they fear their questions will cause emotional pain. As a result, organ recipients and, even more so, donor kin learn in their daily lives to stay silent when in the company of others, holding their sadness and grief inside. When donor kin and recipients ask these questions of one another, they understand them not as invasive but, rather, as attempts to communicate across the divide with the few whom they can trust. In this sense, they are all survivors of a shared trauma, bound together by a highly unusual form of embodied intimacy.

Defying Transplant Decorum: The Taboos and Consequences of Communication

Since the onset of my research, I have been struck consistently by the strong taboos imposed by transplant and procurement professionals that forbid communication between recipients and donor kin in cases involving cadaveric donation. It is important to realize, however, that strong sanctions against communication define one aspect of a much larger trajectory of shifting trends. Renée Fox and Judith Swazey, whose sociological research extends back to the 1950s (Fox 1959), reveal that organ transfer in the United States did not in fact begin as an anonymous affair. As they explain,

> During the early years of human organ transplants, medical teams were inclined to reveal the identities of the donors of cadaver organs, their recipients, and their families to one another, and to provide them with details about each other's backgrounds and lives. Physicians believed that [these parties] were entitled to such knowledge. Moreover, they thought that it would enhance the meaning of the transplant experience for the recipient and recipient's family and afford consolation and a sense of completeness to the donor family. [Such policies

changed] with the passage of time and increased clinical experience.
(Fox and Swazey 1992: 36)

In short, the ideology of communication shifted from assumed intimacy to enforced anonymity, the latter remaining firmly in place and guiding official protocol well until the end of the twentieth century. During the early 1990s, when I began my research, transplant professionals regarded written communication and, even more so, personal encounters as subversive acts. At this time there were very few avenues that might have facilitated initial contact. Whereas today organ recipients are strongly encouraged to write anonymous thank-you letters to their donor families, ten years ago this was highly unusual, and little structure was in place bureaucratically to facilitate the forwarding of correspondence. Some professionals even considered attempts to communicate as evidence of pathology—that is, that the recipient was unable to come to terms with his or her altered life course.

In the context of my own work I have found that regardless of the transplant event—be it in celebration of transplantation or a commemorative affair designed to honor donor families—tales of personal encounters always generate spontaneous responses of joy and celebration from the audience. Recipients and donor kin who have met one another are held in awe by others, who respect their courage in tracking down one another. Over the years, tales of encounters have occurred more frequently, and today they are more readily embraced by professionals, some of whom may now orchestrate initial meetings. For instance, if, in 1992, an organ recipient spoke publicly of having met his donor family, he generally raised the topic without the approval of transplant staff. This would be true even if his transplant unit's social worker had assisted him in his original efforts.

In some cases donor kin and recipients have learned of one another or met surreptitiously. As Dale Sabrinski revealed in the previous chapter, a nosy neighbor who liked to follow the obituaries took it upon herself to tell him who his donor was. Knowing the date and time of his transplant, she was able to link his lifesaving surgery to a suicide by hanging committed by a young man in his area. This news marked a double blow for Dale because he had not been told the cause of his donor's death (transplant staff rarely report violent donor deaths to organ recipients).[4] A far more typical approach involved the chance encounter in the hallway during a conference or celebratory event. As one woman explained, after hearing a donor's mother speak publicly of her son's death, she matched the date to that of her own liver transplant. When the conference adjourned temporarily midmorning, she took advantage of the moment and sought out the donor's mother on her way to the bathroom.

The two woman exchanged further details of their stories and concluded that they were, indeed, linked to one another through organ transfer.

From a professional point of view, such tales only underscore the importance of withholding donors' full personal names and the precise dates of their life spans. This became all too clear when the NDFC displayed its Patches of Love quilt at the 1998 Transplant Games, the first time the quilt was available for open viewing by large numbers of transplant recipients. Quilt squares often displayed photographs of organ donors transferred onto cloth, and many in turn bore donors' full names and dates of birth and death (similar to what might appear on a tombstone). NDFC staff had lobbied hard for the right to mount the quilt in a public venue frequented by recipients. They were outraged when they learned of an attempt by one state's OPO to start its own donor quilt, where submissions were restricted to including either donors' full names *or* dates of death, but not both. As I have argued elsewhere (Sharp 2001), virtual donor cemeteries posted by Transweb are perhaps the most subversive acts of all. Here one can conceivably type in the date of one's transplant and then read the life and death story of one's personal organ donor as written by his or her surviving kin.[5]

First Contact

The shift in attitude toward communication among professionals began in the middle to late 1990s. When and where this occurred depended on the region of the country in which one lived, with unofficial approaches and more official policies resulting from the stance advocated by individual OPO directorships. Evidence of this shift is exemplified by a presentation given in 1998 before a recipient support group based in a major East Coast city. Dora Tuckerman, the evening's speaker, had experience in trauma work and had been hired less than a year earlier by her local OPO to oversee the exchange of correspondence between recipients and donor families. During her presentation Dora distributed handouts that explained how a newly instituted communication process worked, as well as guidelines on how to begin planning a letter, and suggestions on what sorts of messages might be appropriate. Recipients attending this meeting voiced a range of anxieties in response, involving three dominant themes. First was the concern that by writing to donor kin they would only reopen wounds, reminding these families of their losses. The second focused on resistance to a policy that did not honor letters as confidential documents because, as Dora explained very clearly, to protect the privacy of all involved parties, she was required to read and, when necessary, edit the contents of all letters that passed through her office. The third concerned the deep sorrow of those who in the past had attempted yet failed to communicate with donor kin. This was expressed especially strongly by two men (both of whom had received liver transplants between seven and ten years earlier), each of whom had written to their donor families following their surgeries but had received no answers. One of these men asked Dora if she could find out what had happened to his letter, one sent to a donor family in yet another state. Dora explained, with a hint of frustration, that no channels were in place that would allow her to track such aged correspondence; further, at that time bureaucratic links across state boundaries were extremely weak. In response, the man became even more agitated, accusing Dora under his breath of being obstructionist.

Certainly Dora should not be faulted here. As she later explained to me, she had taken the job only a few months earlier and was still feeling her way in a world where essentially no policies existed, except those that denied the legitimacy of contact. Dora felt compelled to proceed with great caution, too (and this extended even to conversations about her work), because her activities were heavily scrutinized by a director fearful of any bad publicity targeting her OPO. Nevertheless, the agitated response offered by this male recipient was legitimate. After all, at the time (and, as we shall see, currently as well), many OPOs and transplant units deliberately blocked communication. OPOs like Dora's, which have defined the vanguard for this movement, now oversee a steady flow of correspondence and are proud of the encounters they have subsequently orchestrated. Whereas donor kin and recipients may be anxious to learn more of each other, some transplant unit staff may be less willing to embrace new OPO policies.

This is best illustrated by events that occurred during a more recent workshop specifically on donor kin–recipient communication, one organized by yet another East Coast OPO in 2003. Following a presentation by Suzanne Winkler, a social worker trained in grief counseling who runs her OPO's communication program, a heart recipient in her fifties told the story of having recently received a letter from her donor family, one forwarded to her by Suzanne's OPO office. She gleefully offered the letter to staff in own transplant unit to read, hoping to share the joy she felt in hearing from these special strangers. Instead, transplant unit staff responded by telling her this had been a mistake, and they confiscated the letter. The woman was especially distraught because the letter had been an original, not a photocopy. The shift in OPO policy was reflected in Suzanne's immediate response that "they [the transplant staff] are not supposed to do that"; this was followed by a question from a donor mother who asked what sort of work could be done to "educate" transplant staff on updated procedures. The recipient then continued her story: her transplant unit had a formal policy stating that absolutely no communication should occur within the first year after surgery. At this point Suzanne reiterated that such a decision was outdated and defied current policy set by her OPO in conjunction with its local network of transplant units. Suzanne then promised she would look into the matter and try to track down a photocopy within her own files for this distressed woman. Such events never would have occurred, or been discussed so openly, even five years earlier. In most parts of the country the recipient would have been afraid to tell this story publicly, even if she or he had been assisted by a sympathetic professional (for one, to do so might endanger a professional's job). The few cases I encountered in the early 1990s generally occurred through chance encounters or as a result of the bold actions of a handful of sympathetic professionals, often based within transplant units.[6]

Ralph Needham offers a rare glimpse at early and professionally sanctioned communication efforts. In 1988, when he was in his late thirties, Ralph received a double lung transplant in a western state after nearly dying from idiopathic pulmonary disease. A year after his surgery he received a letter from the wife of his donor. The donor was a twenty-five-year-old man who had suffered a severe head trauma and had left behind a family that included three children (the third was born following the father's death). The donor's widow (who had since remarried) had contacted the local OPO and asked if she could write to Ralph, who was the only recipient of her husband's donated organs. Staff from Ralph's transplant unit then asked if he would like to see the letter, and he agreed. When I asked him if he felt any connection to his donor, or how his feelings might differ from those of the donor's wife, he answered thus:

> Her husband gave me two good lungs. . . . She thinks that her husband lives on in me; but I feel uncomfortable about that—I feel they are *my* lungs now. . . . They are good lungs. After the transplant the doctors said the lungs were in very good shape. . . . My job is to take care of them, because *he* took such good care of them, too. . . . I continue [to correspond with my donor's wife]—my wife is the kind of person who likes to keep in touch with people, she thinks this is important. So when she receives a letter from someone she always writes back. . . . I sent her [the donor's wife] a Christmas card last year, and then she wrote back. (cf. Sharp 1994: 379)

When I later asked staff from Ralph's transplant unit how the decision was made to transmit the letter to Ralph, Delia Boxer, an outspoken social worker, responded as follows:

> Ahh, look, we've known Ralph an awful long time, and he's a special person—he's one of the first and only lung transplants we've ever done,

and he's an incredibly level-headed kind of guy. I guess you could say we don't always do things by the book around here—[our director]—you know her, right? She's different in this way from others [who work in transplant elsewhere]—she's not one to get all bogged down by official protocol—we like her because she's such a renegade. On top of it, this is basically a rural state, and so there's this small-town idea that guides how we [who grew up and live here] are with other people [in our daily lives]. Besides, the donor's family lives pretty far away and so there's not much to worry about their crossing paths. Besides, Ralph's wife is a [pediatric] nurse, and she understands that privacy matters. And so does Ralph. He's not the busybody type, you know. He's not going to jump in his car and drive out there and ring her doorbell or anything like that.

Far more often, though, encounters throughout the early 1990s occurred less in response to professional compassion than from the institutional desire for local fame. In cases involving especially dramatic surgical feats or highly publicized local tragedies, public relations professionals for local hospitals would at times release the identities of donors and recipients to the press. In such instances, reporters arrived and publicized the event, generally offering full names and even photographs of recipients, the deceased donor, and the donor's kin. Usually this was the first time these parties learned of one another's identities. This is in fact what happened at a local hospital in Indianapolis in 1990 (just before I started my research), when a single organ donor saved the lives of several patients. After reading the story in the statewide newspaper, much to the chagrin of recuperating patients (not to mention transplant staff), the donor's family showed up unannounced at the bedsides of several recipients, asserting ties to their newfound kin (Sharp 1994: 369; see also B. Smith 1994).

Close Encounters

Among the most striking aspects of donor kin–recipient communication is the manner in which face-to-face encounters insist on this sort of reordering of community in everyday life. This communication takes several forms. Today many transplant recipients write anonymous thank-you notes. (One OPO that encourages this practice estimated that fewer than 50 percent of all recipients within its region do so.) Some OPOs insist that recipients should at least try to write such notes. In the words of one staff member, "If someone gave you pajamas for Christmas, you'd write a thank-you note. Someone gave you life—you have to [write]!" Longer written exchanges occur far less frequently and usually not until several years have passed.

There are no statistics available on this practice because exchanges remain confidential and may not necessarily involve OPO or transplant unit staff. I estimate that perhaps 15 percent of recipients alive today nationwide have received a letter from their donor families, and even fewer have had face-to-face encounters. As explained earlier, however, stories of communication and encounters now form an important part of conferences and commemorative events for recipients and donor kin. The positive outcomes of these stories give others the courage to try to make contact themselves.

Encounters, when they do occur, are rarely singular affairs. If parties decide to meet one another, this usually is merely the first step in what slowly evolves into a highly intimate social relationship that will persist for years. Donor kin and recipients readily adopt creative strategies for defining their relationships with one another. Fictive kinship—or the strategy of rendering those unrelated to us either by blood or marriage as close kin (Schusky 1965: 76)—emerges as a familiar and, in the words of several research participants, "natural" strategy. The idiom of friendship fails to embody the level of intimacy that organ transfer engenders, and thus organ recipients and donor kin readily incorporate one another as mothers and fathers, sisters, brothers, and children. In addition, the natural intimacy of blood ties negates the strangeness of the hybrid body. The fact that donor flesh coexists (and, literally, bonds) with the recipient's through successful transplant surgery facilitates the literal reading of this bond as a "blood" tie.

The social ties donor kin and organ recipients establish with one another are mediated by several important factors. Most important, these are the identity of the deceased donor (where age and gender matter especially), the varying symbolic weights assigned to different organs, and, finally, a specific participant's longing to meet certain categories of recipients or donor kin over others. Organ recipients and donor kin, though they lack any official guidelines on how to do so, forge these new bonds in remarkably similar ways, following with great regularity a particular set of rules intrinsic to American concepts of fictive kinship. Fictive kinship lends itself well to American practices that privilege blood ties; in the context of organ transfer, this form of sociality reinforces the idea that to embody a transplanted organ is to embody some essence of the donor, too (cf. Fox and Swazey 1992: 36; Crowley-Matoka in press).

To begin, if we embrace the idea that a donor's identity is harbored in his or her transplanted organs, then organ recipients represent, at least in part, the donor self. The response, then, is to assign to the recipient an intimate kinship category that parallels the donor's original relationship to his or her surviving natal or nuclear family members. Consider, for example, David, a

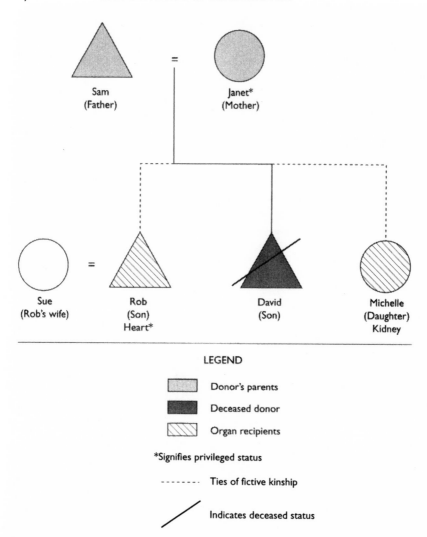

Figure 9.   Organ transfer's fictive kin.

young man of twenty-two who died in a car accident, and whose parents, Sam and Janet, donated his organs for transplant when he was declared brain dead. If and when these parents meet Rob, the man who has received David's heart, or Michelle, the woman who now has one of David's kidneys, David's surviving parents will incorporate these two recipients into their own family as their son and daughter (figure 9). It is especially noteworthy that these fictive ties of kinship are reserved exclusively for the recipients themselves:

they do not extend to, say, a recipient's spouse or offspring. Thus, Sue remains simply Rob's wife. In addition, I have found that only a donor's previous blood ties to his or her parents or siblings are reactivated, and not those to a spouse (or, it seems, children).

As noted earlier, following their transplants, recipients frequently celebrate dates that mark birthdays and rebirthdays. In turn, through the process of incorporation involving donor kin, they may recognize two sets of parents: those who raised them, and those of their deceased donors. It is important to realize, too, that these newly established relationships are defined in *structural* terms, regardless of age. That is, even if the heart recipient is the same age as, or even older than, the donor's parents, the recipient will still be thought of as a new son or daughter. Fictive kinship in this context also activates strong sentimental bonds, as expressed in the words of a donor mother who, in writing to the recipient of her daughter's kidney, stated: "Meeting you is like finding a long-lost child." As we shall see, the potentially humorous dilemmas generated by this form of structural readjustment escape neither donor kin nor organ recipients. Involved parties playfully acknowledge the peculiar nature of their newfound relationships while still guarding them as precious and even sacred strategies that allow them to redefine and realign their social worlds.

Blood Ties and Brotherly Love

Not all are created equal in the world of organ transfer. In attempts to locate either donor kin or organ recipients, greater weight is placed on certain categories over others. First, whereas all organs bear the potential for harboring the essence of their donors, certain organs matter more than others. Thus, donor kin most frequently express the strongest desire to encounter the recipient who received the donor's heart. Furthermore, far less weight (and thus longing) is assigned to donated tissues, particularly bone, skin, and muscle fragments. Sometimes during interviews donor kin express embarrassment or shame when they offer information on which body parts they declined to donate, perhaps asking me to hazard a guess as to which of these it might have been. In response, I always suggest the heart, eyes, or the long bones: heart and eyes (or, more appropriately, corneas) because they are most frequently understood by donor kin as harboring the self, and eyes and limb bones because their procurement inspires the most graphic and disturbing images of body mutilation. My guesses are invariably correct. In the search for particular organs (and their recipients), for donor kin it is the encounter with the heart recipient that is by far the most highly charged emotional experience. As other authors report, donor kin may long to hear the sound of the beating heart, and some ask permission to press their ear to the recipient's chest, hoping to sense their loved one at work inside another's body (Gutkind 1988; Selzer 1990). What this means, too, is that some donor kin might actually prefer that the first encounter be with a kidney or liver recipient, because their transplanted organs are imbued with less symbolic weight. In essence, such donor kin are steeling themselves for a potentially more wrenching experience with the heart recipient.

One of the first examples I collected where an encounter had generated ties of fictive kinship emerged during interviews I conducted at the 1992 Transplant Games in Los Angeles. As in Ralph Needham's case, the involved parties were able to meet through the efforts of sympathetic transplant unit professionals. This relationship involved two men, Bob and Ray, who were linked to one another by a "domino procedure," where one recipient, whose lungs are dysfunctional, nevertheless receives a pair of lungs *and* a heart; his healthy heart is then transplanted in another recipient (figure 10).

As close friends of the two men explained, Bob required a lung transplant, but his surgeons opted to give him a new heart as well. The rationale that drives the domino procedure is that it is easier—and safer—to transfer a set of lungs still attached to a heart than to excise only Bob's damaged lungs and then attempt to reattach a new set to his original heart. Bob's compromised lungs were similarly removed along with his heart; the former were discarded, but his heart was then transplanted in Ray. In essence, then, this example of organ transfer united three bodies through two transplant surgeries: (A) an anonymous brain-dead donor who provided a heart and pair of lungs; (B) Bob, who received these organs but then passed on his own heart to another; and (C) Ray, who received Bob's heart. Bob and Ray were anxious to meet one another, and their respective transplant teams assisted them in doing so, an effort that was coordinated by their state's OPO. When they met, Bob said he felt the same pain in his new heart that he used to feel in his old one. Bob and Ray's relationship has slowly evolved into one marked by great emotional closeness. As reported in 1992, these two men and their wives regularly vacationed together. Bob and Ray think of themselves as being more than friends: instead, the bond established through organ transfer ties them to one another as a reunited pair of beloved brothers.

A Fateful Homecoming

As subsequent case studies in this chapter will show, transplantation is most often understood as generating inseparable ties of blood kinship between organ recipients and their respective donors' kin. Whereas my own data reveal that social rejection by either party is rare, occasionally there are

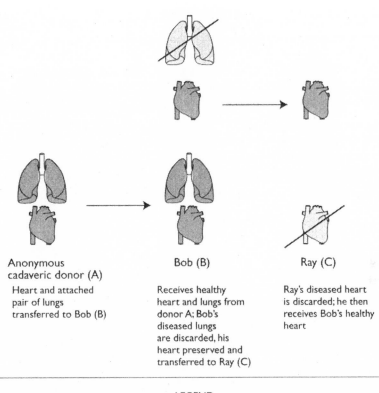

Anonymous cadaveric donor (A)	Bob (B)	Ray (C)
Heart and attached pair of lungs transferred to Bob (B)	Receives healthy heart and lungs from donor A; Bob's diseased lungs are discarded, his heart preserved and transferred to Ray (C)	Ray's diseased heart is discarded; he then receives Bob's healthy heart

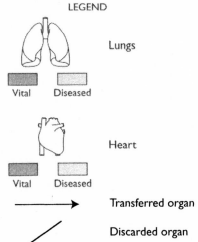

Figure 10.   The heart-lung domino procedure.

terrible failures. Those most likely to end in tragedy inevitably spring from the period that predates the careful and systematic policies that now guide the actions of communications coordinators based in various state OPOs.[7] A rare instance I offer here was driven by the desires of professionals perhaps a bit too anxious for publicity.

Mrs. Cruise's troubled teenage son died from a self-inflicted gunshot wound to the head during a standoff with police. Soon after her son's death, she and her husband were pressured by their local OPO to make contact with their son's recipients because it might generate a story of love and sharing across a racial divide. OPO staff were, however, dead wrong in their calculations. As Mrs. Cruise explained during a 1998 workshop on donor family–recipient communication:

> We lost our [teenage] son four years ago. We met his [heart] recipient— we lived in the same city [in the Southwest]. I tried my best [to make this man feel] welcome in my home. [I told him] my son committed suicide [when cornered by police]. He [the recipient] was carrying a lot of guilt. The OPO really exerted a lot of pressure on us—we have tried to promote the minority issue—we're Hispanic. They later arranged a meeting but he had something else to do! His children were really grateful, he said. [We had attended an event where] donor families gave medallions to their recipients but he didn't come. [After that], three times events were arranged [where he agreed to come] but he didn't show up. Our culture is different—he's not Hispanic. I'm a Christian; we were told that our son saved forty lives, but we've only met one! [This man is] the only [recipient we've met] . . . [but] he doesn't want to have anything to do with us. . . . When [finally] we met, it was clear he was shocked—he didn't know about our background—our name doesn't make this clear, you know . . . and he [was clearly agitated by being in our house and he] wanted to leave right away. . . . [But there are] kind people *here* [at the Transplant Games]. . . . That man over there—he gave us his [Olympic] medal! He has the heart of a Hispanic girl and so he said "this [pointing to herself and her husband] is my Hispanic family." But [our son's other recipients]—none of them ever wrote back.

In response, an unidentified recipient shouts out. "Every breath we take is because of your decision!"

Two days later, at the end of this conference, Mrs. Cruise stood up and explained that she had reached another level of understanding as a result of subsequent conversations with other donor families and recipients who had approached her after hearing her story. Two experiences proved cathartic in changing her thinking. The first involved coming to grips with the fact that, as others repeatedly explained to her, her son's heart recipient was quite plainly a racist, and his behavior toward her was abominable and was considered anomalous in the transplant world. This is because transplant professions strongly embrace what I have referred to elsewhere as the democratization of organ transfer. As professionals like to explain, organ transfer is "color blind." Those who work in transplant units may avoid assisting prospective patients who say they would refuse an organ from someone whom they consider racially inferior. I know of several transplant programs that deny such patients access to waiting lists if they express blatantly racist and even exclusionary class sentiments (Sharp 2002b). Mrs. Cruise's second source of catharsis was the overwhelming response she received from recipients who had never met their own donor kin. In her closing remarks during a final workshop, Mrs. Cruise spoke in moving terms of "a dozen newly adopted recipients." By the end of this public event, Mrs. Cruise's troubled son had finally come home to her through this large and newly established web of fictive kin relations.

Mother Love

Whereas donor kin may search fervently for the recipient who received the transferred heart, organ recipients are united in their own particular search. The greatest emotional weight is assigned to a donor's birth mother, a woman who may now potentially fill the role of a second, albeit fictive, mother for the organ recipient. Today at transplant events a small crowd may roar with approval when a recipient steps up to the microphone, tells his story of sickness and recovery, and then with great joy introduces his "donor mother" to the audience. Also, mothers may be quick to form social bonds with one another, in part, as two of the following case studies reveal, because donor mothers may be more receptive to embracing strangers as kin than are their husbands, and they may be more willing to talk openly and in public about their losses. Although the data are sparse at this point, I posit that donor fathers typically turn inward or prefer to work behind the scenes, and donor mothers turn outward, assuming the public face of donorship, marking equally legitimate ways to struggle with their shared source of grief. Organ recipients, in turn, associate warmth and kindness with donor mothers over all other potential kin. Although I can only hypothesize here, this might very well be because recipients equate their harboring of others within their own bodies with the gestational experiences of their donors' birth mothers. (I will return to this theme at the end of this chapter.)

Kelly McCarthy, a towheaded blonde in her midthirties, offers a poignant story that exemplifies a mother's actions. Kelly's daughter, Kirsty, died at age twelve from injuries sustained in a school bus accident when she was on her way back from an overnight athletic event in New England.

> Soon after Kirsty died I called [the director of the local OPO] and explained I wanted to write to [Kirsty's recipients]. I kept getting the runaround from their PR person! When she finally got a letter [to me] it wasn't from her [recipient] at all—the dates didn't line up. I thought, "Someone else needs this letter!" and so I sent it back. [Over the years I've become more insistent] about meeting recipients—I think that if they want to, [it should happen], and it makes me angry how the letters are edited and how I have to go through [someone at the OPO] to do this. I finally [cornered] an [OPO staff member] at [a transplant event], and she got [the OPO] to do something. . . . When Kirsty died I received really limited information on [her recipients]. I knew their ages, for the recipients for each of her organs. . . . I finally got a letter from a mother whose son got a kidney [but meeting was nearly impossible because we lived so far apart]. A little girl got her heart, another man a lung. . . . They told me they were all [local but meeting was actually very hard]. I knew her [other] kidney went to a teenage girl. I had to push and push until they would help me locate her!
>
> Then, last year, we invited them to our house for a cookout. They live about four hours away and they're [originally] from [St. Lucia]. When they came they brought all sorts of family with them, and they had to travel by bus so [my sister and a friend of mine and I ran carpools] to pick them all up. They had so much fun they want to come back this year!
>
> I was surprised, I thought I'd be drawn to the daughter—she is in fact my [oldest] daughter's age, and the two of them hit it off—but instead [for me] it was the mother. We just had a lot more in common— we really understood each other, it was so natural, because we both knew what it was like to live with the fear of losing a child.

Bureaucratizing the Encounter

The hard-won battles led by Kelly and other surviving donor kin (marked particularly well by the concerted efforts of NDFC staff) have forced a number of OPOs to reconsider their policies concerning donor kin–recipient communication. One of the most influential moves by NDFC springs from its forging the Donor Family Bill of Rights. First issued in 1994, this document defended the right of donor kin to "receive timely information" about the placement of organs and tissues and, if they so desired, to communicate anonymously with recipients and receive regular updates on their status (Corr et al. 1994; NDFC 1994). Three years later, the NDFC issued a detailed communication guide which underscored that letters should not be edited or altered without permission (NDFC 1997).[8]

As exemplified by the work of communications coordinators such as Dora Tuckerman and Suzanne Winkler, several OPOs have established their own official guidelines that shape correspondence, and they have standardized policies for face-to-face encounters. Most noteworthy is the current practice of hiring social workers and/or grief counselors to fill the official role of gatekeeper. This approach underscores that OPOs are highly sensitive to the emotional needs of donor kin in particular, and they anticipate that a desire for contact across the divide is conflated with a sense of loss and, potentially, terrible personal pain. The evidence offered here reveals that a number of OPOs had mediated encounters as early as the late 1980s, yet only around 1998 was this role first institutionalized. Before then, it generally fell to local donor mother volunteers or OPO staff members who handled correspondence in their spare time.

The effects of hiring specialists to oversee communication are varied. I have found that the incidence of encounters appears to be on the rise, in part because of the loosening of taboos, so that donor kin and recipients are now more willing to speak openly about how they met one another without fear of subsequent censure from transplant officials. This then inspires others to do the same. Another reason for the increase is that bureaucracy sometimes contributes to greater efficiency. Whereas ten years ago no one was in place to establish policies and protocols, the specialists now employed by some OPOs serve as a nexus of communications, working closely with a wide network of local and regional transplant units. The now regular institutional reliance on patient and family databases (within the OPO, transplant units, and UNOS itself) further facilitates the process. The downside, however, is that donor kin (and recipients) may have no choice but to accept OPO employees as official gatekeepers, and to comply with their guidelines if they want their correspondence to be forwarded.

As the experiences of Mrs. Cruise reveal, although the principle of egalitarianism may drive an OPO's effort to orchestrate an encounter, such efforts can also be exploitative. Further, some participants are displeased with the common OPO policy of opening, reading, and editing letters. Rather than viewing such efforts as methods for protecting privacy, they perceive them as invasive tactics that degrade the intimacy of personal correspondence. The ability of communications coordinators to withhold addresses and then determine on a case-by-case basis whether personal encounters should occur further outrages some parties. The distinction between the harm an encounter might cause to a donor parent or recipient, on the one hand, and to the public image of the OPO, on the other, is invariably blurred. Shifts in policy are neverthe-less revealed through a comparison of Dora Tuckerman with Suzanne Winkler. Dora's role in its early stages was predominantly that of gatekeeper, and the problems voiced during her presentation expose older (and probably unsol-vable) communications problems. Suzanne, whose concerns are more closely aligned with the needs of involved parties, exemplifies more recent trends. In essence, then, by 2003 some communications coordinators had begun to play the role of advocate both for the donor family *and* for the transplant patient.

The bureaucratization of donor kin–recipient communication marks a dramatic shift from renegade acts of personal contact to more carefully, and professionally, orchestrated encounters. In essence, within the realm of or-gan transfer, personal encounters have become part of the program. (This process has much in common with the adoption industry, where it has be-come common practice for adoptees and birth parents to seek out one an-other. Particularly striking is the concept of the "searcher," an issue I will address at the end of this chapter.) The efforts of OPO communications co-ordinators inevitably shape the nature of written correspondence, guarding practices at least within their own area. At issue is the question of these in-dividuals' allegiance. After all, they are housed within and are on the pay-rolls of their local OPOs, and thus they are inevitably most deeply com-mitted to guarding the emotional needs of donor kin. In the words of one coordinator, "Donor families *always* come first." This is especially true if they specialize in grief counseling. Some communications coordinators, like Suzanne, nevertheless run workshops for recipients, too, and the written guidelines they provide parallel those given to donor kin.

A general set of standards is now followed by a number of OPOs. First, written guidelines frequently offer suggestions on how to compose letters or choose appropriate greeting cards for donor kin. They also always underscore what must be left out of a letter: most important, this includes surnames, ad-dresses, and details about a recipient's illness or a donor's death. Letter writ-ers may also be discouraged from mentioning the specific area of the coun-try or state in which they live, and from offering statements that assume the other party shares similar religious beliefs. Policy dictates that a letter be sub-mitted in an unsealed envelope, with personal information supplied on a sep-arate sheet. Thus, contrary to policies advocated by the NDFC, nearly all com-munications coordinators read and, where necessary, cut out or cover up inappropriate material before forwarding the letter to the intended party. Often a photocopy of an altered letter is forwarded. As Suzanne Winkler ex-plained, "People are very clever—they'll scrape off the White Out or hold up crossed-out text to the light to see what was written underneath." (I have encountered only one coordinator who refuses to edit letters from donor kin, and who forwards them unaltered, although the same policy does not apply to letters written by recipients.) Whereas donor kin work directly with the coordinator, organ recipients generally offer their correspondence to staff from their transplant units, who should then forward letters to the OPO for screening and final mailing. All subsequent correspondence passes through the coordinator's hands and remains anonymous unless both parties express a clear interest in meeting one another. Whether or not this ultimately happens is up to the coordinator, who makes decisions on a case-by-case basis.

Today procurement professionals are more likely to support attempts to communicate because they realize that at least under some circumstances it may ease the pain of the mourning process. In a strict sense, then, Kübler-Ross's notion of acceptance has fallen by the wayside. As a grief counselor employed by an OPO explained, "No, we now know there's never true closure. What we now acknowledge is our understanding that life will never be the same." Transplant staff, on the other hand, are less likely to support these new communication initiatives because of the still dominant assumption that a recipient's identification with the donor is pathological. From their point of view, the desire for contact offers evidence that a recipient is resisting the push to get on with life, to start afresh, and to view his or her own experience as a surgically orchestrated and miraculous form of rebirth. After all, from the perspective of transplant staff, organ donors are nearly always anonymous beings, and only surgeons have any direct contact with donors. Even then, however, donors are brain dead (and anesthetized) strangers whose passive bodies yield to the scalpel and clamp. Potentially, then, open communication is deeply troubling for transplant professionals. Face-to-face encounters with donor kin may force them to ponder at a deeper level that that their work is not simply about saving lives. It also relies on the sudden deaths of known, and often beloved, individuals who have names and histories, and whose kin remain behind, caught in a perpetual state of mourning. As the two case studies in the following section reveal, however, some organ recipients willingly risk exposure to this pain in their search for their respective donor kin.

THE TIES THAT BIND

Here I offer two extended case studies that uncover a number of themes common to donor kin–organ recipient encounters. First, they underscore the significance—and, in the words of several research participants, the inherent *naturalness*—of fictive kinship as an appropriate idiom of sociality. Second, they reveal a preference for meeting, or the special position reserved for, the donor mother. Third, both cases involve sudden and unexpected deaths of children, the first a frail newborn, the second a teenage son. They thus challenge the public assumption (promoted through donation campaigns) that donors are young adults who nearly always die from car and motorcycle accidents. In contrast, the majority of the donor kin I have encountered lost children, approximately half of them from gun violence. Fourth, these two cases reveal common strategies employed by surviving donor kin for coping with sudden, unexpected deaths. A response they share is the desire to meet recipients who have received their children's organs. The nature of their encounters reveals the contradictions that arise when disparate parties confront one another's personal understandings of the donor, now embodied in the recipient's body. Finally, they underscore that such encounters must not be idealized, a fact that all interviewees recognize. The decision to meet one another is never approached lightly, and, as both donor kin and recipients stress, this is only the beginning of a long-term commitment to remain involved in one another's lives. As such, then, donor family–recipient communication is not for the weak of heart.

A Precious Jewel

Sara Carter is among the first donor parents I interviewed, and she remains among the most memorable, too. Sara had actively sought me out for reasons that struck me as unusual. As she stressed in a note she wrote to me, her purpose was not to promote donation (although she strongly supported it) or simply to share a tale of hardship and joy. Rather, she wanted me to understand how problematic encounters with recipients could be. Sara lives in a predominantly white, rural town in a northwestern state, and she considers herself a housewife by profession, although she occasionally assists her husband in keeping track of the accounts for his landscaping business. Sara described herself as a married thirty-six-year-old Christian (Lutheran) mother of three.[9] When we met, she was carrying her youngest child, a baby boy, in her arms. Her oldest child is now deceased, an infant who stopped breathing on the second day of life. At the time of our interview he would have been more than six years old; Sara's second child, a girl, was two years younger. When I interviewed Sara, she told her story very calmly while eating her breakfast and holding her sleeping baby in her lap.

> [My husband and I] had wanted a child for a long time—Mathew was a beautiful little boy. Half an hour after we'd returned home with him

from the hospital I was sitting and nursing him and my husband asked, "Is he OK? He seems limp." We both looked at him and realized he wasn't breathing. My mother was there, and [she] knows CPR, so [she tried this, and my husband] called 911. My [mother kept saying], "Oh [Lord, am I] doing this right?"

We live in a relatively isolated part [of a largely rural state], and so they took Mathew in an ambulance some distance to a hospital in the nearest large town. He had a pulse but he was unable to breath on his own. They were wonderful at the hospital—everyone told us we had done nothing wrong, and everyone was praying with us. I [soon] gave it over to God. I said, Lord, I have no control over this. His will be done—whatever happens, I will accept it. I won't be angry with you. I felt peace—a wonderful sense of peace; [this is something my husband still cannot feel]. . . . They decided to fly our baby to [another larger urban hospital in a regional city], and all of our family [drove the lengthy distance to be there]. But the next afternoon they told us our baby was brain dead. There was nothing they could do.

A pediatric nurse came and talked to us and brought up donation— she had worked [in experimental xenotransplantation in the past]. She said, "I have worked with many heart babies, and I can tell from across the room that your son has a beautiful heart." . . . We prayed together and then we said, could we donate something? Could some good come out of this? The coordinator came, everyone was crying, and she, too, was so compassionate. [My husband and I granted consent, and Mathew's heart was later flown to a hospital in a neighboring state.] Mathew's heart saved a [four-month-old] baby who was nearly dead. . . . [We did it] because we knew it would help another family. It gave meaning and purpose to Mathew's life.

A short while later we got a card from the recipient.[10] The boy's name is Jules, [like something very precious]. He had that name *before* [they knew he needed the] transplant—and we gave him a second . . . life. A year later we got [a] picture [of him]. The coordinator then told us [Jules's parents would] like to talk to us sometime. So we talked over the phone, and eventually we all met each other [through the help of a minister]. It was then that we heard their story . . . [and when we met Jules for the first time].

. . . We spent all of the next day with them, getting to know them, and we learned that our two babies had been in the same [hospital]! . . . Everyone on the staff knew this, but they didn't tell any of us at the time. We figured it out together [and we later asked]. It was an amazing experience, really, to meet them . . . [but it was a shock, too—it wasn't quite what we had expected]. He's a healthy baby,[11] but he's a little developmentally delayed. And he has, you know, the side effects of the drugs. [For one,] he's really hairy! And he has really dry lips—I'm always wanting to put some Chapstick on the poor little guy. And he has a cough or a cold most of the time, so he has a really snotty nose. And his gums are overgrown over his teeth.[12] His talking is not fully developed, and he [now walks in a jerky sort of way]. They later did a heart cath[eter] on him [to check his heart function] and they nicked a blood vessel that then constricted—this will shorten his life.

We've [stayed in touch] and we've [even vacationed together for several days; then] they came and [stayed with us, too]. There are good things and bad things—my husband is reluctant to keep [in] contact, but I just have a lot of love for them. To me, this family, they're my distant cousins. OK, we've extended our family! There's Mathew,[13] he's their child, but the mom doesn't have a lot of friends and they [struggle because they are poor]. . . . What troubles me is they haven't disciplined him. If he does live longer, he's going to have [social] problems. And then there's the jealousy. We have two healthy children, and the father doesn't want the mother to [visit us] here. But if the roles had reversed. . . . Maybe it's better if the relationship is mom-to-mom.

As for Mathew, [no, he doesn't live on in another, but] Mathew left a legacy. He lives on in part. But that's not Mathew [inside Jules]— it's just a part . . . something bequeathed. That's exactly it. He's a . . . [precious jewel] . . . that's [graced] our lives.

In a sense, the trajectory of Sara's story is propelled by its assumed im-possibility: babies do not die at home the day they have been discharged with a bill of health from the hospital, and certainly not when cradled in the safe embrace of a nursing mother's arms. Against the shock and horror of this experience, Sara paints a tale of how she struggled to come to terms with her loss, finding strength in her Christian faith to place her baby in God's hands. The desire to designate a baby as an organ donor is not so un-usual, for as Sara and many other parents explain, organ donation enabled some goodness to emerge from a terrible tragedy. The fact that Jules, who received Mathew's heart, not only was a baby but also, coincidentally, was being cared for in the same hospital as Mathew, helps to confirm that this was the proper decision, as if it were a miracle meant to happen all along. As Sara suggests, however, her husband has not found the same sense of peace as she.

Much of Sara's calm is embedded in her decision to meet the heart re-cipient and his parents. As she recounts her tale, it becomes clear that Sara sees much of her own life reflected in that of Jules's family, although in cer-tain ways it is a negative reflection, one that helps to reconfirm that she her-self has been blessed. Whereas Sara is economically comfortable, Jules's par-ents are poor; and whereas Sara's two living children are healthy, Jules is a sickly child in need of constant medical attention. Sara also merges the two boys in her mind, so that at times she refers to Jules as Mathew, as if her own child were still alive but living in another household. It is even difficult to know whether the precious jewel in Sara's life is Jules or Mathew (or both). The slip she makes in referring to Jules as Mathew is striking, offering poignant evidence of a mother's ability to merge the two children in her own mind. It marks, too, a reluctance to view Jules's body as an unnatural hybrid made up simultaneously of two children at once. In her speech, then, she struggles with competing images of the heart "bequeathed" to another child with the sense of the persistent, overpowering presence of her lost son. Although this idea is only a hypothesis at this point, mothers like Sara and Kelly, described earlier, may well struggle at some level with a broader social discomfort with the idea of a mother giving away parts of her dead child's body. The act of befriending the recipient's mother offers a means to confirm that her own deceased child's parts are well cared for, and that she herself may well be offered fleeting opportunities to mother a child who has survived his or her own life-threatening ordeal. As the donor's mother befriends the recipient's, the two mothers in turn are merged through bonds of intimacy.

Among the most compelling aspects of Sara's narrative is the manner in which she draws on new forms of sociality to reconstruct a shattered world. With her relationship with Jules's mother comes a strong sense of obligation to stay in touch, and to reach out and care for someone else's suffering child. Sara speaks, too, of Jules's family as her new "distant cousins": as she states, "we've extended our family." Most striking here is the fact that two mothers emerge as pivotal figures in this newly created network of fictive kin. Sara describes the bond she shares with Jules's mother as if they were two close sisters, or perhaps a pair of mothers sharing in the care of a single sickly child.

The Telltale Teenage Heart

Sally Duster and Larry Merrill, both of whom are Euro-American and from the South, consider themselves to be dear old friends, having met face-to-face seven years before I encountered them in 1998. Sally has worked for the last ten years in the personnel office of a large accounting firm, and Larry (now retired) was a middle manager for a company that ships machine parts worldwide. Both are active in promoting organ donation in their southern state, and they had in fact worked together at health fairs and other events for even longer without knowing of their shared history. Instead, they only came to realize very slowly that Larry had the heart of Sally's son inside of him. As Larry explained, "It was hard not to find out—as one friend [of mine] finally said [to me] one day, 'Hell, Larry, everyone in the county knows who your donor is!'" This was because the story of Sally's son had been a high-profile case in the news, and because her son's death coincided so neatly with the timing of Larry's transplant. When I conducted this joint interview Sally was a widow of three years; although she was only in her mid-fifties, she looked considerably older. Larry is twelve years her senior, but until I asked how old they were, I assumed the two of them were approximately the same age. Both grew up in the same midsize town that is now a satellite of a major southern urban center.

At their request, I interviewed them together. This was a difficult and rocky interview for me. For one, Larry wept openly several times. Although Sally assured me not to worry, that "it's just the steroids talking—he always does that," I was especially shaken the first time Larry reacted this way. Although by this point they had known of each other for over seven years, I soon learned that Larry had never heard the full story of how Sally's son had died. At times I felt as though I were a confessor of sorts and suggested more than once that we terminate the interview. Interviews with donor families in particular are exhausting affairs; when I have conducted paired interviews with recipients and donor kin, the interview typically spans several hours to half a day, as each party takes a turn telling his or her story (or, in the words of some, offering a testimonial). There is, nevertheless, an intense need within these pairs to tell their tales in tandem, and so, out of respect for Sally's and Larry's wishes, the interview continued in spite of Larry breaking down and crying. Because this chapter focuses on communication between donor kin and recipients, the excerpt here is drawn from the second half of the interview, in which Sally speaks of her son's death, and Larry and Sally talk about the relationship they share as a result of organ transfer.[14]

Sally spoke first of her son:

> SALLY: Charlie was almost seventeen years old [when he died] . . .
> [and he had been left] alone in the house [for only a few hours].
> The doctors [later] said he was brain dead. They did this I felt
> because it was just the easiest way for them to say he's going
> to die. He was shot at home—they said it was a suicide . . . [but
> I didn't believe it]. That's just what the police said. I've never
> been sure, though. You see, there's a woods behind my house
> and cars used to drive in and out all the time. There was a lot
> of drug [activity] going on in there. The thing is, the day [after]
> Charlie [was shot], the cars stopped coming.

At this point Larry burst into tears and began to sob. Sally put her hand on his and replied calmly, "We don't talk about Charlie's death." I suggested we stop the interview, but they both insisted on continuing.

LARRY: I wrote to Sally when I was [still] in the hospital even though my doctors didn't want me to. Then I wrote a Christmas card. I looked everywhere! I wanted a Christmas card with a heart on it. Damn if that isn't a hard thing to find! All around me everyone was asking, do you know your donor? No, I'd say. [It turned out] that one of the members of my [church] was Charlie's [relative]. I was afraid to meet [Sally] because I was afraid I couldn't stay composed. But there were connections everywhere! My wife "Bulldog" [is an administrator] who works [for the county] and she had [actually met] Charlie at his school.

L. S.: Bulldog?

SALLY: . . Everybody calls her that. She's a real pistol . . .

L. S.: What happened then?

Sally and Larry explained that they had met three years later, after they had exchanged several letters; they were assisted in their endeavors by a procurement coordinator.

LARRY: I went to her house for lunch.

SALLY: I wanted to know, how's he doing? I was so afraid he was going to die!

LARRY: Her daughter was there—she had a dream she'd meet me [one day]. Sis—that's what I call her, [Sally's daughter]—came right over and put her head on my chest to hear the heart!

SALLY: It was a really good idea to wait three years to meet, but I really wanted to meet. I was afraid he'd die before I met him. Someone told me [one night that Larry] would be on the news. I watched but I still needed time—and before we met I made Larry ask Bulldog . . . he had to ask her first—I wanted him to make sure she said it was OK before we met.

LARRY: [With a romantic air] We met at a tree planting ceremony to [commemorate donors]. We planted a large magnolia tree with a bench and plaque so people could go sit there and meditate. I looked over and there she was—

SALLY: [Interrupts]—But you called up and invited us to come!

LARRY: [Continues in the same dreamy tone, as if oblivious to Sally's correction] I was fine until I made eye contact with her, and then I lost it. [Larry lets out another sob and then wipes his eyes.]

Sally and Larry then explained that they now work regularly together at donor campaigns, and they celebrate major holidays together in some form. Larry and Bulldog usually stop by Sally's home for cocktails on Christmas Day, and he has surprised her on several occasions on her birthday. The one day they avoid—and that they rarely speak about—is the day of Larry's transplant. This is a day of joy for him, when he typically has a "rebirthday" party, for which Bulldog always bakes him a heart-shaped cake. For Sally, though, it is a very dark day when she prefers to be alone. As they explained, at first these encounters were difficult.

LARRY: Her house is full of [mementos] of her son, and there are photos everywhere!

SALLY: There's only one in my house!

LARRY: I later helped Sally meet Paul [who is in his forties and has] Charlie's kidney. She asked me to try to find him for her [so I did]. [I thought it would be best] if we met on neutral territory—so we went to a restaurant [we both love to go to] and where I know the owner [really well].

SALLY: Everyone knew what was going on.

LARRY: The owner's a good friend of mine. Everyone was crying, even the cook! And we all stood around together and played a favorite song of mine [about miracles and impossible dreams] that come true.

Next Sally and Larry explained how they understand their ties to one another. As I soon learned, they have developed an elaborate array of fictive kin terms for incorporating each other in their lives. For example, Larry addresses Sally's daughter as "Sis," and she calls him "Bro." After Larry's own birth mother died, he then began to address Sally as "Mom," and she now calls him "Son" (it matters little that Larry is twelve years older than Sally). As Sally explained, Larry now sends her a Mother's Day card. These terms have facilitated the establishment of an elaborate joking relationship, one that simultaneously underscores their devotion to one another while allowing them to make light of the potential trespasses such intimacy may engender. One need only consider Sally's insistence that Larry acquire his wife's permission to meet with her for the first time, set against Larry's romantic tone as he describes their initial encounter. They are mildly troubled by the adulterous overtones of their relationship, one laced, too, I would assert, with the incestuous, given that Larry now harbors part of Charlie inside his body. The playfulness of their bond was especially evident when I asked Larry about his religious faith, to which he replied:

LARRY: I'm a Whiskeypalian! I told Sally that when the heart [reaches twenty-one] I'm gonna take him out on the town!

SALLY: So I called him up on Charlie's twenty-first birthday and I said, "Now, Son, you're twenty-one, so you can go out and have *two* drinks [tonight]!"

The intimacy of fictive kinship guides behavior at those moments when the merging of bodies might signal social transgression, as well as at other moments of personal crisis. When Sally suddenly found herself a widow, Larry and Paul assumed roles generally reserved only for close kin. As Sally explained, "When my husband died, Paul came and stayed at Larry's house and they spent two full days at the funeral home with me. They said they were there to represent Charlie." Throughout the funeral, Larry and Paul hovered about Sally, assuming the combined surrogate roles of older and younger son (with Larry, in turn, perhaps standing in as a surrogate spouse, too).

This case study offers yet another example of a mother who has lost her child, again under what would seem impossible circumstances. A teenage son raised in a suburban setting should be safe when left alone at home and not be murdered inside or in the woods behind his own house. Charlie's death remains an inexplicable one, and this, combined with his youth, renders this an experience for which no closure or peace is truly possible for Sally. Sally and Larry are united in their love for Charlie, who is now embodied in the heart that beats within Larry's chest. In knowing Sally, Larry must learn to merge his idealized version of Charlie with the realities of a life-and-death story supplied by Charlie's mother. As in Sara's case, fictive kinship provides the most appropriate and natural idiom for expressing the intimacy of their social bond; this then shapes their ongoing obligations to each other. As Sally and Larry reveal, their relationship has evolved elaborately and creatively, a process marked by wit, humor, love, and devotion, growing over time until they now respond to one another as mother and son. This is especially clear in Larry's decision to stand in for Charlie during the funeral for Sally's husband. Larry, like Sara, shares the strong sense of obligation to assist newfound kin, especially during deeply troubling times.

The pivotal role of the donor mother is exemplified, too, in Sally's sense that forging a relationship with Larry would be unnatural, or an adulterous trespass, and thus she insisted on having Larry obtain Bulldog's permission before agreeing to a personal encounter. In assuming the role of donor mother to Larry, she eliminates the discomfort that arises when one considers their proximity in age. In essence, the mother-son bond trumps age. Today Sally, Larry, and Bulldog are dear to one another. They not only gather during holidays but also traveled the long distance together to the 1998 Transplant Games. Because of Larry's disabled status, Bulldog drove the entire way. But whereas Sally and her daughter consider Larry to be their son and brother, respectively, there is no special term of address reserved for Bulldog (see figure 9). Instead, she remains connected through affinal or marriage ties: structurally she is simply "Larry's wife," whereas Larry, in embodying Charlie's heart, is now embraced as blood kin.

CLAIMING THE DONOR BODY

All the parties described here struggle on some level with the question of how to cope with issues of donor ownership. What rights do surviving kin have to trace the whereabouts of the remains of the lost loved one? Can one, for instance, assert claims of access—or postmortem visitation rights? How invasive is the desire to hear the heart beat again in someone else's chest? How much of the donor's tale should be revealed to recipients during face-to-face encounters? A shift to the recipient perspective encourages yet a different set of questions. Where lies the boundary between self and other? Should recipients squelch any sense that some essence of the donor persists within them? If they do embrace the idea that the donor is more than a mere body part, then, what precisely is the donor now?

As Sara states at one point, she has "bequeathed" parts of her son to others. Yet as her and others' narratives reveal, donor kin and recipients alike share the understanding that transplanted organs, as donor fragments, carry with them some essence of their former selves, and this persists in the bodies of recipients. The donor then becomes a transmigrated soul of sorts, one that generates compelling dilemmas for involved parties. Are donors mere phantoms for donor kin, their memories fed only by past experiences? Can recipients integrate their imagined donors as part of their now repaired selves? Face-to-face encounters simultaneously feed these imagined possibilities and confound them, especially when each party becomes familiar with the other's tale. The creative playfulness of fictive kinship enables these once disparate and now intimate parties to reconstruct together the trajectory of the lifetime (and postmortem) experiences of the donor. At risk here is the further shattering of each person's world; yet, as successful encounters reveal, potentially each party is partially healed by the process.

Both transplant and OPO professionals regard the bonds of fictive kinship as pathological in part because they can anticipate so readily the emotional dangers of social intimacy. On one level, one cannot help but respect professional gatekeepers who strive to protect the psychic health of recipients or donor kin. On yet another level, though, so paternalistic an attitude may infuriate recipients and donor kin, for these are individuals who have already endured exceptional levels of professional intrusion in their lives. After all, each of them has confronted death and survived the trauma. As the examples offered here reveal, the decision to meet face-to-face is never made in haste. Although the number of encounters is small, the desire to meet is slowly growing. I do not advocate that encounters *should* occur; nevertheless, the data generated from my research contradict professionals' fears. Of the more than thirty cases I have recorded, the only encounter to fail involved Mrs. Cruise and her husband, and this couple felt that it had been foisted upon them by an overzealous OPO.

At this point, then, I wish to explore the theoretical implications of the encounter as a social process. How might we understand the cultural logic that drives donor kin and recipients to embrace one another as family? The search for intimacy and its associated dilemmas in organ transfer are mirrored in other social contexts, especially in anonymous adoption and gestational surrogacy. Of particular concern to me is the predominant notion that blood—that is, biological—ties are intrinsic to forms of sociality in all three contexts. Organ transfer is particularly intriguing because, as we shall see, it is the quite literal sharing of organs and even smaller body fragments that so quickly enables recipients to become the intimates of surviving donor kin.

Biogenetics and Sentimentality

As David Schneider argued several decades ago, a dominant principle guiding American kinship is the assumed "biogenetic" property of relatedness. More specifically, American kinship, as a bilateral system, views mother (genetrix) and father (genitor) as sharing equally in the process of creating a child (or, as we would say today, a fetus). This concept of family rests on the assumption that a child is equally related by blood to the maternal and paternal sides.[15] Indeed, this concept of shared blood offers an intriguing framework for deciphering how distinctions are made between kin and nonkin, first in everyday practices, and then in organ transfer and other specialized arenas.

As Schneider asserted, the biological and thus "natural" connections rendered possible by blood ties operate in ways quite different from the social rules sanctioned by legal codes. For example, regardless of our actual natal home arrangements, in a host of bureaucratic contexts we are expected to supply the names of our mother and father because they in essence define who we are. The inherent natural character of blood also renders such ties permanent: in Schneider's words, blood's "nature can not be terminated or changed." Whereas marriages can be dissolved through divorce, blood ties between parents and children are permanent. Although one might attempt to sever one's *legal* obligations to a child through disinheritance, the child (unlike the ex-spouse) remains forever linked *biogenetically* to his or her parent(s). Also, it would be ludicrous to speak of having an "ex-mother": even if she is deceased (or no longer on speaking terms with us), she will always remain our own because she is intrinsic to our biological origins. In short, blood is a "natural, genetic substance" shared by individuals by virtue of their births (Schneider 1980 [1965]: 24, 1–27; see also Schneider 1984: 165–77).

These biologically determinist arguments are so pervasive in our society that they are embraced as scientific truths. Schneider also recognized that the genetic logic of kinship is remarkably flexible: as science generates new theories of relatedness, principles of American kinship adjust so as to integrate these, too, as social facts. Current public fascination with the new genetics, for instance, validates his assertion. Whereas thirty years ago one spoke of "blood kin," today blood relatedness is understood to operate even beyond the cellular level to include DNA. Finally, and of great significance to my work here, is Schneider's assertion of how inherently sentimental blood ties can be. As reflected in the rubric "blood is thicker than water," the sense of shared blood inspires strong "bonds, feelings of kinship, [and] instinctive affection" (Schneider 1984: 167). In short, the concept of biogenetics enables strangers (such as distant cousins) to embrace each other readily as intimate kin.

If biogenetics is the linchpin of American kinship, how might this concept assist us in deciphering sociality in contexts mediated by transplant medicine, where there is no fetus or conjugal pair, but where donor kin and recipients nevertheless assert they are family? In what ways does the peculiar overlapping of bodies, so intrinsic to organ transfer, augment or challenge Schneider's premises of more than two decades ago? As I will argue, organ transfer has much in common with other (frequently medicalized) contexts where blood ties remain murky at best. In turn, organ transfer also emerges as a unique example, and thus one that uncovers radically new ways of thinking about sociality. In the realm of organ transfer, biology, embodiment, and sentimentality define an inseparable triad.

Today, reproductive technologies raise deeply troubling questions about the boundaries of sociality (Franklin 1997; Franklin and Ragoné 1998; Ginsburg and Rapp 1995; Layne 1999; Ragoné 1996; Strathern 1992a, 1992b). Within the literature on prenatal genetic testing, cloning, and surrogacy, for instance, one frequently encounters a melding of Schneider's ideas with more contemporary arguments posited by Paul Rabinow, for whom burgeoning genetic technologies foster new forms of "autoreproduction." Reminiscent of Schneider's older concept of biogenetics, Rabinow speaks specifically of *biosociality*, a term he offers as a means to underscore the (at times insidious) capacity of technological innovations and knowledge to reshape social processes.[16] Rayna Rapp's recent work on amniocentesis provides a compelling illustration of this point. As her fieldwork on Down syndrome and other genetic mutations attests, parents drawn together by support group and lobbying efforts may express extraordinarily strong bonds of sociality by virtue of their children's shared genetic traits (Rapp 2000). As Rapp's examples reveal, the sharing of blood (understood here specifically as shared genetic characteristics) offers a potent symbolic idiom for expressing both similarity and intimacy among strangers.

Rabinow warns us as well that "the new genetics will carry with it its own distinctive promises and dangers" (1992: 241–42). The case of organ transfer most certainly bears this out. As will become clear in the following chapter, the experimental, hybrid domain of xenotransplantation offers extraordinarily promising—yet monstrous—possibilities. As Rabinow further asserts, the power of biosociality lies in its ability to worm its way into "the social fabric at the microlevel by medical practices and a variety of other discourses" (241–42). What troubles me, however, is the haste with which some contemporary authors embrace Rabinow's warnings, while ignoring the wondrous potential of biosociality. As the case studies offered earlier in this chapter reveal, intimate ties between former strangers emerge as subversive acts that challenge professional ideology head-on.

Most certainly one could argue that the bureaucratization of donor kin–recipient communication marks an early step in the professional co-optation of lay practices. Nevertheless, something far more profound is also at work here: as Schneider himself explained, blood ties incorporate strong sentimental qualities. In the realm of organ transfer, the sharing of body fragments overrides an aversion to hybridity's monstrous qualities, generating instead not only a strong sense of sameness but strong emotions, too. What we are witnessing here, then, is a set of practices more radical than what Rabinow himself imagines. For this reason I offer as an alternative the term *biosentimentality* as a means to move beyond Rabinow's warnings. With this in mind, I intend to explore the relevance of biosentimentality by comparing organ transfer to anonymous adoption and gestational surrogacy. As we shall see, organ transfer's uniqueness lies in its ability to transcend normative (or natural) forms of human coupling, where the notion of sameness is at once about shared human fragments and about sentimental kinship structures.

Bureaucratic Secrecy and Adoption Searches

Organ transfer bears an uncanny resemblance to anonymous adoption in this country. Particularly striking are the similarities that emerge when encounters between organ recipients and donor kin are compared to reunions involving adult adoptees and their birth parents. Adoption reunions are a relatively recent trend in the United States, yet they predate organ transfer encounters by at least a decade, and thus I suspect that the actions of adoption activists in part inform how donor kin and organ recipients understand their own encounters. Once considered highly subversive and taboo acts, adoption reunions have since attracted the attention of researchers, whose writings have led many adoption agencies to accept (albeit reluctantly) that reunions define an inevitable component of their work. A brief history of adoption policy exposes shifting perceptions of blood ties and the emerging relevance of biosentimentality.

As Elizabeth Snider explains, the policy of sealing adoption records in the United States dates back to the early 1900s, a practice driven by the assumption that illegitimate children had "bad blood," and adoption provided them with an opportunity to be "reborn, with a new life and new identity" (1997: 3; see also Branton and Snider 1990). This policy and associated assumptions remained in place for much of the century. During the 1970s, however, some adoptees began to assert publicly their desire to learn more of—and perhaps even meet—their birth parents. By the 1980s, many adoptees were asking more open and pointed questions about the circumstances leading to their adoptions, so much so that the action referred to as "searching" (and involved parties as "searchers") slowly became a more accepted aspect of adult adoptee experience. By the 1990s, the topics of searching and reunion outcomes defined a viable field of study for a host of researchers within the United States (and elsewhere), and adoption reform organizations had emerged as a stabilized site of activism. At this point many experts no longer viewed the desire for reunions as renegade or pathological but instead saw it as a "legitimate" and "existential need [among adoptees] to know their origins" (Snider 1997: 45; Campbell, Silverman, and Patti 1991: 329; cf. Lifton 1988; Simpson, Timm, and McCubbin 1981; Triseliotis 1973).

As with OPOs, American adoption agencies have resisted attempts by both adoptees and birth parents to locate one another, carefully guarding their original (and highly confidential) records. In response, reform groups have enabled searchers to circumvent the agencies that originally handled the adoptions of surrendered children, offering search assistance, emotional support, and precontact counseling (Feast et al. 1998; Howe and Feast 2000). Such groups have, in Judith Modell's (2002) words, successfully challenged the "sealed and secret kinship" of stranger adoptions, and their lobbying efforts have even transformed state policy. Recent legislation passed in Oregon, for instance, now grants adoptees access to their personal records (Modell 2002: 1–2, 53, 69). By the 1990s, some adoption agencies had even begun to assist searchers, helping to orchestrate encounters. Typically, though, they persistently advocate pre-reunion counseling, and they view social workers as crucial intermediaries (Campbell, Silverman, and Patti 1991; Sachdev 1989). Similar bureaucratic responses have emerged in the realm of organ transfer. Through the concerted efforts of the NDFC, OPOs have begun to hire communications coordinators. As presentations made by Dora Tuckerman and Suzanne Winkler reveal, they not only oversee but also censor correspondence, and they determine whether certain encounters should occur at all.

Anonymous adoption and organ transfer share other similarities, particularly when framed by the concept of biosentimentality. As researchers based in both the United States and the United Kingdom report, adoptee searchers are driven by the conviction that their sense of self remains incomplete without knowledge of their origins, and this longing can be answered only by locating those with whom they share biological, genetic, or blood ties. Even among those separated at birth, the language of blood prevails as a means to underscore permanence. For instance, birth parents are regularly referred to as "natural" parents, as opposed to the adoptive parents who raised the child. This overwhelming desire for "genealogical and genetic connectedness" is driven by the necessity of locating others who, in the words of one respondent, are "just like me" (Howe and Feast 2001: 357, 364–65).

Indeed, adoptees may speak of "feeling more 'complete,'" or as if they had been pieced back together "like a puzzle" following their reunions (Campbell, Silverman, and Patti 1991: 332–34). Such expressions translate well to the realm of organ transfer: after all, transplant patients experience radical forms of body repair as a result of their surgeries. Medical professionals frequently recognize this too and may even employ similar metaphorical expressions. Preeminent transplant surgeon Thomas Starzl (1992), for instance, has gone so far as to describe his patients as "puzzles" or as "the puzzle people."[17] Reunions in both realms also serve to confirm the sentimental structuring of blood relatedness. Adoptees and birth parents, like donor kin and recipients, speak of experiencing a strong sense of belonging and immediate love for one another at the time of their first encounter (Howe and Feast 2001: 352, 357, 364–65; Campbell, Silverman, and Patti 1991: 332, 333). In essence, then, assumptions about blood relatedness drive the shared belief that sentimental feelings are a natural response.

However, whereas reunions assist adoptees in answering crucial "identity needs," once they are met there may be little more "than the blood tie to sustain the relationship" (Howe and Feast 2001: 365). Researchers on adoption reunions offer a range of explanations for why this might be so. A dominant assumption is that long-term relationships are ultimately dependent on compatible personalities (Howe and Feast 2001; Plomin 1994). Yet another argument holds that adoptee searchers are driven primarily by the need to learn of their origins, and birth parents by the desire to learn what happened to the surrendered child (Campbell, Silverman, and Patti 1991; Silverman et al. 1988). Face-to-face encounters answer these troubling questions. Relevant answers offer a sense of completeness, or closure, to a paired set of severed lives or histories.

As such, long-term relationships between adoptees and birth parents may be unnecessary. As David Howe and Julia Feast suggest, too, the very "lack of a shared history" might account for an inability among adoptees and birth parents to sustain their relationships over time (2001: 364). I stress, however, that this inability should not be taken as evidence of failure. Rather, adoption searching involves uncovering secret details about the past, but not attempting to generate a future, intertwined life history. Adoptees and birth parents strive to *salvage* the past, and thus their individual histories merge and then terminate (or are brought up to date) at the moment of the reunion. The fact that involved parties are alive, too, certainly facilitates this process: upon learning of one another's pasts, they can then move on with their own lives. In this sense, adoption searches should be understood as reflective or retrograde forms of memory work.

Postmortem Memory Work: Constructing a Unified Donor History

Organ recipients and donor kin likewise consider themselves bound to one another through shared biogenetic properties, among which the dominant aspect is the quite literal sharing (or embodiment) of donor blood and flesh.[18] At several junctures of this chapter, research participants comment on how their own experiences parallel those of adoption. Particularly compelling is the manner in which organ recipient–donor kin encounters are idealized as the successful reunification of family members. One donor mother cited earlier, for instance, speaks of locating an organ recipient as akin to finding a long-lost child. An underlying assumption is that such encounters are less problematic than those in adoption, so that donor kin–recipient encounters emerge as quintessential miracle stories of parent-child reunions. Such ideas are informed by a dominant cultural misconception that most adoptions result from child abandonment, as opposed to organ transfer, which is defined solely as a selfless act of giving.[19] Such sentiments were expressed quite clearly by twenty-six-year-old Martha Gates, who, as I learned during the course of an interview, is both an adoptee and a kidney-pancreas recipient:

> L. S.: Do you think that the wish to meet one's donor family has anything in common with someone who has been adopted wanting to meet their birth mother?
>
> MARTHA: [With some bitterness] I'm adopted . . . [but] I'm not interested in meeting my biological parent—you made a decision, for whatever reason, hopefully for a good one, to give up a child. I tell my mom, if any such person ever shows up you invite them in, you get as detailed a medical history as possible, and then get them out of there.
>
> L. S.: What about looking for your donor [family]?
>
> MARTHA: It's not the same. I wrote a letter on my one-month anniversary but I never heard back. But I know [from the OPO that] it went through. My husband and mother want me to [contact them] but my dad says don't. My parents say if they ever had to make the decision to donate my organs my dad says he wouldn't want to know the recipient, but my mom says she would.

In contrast to the shared desires of adoptees and birth parents to reconstruct their separate pasts, within the realm of organ transfer origin stories mark only the beginning of donor kin–recipient histories. That is, encounters involving donor kin and organ recipients are not about closing a chapter of one's life, or filling in the lost details of an otherwise nearly complete personal history. Instead, donor kin and recipients initially search for one another to *recover* the history of the donor. Or, put another way, both wish to learn of the donor's fate. The initial encounter is therefore only a first step, one that facilitates the long-term possibility of eventually generating a unified, future history through prolonged intimacy. Donor kin and recipients therefore search for one another to recover and link their past *and future* histories, as mediated by the donor as a third, missing party. The possibility of forging a shared history is enabled in part by the unending (and thus open-ended quality) of donor kin grief, as well as by recipients' understanding that their surgical transformation is a form of rebirth. Their ability to forge a shared history hinges, too, on their combined understandings of embodied intimacy, and the preciousness of gifts generated from a donor's body.

Long-term relationships enable donor kin to bear witness to the donor's new accomplishments. This idea was expressed clearly in a speech delivered by a donor mother at the 1992 Transplant Games. As she explained, "Not a day goes by when I don't think of my son. . . . He was always active as an athlete; after [he saw] the 1984 Olympics he said, 'Mom, I'm going to be at the Olympics.' I know he's here now, too. . . . There's thirteen of you out there [who have received organs and tissues from my son]. . . . You're helping my son become a star." No one sitting with me in the grandstand considered this statement strange; rather, it inspired a loud round of applause from the crowd of recipients gathered in the stadium. On that day, the Transplant Games enabled this mother to bear witness to her son's latest accomplishments. This seemingly unorthodox way of talking in fact offers naturalized ways to speak of the dead and, in partnership with others, generate a rich array of postmortem memories.

Clearly, transplanted organs harbor the potential for generating long-term personal histories. The making of postmortem donor histories necessitates that donor kin and recipients initially share private stories when they are still strangers to one another. The donor's story is pivotal to this process in several ways. First, it assumes a privileged stance in relation to the recipient's tale of sickness and recovery. The possibility of recovery, however, hinges on the decision of donor kin to offer new life to another when faced with the donor's tragic death. If recipients are to experience a sense of catharsis in meeting donor kin, they must bear witness to the latter's suffering as they speak of the donation experience. As a result, both parties brace against renewed forms of grief, because neither can forget the donor's death. During face-to-face encounters these parties share stories of intense personal suffering. This intimate form of exchange facilitates the possibility for redemption, far more so than that offered by impersonal, public memorials. When donor kin and organ recipients take turns speaking (and listening), their private narratives merge into one seamless tale, the donor's death marking the threshold between loss and subsequent rebirth. As such, all may bear witness to the cathartic notion that death may indeed beget new life.

How the Body Remembers

Encounters between donor kin and organ recipients thus generate shared understandings of unusual forms of embodied intimacy. At work here is the literal reading of biosentimentality, for organ recipients are frequently understood as experiencing remarkable transformations by virtue of their harboring within them the body fragments of organ donors. This extraordinary development bears the potential for transforming the recipient's sense of self into a gestalt composed of the ego merged with another.[20] The logic of biogenetics renders this process possible.

If we return to Rabinow's assertion that the new genetics generates new forms of sociality, we find that in the realm of organ transfer even cells can possess properties that enable donors to assert their presence beyond the grave. As Emily Martin (1994; cf. Haraway 1989) illustrates, immunological principles now occupy a prominent position in quotidian understandings of the body and society in American culture. This has taken an especially curious turn in the realm of organ transfer, where the language of immunology now supplies new and potent metaphors for the preexisting biogenetic determinism of social intimacy. More specifically, by the mid-1990s, and in the context of my own work, some research participants had begun to speak of "cell memory" as a compelling explanation for why recipients could experience a donor's presence; this argument has persisted a full ten years later. Cell memory is an immunological concept that refers to the body's ability to code and later respond to pathogens. Vaccinations, for instance, may be understood in this way: T cells in the body can learn to recognize and thus "remember" diseases based on exposure through prior inoculation. The metaphorical language of cell memory, when applied in the realm of organ transfer, is taken quite literally to mean that *cells retain memories of their origins*. Because many lay informants think of the cell as among the smallest units of the human body, this means that no level of body fragmentation can destroy the transmigrated essence of an organ donor. As two OPO employees explained to me on separate occasions, even T cells of unidentified (and thus assumed donor) origins have been detected in transplanted hearts.

Donor persistence at the cellular level is representative of a wider body of folklore that pervades the realm of organ transfer. Recipients have long spoken of experiencing radical transformations to their private sense of self following their surgeries. For instance, men often speak of being gentler or more intuitive because they now have the hearts of female donors. Television talk show hosts never tire of interviewing recipients who claim to have acquired new tastes for foods (such as broccoli), drinks (like soda pop or martinis), or activities (perhaps motorcycling or painting). Recipients, donor kin, and professionals all tell such tales, offering anecdotes of individual recipients who learned from surviving kin that these were in fact their donors' passions. Such understandings are further legitimated through the weight of (albeit misunderstood) biologically reasoning: if cells have "memories," then they must be able to "remember" their origins, too.

Whereas those who counter these arguments generally view them as preposterous, it is not because they assert that they are based on flawed understandings of a scientific model. Instead, challengers regularly embrace *competing* metaphors, among which the most popular is that of "cell replacement." Within this alternative framework, the human body is understood as being in a constant state of regeneration. As such, the essence of the donor cannot survive because the recipient's body slowly and methodically erases every trace of the donor's origins, transforming the transplanted organ, cell by cell, into a part of itself. In this competing model, the human body resists sociality and instead exhibits cannibalistic tendencies. In other words, whereas the donor's presence is initially acknowledged in the form of a transplanted organ, over time each donor cell must die, only to be replaced by new ones generated by the recipient's own body. The fact that a heart recipient's body is understood to be in a constant state of (low-level) rejection helps support the logic of this argument: that is, graft rejection supplies yet another potent metaphor for confirming the impossibility of the donor's sustained presence.

As Schneider himself emphasized, "If science discovers new facts about biogenetic relationship, then this is what kinship is and was all along, although it may not have been known at the time" (1980 [1965]: 23–24). As the competing logics of cell memory versus replacement show, participants in organ transfer most certainly continue to draw on the language of blood, genetics, and, now, immunology in their search to comprehend the limits of sociality. As intensely metaphorical ways of thinking, such arguments, of course, are not really about biology at all (Schneider 1972: 45, cited in Ragoné 1996: 358). Nevertheless, science clearly offers potent symbolic frameworks for thinking about the highly troubling idea that living human bodies can be sustained by organs taken from the dead. The lay theories of cell memory versus cell replacement rely on literal readings of biology's symbolic language to support or reject embodied hybridity and, in turn, donor-recipient intimacy. For those who desire communication, biosentimentality helps quell the horrors of individual suffering. We are witnessing here a new form of "natural" history, one forged through the sharing of blood, flesh, and, now, even cells derived from the donor body.

Maternal Longing

As I noted earlier in this chapter, the longing voiced by donor kin to encounter heart recipients over all others reveals a hierarchy of value assigned to the body and its parts. The heart, associated with love and desire, emerges frequently as housing the greatest amount of the donor's essence. For those parties who embrace the idea of the transmigrated soul of the donor, frequently the heart then possesses the greatest quantity of donor presence, too.

Recipients also long to encounter certain parties over others, among whom the most prominent is the donor's mother. Within the realm of organ transfer the mother-child bond is perceived as an especially important one. Donor mothers stand out as iconic figures of giving, and thus they are honored more than all others at transplant events. On several occasions, for instance, I have witnessed ceremonies for the Donor Mother of the Year (but not Father of the Year), and crowds always cheer the loudest when a recipient steps up to the microphone, tell his story, and then introduces his personal donor's mother to the audience. Some OPOs even have "MOD Squads," composed of mothers of donors who work in hospitals beside OPO professionals, and who speak at public events about the social value of donation. It is important to acknowledge, too, that donor mothers are assumed by OPO professionals to be more likely than fathers to respond to written inquiries and letters. One communications coordinator phrased it thus: "Donor mothers become activists [but] men go into a cave when they hurt. They're not doing anything that's different for men in their society. . . . [As one donor father told me,] 'I don't heal by talk.'" Data presented in previous chapters challenge such stereotypes. (The coordinator's statement about men retreating into caves is most likely derived from J. Gray 1992.) Regardless of the motivations that may drive donor mothers over fathers to become involved in the pubic sphere of organ transfer, donor mothers define a significant category of desire among organ recipients.

Again, adoption provides some clues for why this might be, for adoptees search far more frequently for their birth mothers than they do their birth fathers.[21] This could easily be the result of bureaucratic realities simply because no paperwork may exist that exposes a birth father's identity. Still, within the realm of organ transfer, a number of factors point to the conclusion that the desire to encounter the donor mother is sentimentally driven, and not simply bureaucratically orchestrated by, say, OPO communications coordinators. Recipients' desires are shaped largely by their obsessive interest in donor origins, a theme that most certainly resonates with adoptees, for whom, after all, origins are equated with biological births.

Some aspects of gestational surrogacy provide additional clues that help decipher the logic of maternal longing in the realm of organ transfer. As Heléna Ragoné's work reveals, a common desire shared by infertile couples is a preference for gestational surrogates. That is, a woman unable to bear children may prefer that her own fertilized ova be implanted in a surrogate who will then bear her child to term, rather than having her male partner fertilize the surrogate (a process known as traditional surrogacy). Reminiscent yet again of adoptee searchers, Ragoné describes this form of maternal desire within the contracting mother (or she who will raise the child) as "chasing the blood tie." This reproductive premise is fueled by anxieties about the primacy of genetic relatedness as a defining principle of parentage. Particularly intriguing here is the manner in which the biogenetic principles of American kinship transcend older notions of reproduction (Ragoné 1996). That is, in the context of gestational surrogacy, the contracting mother can trump the child bearer by asserting her biogenetic parentage.[22] This action reconfirms (albeit in technocratically orchestrated contexts) precisely what Schneider had in mind when he wrote of "the unalterable nature of the blood relationship" (1980 [1965]: 25). Although he could not have anticipated how current technocratic medicine could tamper with human reproductive capabilities, we are witnessing yet again the social fact that *shared blood engenders sameness.*

Clearly, organ transfer is not about human reproduction, yet it still has much in common with gestational surrogacy. For one, organ transfer is frequently described as a form of *rebirth.* Organ transfer also links disparate bodies to one another. Rather than sharing ova, sperm, and wombs, organ transfer relies on the literal movement of flesh (and perhaps even residual traces of the donor's blood) from the body of the donor to that of the recipient.[23] A unique property of organ transfer, however, is that it can create new identities while sidestepping human sexual reproduction altogether. Also, both gestational surrogacy and organ transfer draw anonymous strangers together into potentially complicated forms of blood relatedness. Both are about children as well. Whereas a fetus grows inside a surrogate, in organ transfer the transplanted body fragment nurtures the organ recipient, whose body fosters the postmortem trajectory of the donor. The recipient in turn now supports the vital organ, too.

All these contexts—adoption, gestational surrogacy, and organ transfer— challenge the assumed symmetry of the American system of bilateral kinship because they privilege mothers over fathers and other kin. As noted earlier, according to folk understandings, both biological mother and father are assumed to offer equal portions of their genetic material to create a child. Yet in terms of the biosentimental qualities associated with parenthood, it is the mother, or genetrix, who is the object of organ recipient desire. Just as adoptees search for their birth mothers, similarly organ recipients long most of all for reunions involving their donors' birth mothers. Both kinds of searches underscore that personal origins are intrinsically linked to childbirth. Gestational surrogacy expresses yet another facet of this notion because the rhetoric of "the gift of life" is at work here, as it is in organ transfer. In one context this expression refers to a surrogate giving the gift of a child to an infertile woman (Ragoné 1994); in the other, a donor's mother offers fragments of her lost child to grant new life (or rebirth) to the sick and dying. (It is no coincidence that this expression originated with the blood industry in this country.)

All three contexts discussed here potentially allow involved parties to have two mothers at once: birth and adoptive mother, surrogate and social mother, and biological (birth) and donor's (birth) mother. Yet organ recipients are unique in that they are simultaneously *bound biologically and emotionally* to *both mothers*, once they equate transplantation with birth as an embodied form of intimacy.[24] I hypothesize, too, that recipients might even view their experience as a quasi state of motherhood. Just as the donor's mother once felt her child move within her womb, an organ recipient can sense the donor's presence as a new set of lungs breathes or a heart beats in his or her own chest. Perhaps recipients and donor mothers are drawn to one another because they share this deeply private experience. If so, this is indeed a truly radical and new form of embodied intimacy.[25]

I would posit, too, that new forms of intimacy render fictive kinship simultaneously so natural and essential in the context of organ transfer. When Larry assumes the structural role of fictive son to Sally, together they circumvent the possibility of a more adulterous coupling (a concern voiced clearly by Sally when she insisted that Larry acquire Bulldog's approval before they met). The primacy of the mother may also account for the intimacy that can arise between pairs of mothers, as reported separately by Sara and Kelly. As Silverman et al. report for adoption, birth mothers who have surrendered their children may seek them out later in life. Such mothers are driven by the need to know that their children are well, to express their love, and to explain why they could not keep them as babies (1988: 526). The mothers of organ donors likewise hope in part to heal themselves by tracing the destinations of their deceased children's organs to the now thriving bodies of transplant recipients. They, like adoption's birth mothers, will suffer for years from the sense that the children they once nurtured were suddenly torn from them. These two sets of women define complementary categories of birth mothers who, albeit under radically different circumstances, had to relinquish offspring to the care of strangers. As is true for both, life most certainly can never be the same.

This idea of the two mothers is further naturalized by the widespread understanding that organ transplantation is experienced as a form of rebirth (cf. Lifton 1975 on adoptees' experiences). As noted previously, when organ recipients introduce themselves, they often speak of having two birthdays: the first marks the onset of infancy, the second, or "rebirthday," corresponds to the date of the transplant. Larry, like many recipients, celebrates the anniversary of his transplant with a rebirthday party, complete with a cake shaped like his organ, and he and his guests consume it with gusto. Others, too, are reborn through the process of organ transfer. Whereas the processes of organ donation and procurement necessitate a second or even third death (see chapter 1), transplantation ultimately grants the donor a second (or third, or fourth) chance at life. Through organ transfer, both organ donors and transplant recipients now define categories of the twice-born or reborn.

Final Thoughts: Death and Fears of Secondary Loss

In the end, the creative configurations that characterize donor kin–recipient encounters challenge the darker fears that still trouble those professionals who oppose written communication and other forms of intimacy. Contrary to their persistent fears, I know of no cases where donor kin have demanded gifts or money as reparation from organ recipients, nor do they insist on visitation rights, as if they were the noncustodial parents of lost offspring. Instead, donor kin–recipient communication is about building community in highly unconventional ways. As this chapter reveals, the beauty of fictive kinship lies in the astonishingly flexible ways that such practices create bonds between radically disparate parties, thus undermining the strangeness of the hybrid recipient rejuvenated by parts derived from the dead. Organ transfer can enable an older man to become the son of a woman twelve years his junior; a rural-based Euro-American mother the intimate of another from St. Lucia; and two men, once strangers to each other, now a pair of loving brothers. All parties whom I have interviewed also insist that the first encounter must be approached with caution. As one donor mother put it, "There's no turning back—you're in it for the long haul."

It is for these reasons that many professionals are, understandably, deeply troubled by the potential blow of the double loss. That is, how will donor kin cope with the news that, say, an organ recipient they have come to know has died? This surfaces as a very real possibility in two of the case studies offered in this chapter. Sara herself makes reference to this in her narrative, stressing that Jules's life has already been shortened as a result of a botched posttransplant medical procedure, and Sally might very well outlive Larry, given that he is twelve years her senior. What then? Will these mothers' worlds come crashing down yet again, with second deaths forcing them to relive their first traumas?

These are legitimate concerns, voiced especially loudly by professionals who wish to protect the privacy and assumed fragile emotional states of patients and donor families. At this point I can only hypothesize, but my sense is that whereas a donor mother would most certainly mourn the loss of any recipient of her child's organs, ultimately all donor mothers know deep down that recipients harbor mere fragments of the body, self, or soul of the original donor. Encounters with recipients nevertheless grant donor parents a second chance to watch their children grow and extend their histories beyond the grave in strangely profound ways by building on their histories with organ recipients. I believe, then, that most donor kin will be able to cope with the inevitable deaths of recipients more easily even, perhaps, than recipients cope with donors' deaths. This is because recipients frequently suffer from what one communications coordinator labeled "survival guilt." Larry sobs when he thinks of Charlie because he finds it impossible to shake the sense that Charlie had to die so that he himself could live.

So, what of the loss of the now recipient-intimate? Will the donor mother experience this yet again as her outliving her own son, thus forcing her to bear witness to his second death with the recipient's passing? We must not forget that multiple encounters with different recipients mean that transplanted donor parts can generate *multiple histories,* so that a donor is potentially twice and thrice reborn through the prolonged life of each recipient. My point here is that the anxieties surrounding thoughts about recipients' deaths are those of the overly cautious. I imagine instead that donor mothers will generate other creative ways to mourn their original losses. At the wake, funeral, or service for a recipient she has known, a donor's mother may well find herself saying good-bye to not one but two sons: one she has known from birth, the other as a result of her decision to donate. Having viewed a pair of reborn lives well lived, perhaps she might then experience some small sense of closure.

4 Human Hybridity

Scientific Longing and the Dangers of Difference

In June 2004, three transplant recipients died after contracting rabies from William Beed Jr., a twenty-year-old organ donor from Arkansas who suffered a fatal brain hemorrhage in a hospital in Texarkana, Texas. Mr. Beed's lungs, kidneys, and liver were transplanted into four separate patients on May 4: a lung recipient in Alabama, who died from surgical complications, and three other patients at Baylor University Medical Center in Dallas, who received his kidneys and liver.[1] These three remaining recipients recovered and returned home following their surgeries, only to develop encephalitis twenty-one to twenty-seven days later. As reported by the Centers for Disease Control and Prevention (CDC), "They became confused, lethargic, lost their appetite and developed seizures, muscle jerking and other problems." By June 21, all three were dead. The *Houston Chronicle* subsequently disclosed the identities of the deceased: Joshua "Bubba" Hightower, eighteen, of Gilmer, Texas; Cheri Jean Wells Biggs, fifty, of Mesquite; and Jimmy Paul Martin, fifty-two, of Oklahoma (AP 2004b). Two and a half weeks later, Baylor acknowledged that yet a fourth patient, who had received an artery from Beed's liver, had also died from rabies (Grady 2004).[2]

No one in either Texarkana or Dallas initially suspected rabies as a cause of death for the donor or any of the recipients.[3] A Baylor-based pathologist, Dr. Elizabeth C. Burton, however, was puzzled by the overlap of neurological symptoms that had caused three organ recipients' deaths. Burton contacted the CDC, and together they determined that all had died from a strain of rabies generally carried by bats (AP 2004b; CDC 2004; Grady 2004). As published reports repeatedly stressed, this was the first known instance in which recipients had contracted rabies from an organ donor. Humans rarely die of rabies in the United States, and thus inquiries about or testing for this disease do not form part of standard protocols for the majority of the nation's OPOs. This rare instance nevertheless prompted UNOS to issue a press release in which it expressed sympathy for the deceased donor and the first four recipients.[4] UNOS also used this opportunity to emphasize that potential donors are screened with great care, and that OPO staff always strive to obtain detailed medical histories from kin before proceeding with procurement (UNOS 2004b).

Although experts emphasized repeatedly that this was an unusual development, the Beed rabies incident is hardly the first time that a donor's transplanted parts have harbored a life-threatening infection. Similar fates involving rabies had been documented for a handful of cornea recipients (although the majority lived outside the United States). By February 2005, physicians in Germany reported a set of circumstances that mirrored those of the Beed case. There, four organ recipients died from rabies contracted from a donor, whom medical personnel assumed had died from a heart attack caused by crack and ecstasy use (Reynolds 2005). These instances also bear much in common with an earlier set of events when a donor's organs transmitted the AIDS virus to several recipients (Altman 1991). With these parallel stories in mind, we might well argue that transplanted organs are capable, in an epidemiological sense, of "remembering" their origins, because they can infect another living organism with undetected pathogens derived from the original donor body. Although in the Beed case the death toll from rabies appears to have stopped at five, the logistics of supplying the nation with transplantable organs inevitably meant that, within a day of William Beed's death, his infection ranged across four separate states. Had Beed's kin donated a wider assortment of tissues, the crisis would be far more drastic. The Beed rabies story emerges as a landmark incident in the United States specifically because organ donation spread a lethal pathogen across the species barrier, thus defying pervasive understandings of organs as lifesaving gifts offered by compassionate strangers.

DANGEROUS MIRACLES

A dominant component of transplant ideology involves assertions of organ transfer's miraculous qualities, a point I have illustrated throughout this work. This sense of the miraculous extends beyond the process itself: as heart recipient Gene Bea (2003) pronounces repeatedly in his upbeat memoir, surgeons are "miracle workers," and, following his own surgery, he himself was transformed into "a miracle man" whose anonymous donor "lives on" inside of him. Physician and medical ethicist Stuart Youngner (1990) cautions, however, that in such celebrations we deny transplantation's "dark side." Indeed, just as forms of private suffering are frequently denied a public face in the transplant arena, incipient epidemiological dangers are similarly hidden from public view. With careful probing, however, it becomes clear that embedded in the symbolic language employed by professional and lay parties are shared anxieties about hybridity or the surgical melding of disparate bodies.

The Beed rabies incident heralds newly imagined, hidden dangers that may well lurk within the bodies of organ donors or, at the very least, within their transplanted parts. The origins of such dangers are varied. As discussed in chapter 1, transplant specialists have greatly expanded the criteria by which dying patients might qualify for donor status, an action driven by the heightened anxieties that characterize organ scarcity. Fifteen years ago Beed would have been excluded as an organ donor because of his history of drug use (a policy that remains true for blood donors). Gretchen Reynolds, in reflecting on this erosion of strict exclusionary criteria, notes that "organ transplanting has become, in fundamental ways, a victim of its own success" as specialists in the field have "quietly [begun] to relax the standards" for determining donor status (2005: 37, 38).

The Beed case exposes how entangled medical and social criteria have become in shaping organ transfer as a precarious surgical practice. Organ donation offered Beed, as a twenty-year-old unemployed drug user, the possibility of redemption through a very particular form of death. If we revisit the language of body "recycling," Beed, as a valued donor, was transformed from "trash" to "treasure" through organ transfer (again, see chapter 1). In this sense he might well be regarded as the quintessential donor of emergent millennial medicine. After all, as explained by Dr. Goran Klintmalm, who oversees transplantation at Baylor Hospital, "What people have to understand is that donors now, except for the seventy-five-year-olds who die of intracranial bleeds, are not part of the church choir. . . . The ones who die are the ones you don't want your daughter or your son to socialize with. They drink. They drive too fast. They use crack cocaine. They get caught up in drive-bys." In contrast to Beed, Klintmalm describes donors of a bygone era as an idealized sociomedical category. As he explains, during the 1980s, organs were derived from much younger, healthier donors whose organs "were pristine" (Reynolds 2005: 38). Beed, then, was "marginal" in terms of both his clinical and his social worth, a man whose organs became acceptable only through the application of what is currently referred to as "extended criteria." The redemptive promises of organ transfer ultimately failed in Beed's case, however, because his body harbored an undetected pathogen that then killed four "innocent" patients in need.

As such, this case uncovers a range of anxieties associated with hybridity. As described in chapter 3, organ transfer necessitates an unusual form of embodied intimacy, as parts from one body are melded to another, and, in Beed's case, four organ recipients died because Beed himself was infected with a lethal disease. Of particular interest to me is how this case heralds the threat of zoonotic infections that can cross the species barrier. At work here, then, is an altogether new hybrid form of merged bodies, where animal is melded to human.

The troubles associated with such radical couplings define the focus of this final chapter. Although zoonoses are most certainly relevant to the discussion that follows, I am especially interested in emergent social responses to imagined forms of human-animal intimacy, forms engendered more specifically by experimental attempts at xenotransplantation. The promises offered by xenografts are many, and the eradication of organ scarcity is paramount. It would indeed be a boon to transplantation if procurement procedures no longer necessitated acquiring consent from surviving kin or, further, the extraction of organs from dead human patients. Special colonies of animals could instead be farmed specifically for human transplantation. In purely pragmatic terms, xenotransplantation makes economic, social, and clinical sense.

As prior discussions within this book reveal, however, the merging of disparate human bodies already generates a range of anxieties about the integrity of the self for donors and recipients. What, then, of the proposal to merge human bodies with whole organs derived from animals? How significant are anxieties over so unusual a form of human hybridity? What of the notion of rebirth, were animal parts to save the lives of dying human patients? Of greatest concern to me is the potentially transformative power of these parts of nonhuman origin. Members of various involved groups are especially troubled by the ways in which a range of experimental alternatives—which currently include parts of animal as well as mechanical origin—transgress the body's boundaries and, thus, threaten the integrity of the human self. Interestingly, although professionals and potential patients express different preferences within the experimental realm of transplant research, all worry about how radical solutions destabilize human nature.

Anthropologists, writing in other contexts, have likewise noted the prevalence of anxieties over the breakdown of the body's boundaries. The threats heralded by a range of invasive forces define a prominent leitmotif.

As both Donna Haraway (1989) and Emily Martin (1992, 1993, 1994) have observed, the field of immunology, for example, is rife with metaphors of invasion, these symbolic constructions shaped by broader social anxieties about the weakening of national boundaries and the dangers associated with immigration and war. But the vulnerability of the human body extends well beyond the threat of such pathogens as polio and AIDS (Martin 1994). Still other dangers are associated with the monstrous quality of human hybrids, evident in literature and film. Cecil Helman, in writing of the human "spare parts industry," equates the process of organ transfer with the making of Frankenstein's monster, remarking that "bodies which are *partially* artificial are commonplace, as are bodies containing within them the organs or parts of *other* bodies." As a patchwork of body fragments, organ recipients herald "a new type of society" where "the images of the coherent body and the coherent 'self' have both fragmented" (Cecil Helman 1988: 15; italics in original; cf. Cecil Helman 1992).

As preceding chapters illustrate, professionals and lay participants express competing ideas about sociality in the realm of organ transfer. Pervasive forms of professional rhetoric insist that donor and recipient bodies are discrete entities. Within such a framework, donors are indisputably dead, and their organs are reified to the point that they are regularly referred to as mere pumps or filters.[5] Medicalized imagery such as this opposes acts of sociality that (re)animate the donor body in peculiar (that is, unnatural and irrational) ways that run contrary to scientific reasoning. In short, when framed by an exclusively clinical perspective, sociality is considered unnatural because it is pathological. Nevertheless, donor kin and recipients regularly circumvent these aspects of professional ideology: by seizing upon the seemingly unnatural merging of donor and recipient bodies, they naturalize this odd relationship by asserting ties of kinship. Once merged, recipients and their donors may then share histories. In these ways the process of sociality transforms the strange (or stranger) into the familiar intimate.

These sorts of conflicts reveal a disquiet that reigns over many aspects of organ transfer in the United States, even after half a century of practice. Within this specialized medical realm, transplanted organs are now by nature polysemic, bearing the weight of a wide assortment of meanings assigned to them by professional and lay parties. Among professionals, donated organs are prized commodities in a world of great scarcity; these same commodities, in lay circles, can spark rebirths within recipients and, further, may possess personalized biographies (Kopytoff 1986) that persist beyond the grave. The recipient body is thus indeed a gestalt of sorts: when conceived of as being greater than the sum of its parts, its problematic lies in the nagging fact that it is a body both wondrous and monstrous. The inventive strategies employed by donor kin and recipients to generate new forms of sociality underscore just how taxing, in socioemotional terms, the transfer of body parts can be. When such transformative strategies succeed, the recipient body emerges as a highly successful hybrid creature. But what of other hybrid forms, when nonhuman species provide organs for human use? The celebrations and anxieties generated by such imagined possibilities define the focus of this final chapter, where I examine professional longing specifically in the transplant arena; explore the ethical debates surrounding current laboratory experimentation; and, finally, contrast professional and lay understandings of xenotransplantation's promises and dangers.

PROFESSIONAL DESIRES TO CULTIVATE NATURE

Current experimental efforts in transplant medicine spring in large part from widespread anxieties over organ scarcity. That is, professional desires and preferences are driven by an incessant longing for an endless supply of replaceable human parts. Given that the human donor pool has failed to match the growing national demand, surgeons, transplant coordinators, and procurement specialists regularly consider the possibilities offered by the hybrid melding of human bodies with either sophisticated machinery or organs derived from other mammalian species. Oddly, this professional stance generates an assortment of contradictory responses to human hybridity. On the one hand, those who work directly with organ recipients often disapprove of patients' attempts to integrate anonymous donors' organs as parts of themselves, and recipients who identify too deeply on a psychological level with their donors will invariably be marshaled off to psychiatrists, who might very well label them as suffering from "Frankenstein syndrome" (Beidel 1987; cf. Cecil Helman 1988, 1992; Youngner 1990: 1015). Nevertheless, these same professionals may celebrate in their language and literature the wonder of other "monstrous couplings" (Haraway 1992), where human bodies are melded in truly remarkable ways with parts of nonhuman origin. As we shall see, whereas experimental research targets both mechanical devices and animals as futuristic sources of organ replacement, it is organs of mammalian origins that generate the most troubled responses. These responses are couched in terms of the utter strangeness of potential forms of sociality, involving the merging of humans with animal flesh and blood. For this reason, my attention throughout this chapter will focus for the most part on organs derived from animals.[6]

Medical science has in fact naturalized the monstrous nature of organ grafting, for a common technical term employed within the medical literature is *chimerism*, which refers specifically to the *successful* integration of immunologically distinct bodies and parts (Jankowski and Ildstad 1997).[7] Studies of chimerism are driven by the specific desire to identify ever more sophisticated and elaborate means for disabling or deceiving the human host's immunological system such that organs, tissues, blood, and cells of foreign origin are read as "self" (BioTransplant, Inc., and MGH 1999) rather than as invading other. The ultimate desire is to be able to eliminate the need for immunosuppressants altogether (Chillag 1997: 70–73). Recent discussions of chimerism concern questions reminiscent of patients' musings over cell memory: How might the immunologist track the transfer or "migration" of cells from a donor to a host body? That is, does an organ acquired from a female recipient, for instance, retain chromosomal evidence of its origins after being implanted in a male recipient's body? The most complex projects today concern attempts to cross the species barrier so that, one day, transplant surgeons might make the radical shift from allogenic (or human-to-human) to xenogenic (or transpecies) grafting of transplantable parts. How, then, might the human host (that is, the recipient body) be fooled into perceiving an organ from a baboon or a pig as being its own? Or, how can a nonhuman species be transformed genetically in the laboratory so that its organs might appear, on an immunological level, as if they were human or, better still, as if made of cells from a specific recipient? Such are the dreams of transplant laboratory science.

Let us consider briefly the range of imagined sources that might alleviate the current organ shortage. At present, professional longing is focused squarely on implants of either mechanical or animal origin that might replace full human organs. Both trajectories have, at various stages, already included human trials. Yet another realm of research involves attempts to grow whole organs from cell cultures; research to date, however, has failed to generate functioning whole organs of relevance to my discussion of organ transfer; thus, I do not address these efforts here (see, however, Sharp in press [b]). Mechanical devices are generally referred to as "artificial" organs because they are of human design, and their current purpose is to offer either a permanent replacement or a "temporary bridge" for patients' failing organs. The majority of designers are bioengineers who strive to duplicate the complex workings of the heart and someday, perhaps, even other organs in portable form. Current solutions are cumbersome and rife with technical difficulties. Nevertheless, efforts have advanced over the course of two decades such that replacement prototypes for the heart, at least, have moved from being dependent on exterior devices as large as washing machines to palm-sized implants driven by portable battery packs.

A second category of research, involving immunologists, is xenotransplantation. This trajectory is dominated by efforts to develop transgenic animals whose organs could then be transplanted in human patients. Again, research goals have shifted radically from the 1970s to the present. Whereas earlier efforts focused on the use of various immunosuppressant drugs to facilitate the acceptance of baboon grafts by a human host's immune system, current experimentation is marked by attempts to transform a "donor" animal species such that its organs are part human in their genetic structure. Furthermore, whereas simian prototypes were previously the focus of research, transgenic pigs now embody the hope of xenotransplantation. Transgenic animals are developed through gene splicing at very early, in vitro, phases of reproduction and through subsequent inbreeding. The goal is for these animals, and their offspring, to bear human genetic characteristics such that their organs might be implanted in patients without stimulating graft rejection. Following a brief overview of responses to mechanical devices, the remainder of this chapter will focus on xenotransplantation, which defines the most popular alternative solution in professional transplant circles.

Currently, the heart defines an area of intensified research in North America, Asia, and Europe. Research includes attempts to develop both fully implantable, total artificial hearts (known as TAHs for short), as well as pumps designed to perform the action of a weakened left (and, less frequently, right) ventricle. Miniaturization and portability define important goals; over the course of the last two decades, experimental prototypes have moved from requiring extensive and virtually immobile external hardware to a portable battery pack that can fit in a camera-sized shoulder bag. Nevertheless, professionals most involved in the daily workings of organ transfer—that is, those who work most closely with organ recipients— overwhelmingly prefer xenotransplantation to efforts to develop mechanical prototypes. In the words of one bioengineer and inventor, "Most MDs, and especially the [transplant] surgeons, . . . are 'biologists'" who are "overwhelmingly suspicious" of any suggestion that a "mechanical device could do as good a job as a body part." Within this cognitive framework, a body of flesh and blood defines a natural source of replacement organs, as opposed to the dehumanized and thus denatured properties of mechanical prototypes.

During interviews, transplant professionals repeatedly emphasized the dangers of mechanical breakdown as reasons for why they preferred organs of mammalian origin over mechanical implants. From this standpoint, the mechanical device, as artifice, offers at best only a feeble approximation of the beauty of our anatomy's complex workings, debasing the humanity of the patient whose life (or, more specifically, body) would be greatly restricted by a machine's requirements. Machines are at best cumbersome; at their worst, they undermine bodily integrity and human dignity. Practically speaking, so far it has proved difficult to replicate, in lightweight, implantable, and permanent form, the human heart, lungs, liver, and kidneys. Transplant professionals agree that, to date, no mechanical device works as elegantly as the real, corporal thing. These same professionals are highly resistant to plans to harness recipients' bodies permanently to complex machines. This attitude springs largely, I believe, from the fact that this is precisely what transplantation currently promises: an end to dialysis, heart monitors, and dependency on either stationary or portable ventilators. Yet mechanical devices trouble professionals on a deeper epistemological level, too. Social worker Tanya Ryder, who, at thirty-four, already had six years of experience in 1992 working with a range of transplant patients, described a model of an artificial heart as follows: "This is another product to try. But it will be a long time before we rely on this. Right now it is only a 'prolonging device.' . . . It's [impractical] as a final solution—you use it while you're waiting for a transplant. It's big—you have to be tied up to a machine that runs it all the time, so you are not mobile. And it's noisy!" She bangs her fist on the table to produce a loud, steady drumbeat. "That's what it sounds like! . . . As one patient put it, 'I would only take it as a last resort because [I] would lose my 'native heart.' It's not natural—and we don't know enough about it right now."

A decade later, much smaller, implantable devices that replace an excised heart still fail to duplicate the elegance so intrinsic to the original flesh-and-blood model. As a result, transplant professionals still consider them inherently unpleasant and impractical innovations. Echoing Tanya's sentiments, those whom I have encountered in recent years still focus squarely on the "unnatural" quality of technological substitutes. Among the more troubling aspects, as described regularly during interviews, is a disenchantment with the necessity of excising a human, fleshy heart to make way for a mechanical prototype. Transplant professionals underscore that this surgical installation permanently transforms the patient into something not fully, or less than, human. References to the fact that mechanical devices generate unnatural sounds and rhythms emphasize even further the foreign quality of the device and its ability to rob patients of their humanity.

In such instances, professionals may express their skepticism by drawing on imagery reminiscent of the Tin Woodman in *The Wizard of Oz* or other contemporary cyborgs who lack humanity because they have no true heart.

During their research on the Jarvik-7 in the 1980s—a device that defines a groundbreaking prototype for current TAH research—Renée Fox and Judith Swazey found that this corner of transplant medicine was in fact rife with celebratory imagery of the Tin Woodman. As they explain, surgeon William DeVries was fond of quoting the Tin Woodman's lines from *The Wizard of Oz* when speaking of his efforts to work with the device (Fox and Swazey 1992: 98, cf. 158). At a 2005 conference attended primarily by bioengineers and other medical inventors, one professional presentation featured an experimental heart device labeled "Tin Man." In other quarters, however, the Tin Woodman emerges as a monstrous figure, as illustrated by one donor outreach campaign. A poster generated through the efforts of an advertising firm featured a photo of the Tin Woodman with text that read, "If Organ Donation Makes You Happy in the Movies, Imagine How Good You'll Feel in Real Life"; in smaller, italic print, a final caption read, "Consider Life after Death." Local procurement professionals found the poster so bizarre that it was soon pulled from a statewide campaign. In the words of one interviewee, the poster was "too weird" and thus counterproductive to their cause because it associated organ retrieval and "real-life experience" with an artificial man made of metal (see Sharp in press [b]).

The Hybrid in the Laboratory

Alongside recent attempts to refine mechanical prototypes stand other equally widespread international efforts to explore the potential of various animal species as sources for organs (CE 2003; Fishman, Sachs, and Shaikh 1998). The scientific desire to render xenotransplantation a reality is, like artificial devices, hardly new. As recounted by David Cooper et al. (2002), we need only consider the history of biomedicine and surgery to discover a host of relevant experimental procedures. Blood transfusions from animals to humans were attempted in the early seventeenth century in England and France; during the nineteenth century, skin from a variety of animals was grafted onto human patients; and the period from the 1890s through the twentieth century is marked by numerous attempts to transfer animal organs to human patients. The most celebrated, recent case involved Baby Fae, who in 1984 (of all years) survived for twenty days with a baboon heart (Altman 1984a, 1984b, 1984c; Jonasson and Hardy 1985; Kushner and Belliotti 1985; Stoller 1990). A decade later, surgical teams in Pittsburgh, working under the leadership of Thomas Starzl (whose attempts at xenotransplantation date back to the 1960s), tested the effects of transplanting baboon livers in adult patients in conjunction with newly developed immunosuppressants (Starzl 1992: 112–14; Starzl et al. 1993). All human subjects suffered serious complications from graft rejection and died.

To date, survival rates for xenotransplantation have most frequently been measured in hours, not months or even days (Cooper, Gollackner, and Sachs 2002), thus paralleling the early developments of allographs half a century ago (Starzl 1992). Organ rejection is extremely complex and not, as one might expect, an all-or-nothing affair. Rather, it can include immediate acute as well as long-term, chronic forms of graft failure, involving the body's immunologic, histopathologic, vascular, and cellular intolerance for tissues of foreign origin. Such responses are especially pronounced if tissues are derived from nonhuman species. Many of the mechanisms involved in graft rejection remain little understood, especially in reference to survival beyond the body's most immediate postsurgical immune responses during the first few hours or days (Cooper, Gollackner, and Sachs 2002; Robson, Schulte Am Esch II, and Bach 1999). An experimental recipient (that is, a xenotransplant patient) is likely to suffer a slow and, potentially, very painful death, but this person's story nevertheless is described as a medical triumph because his or her body, while undergoing intense forms of medical intervention, heroically refuses to die. Baby Fae's brief life is, for example, still celebrated in this way by Loma Linda Hospital, where her surgery was performed (Sharp in press [a]). When other seemingly unrelated parts of the body succumb, medical teams may declare that the transplant was a success, although the patient died, for instance, from a brain hemorrhage.

Pigs now define a prized donor pool thought to offer the greatest potential for relieving the chronic shortage of transplantable human parts. This desire to meld human and porcine bodies is rooted in older, established medical practices. A now highly successful use of porcine parts involves the regular replacement of damaged human heart valves with those derived from pigs (Cooper, Gollackner, and Sachs 2002; Maeder and Ross 2002). In reference to full organ transfer, much attention is now focused on interbred miniature swine—transgenic creatures that harbor human genetic material that was spliced to pig cells during very early stages of reproduction. Transgenic pigs have been produced within laboratory settings for more than twenty-five years (Cooper, Gollackner, and Sachs 2002), which underscores that such practices have indeed become routinized at least within experimental realms of science.

As I will illustrate later in this chapter, the scientific value placed on porcine bodies is altogether peculiar from a lay point of view, especially when considered from the perspective of the organ recipient. As anthropologists have long argued, pigs are regularly devalued because they are viewed as a source of filth, as is evident, for example, in the dietary prohibitions honored by adherents to Islam, Judaism, and various Christian sects, as well as idiomatic expressions concerning the "slop" pigs eat or the messiness of "pigpens." Yet pigs are also highly valued in some quarters for their intelligence, and more widely still as domesticated creatures that humans can eat (Douglas 1966; Harris 1985; Leach 1964). Such cultural constructions offer little, though, by way of explanation for why science is so intent on melding human and porcine bodies when, as we shall see, individuals in need of transplants reject this possibility. Answers to this riddle are embedded in how science categorizes experimental creatures. The pig bears tremendous potential in terms of its immunological compatibility; in turn, it is also valued for what it is not. It is not simian.

Pigs are favored over chimpanzees and baboons for a range of utilitarian and economic, political, and symbolic reasons. As argued by the very scientists engaged in xenotransplant research, pigs are much cheaper to raise because they mature quickly (within four to six months); they have larger broods than apes and monkeys; their potential supply is assumed unlimited; anatomically they offer a close match for human bodies (the heart, for instance, is just the right size); and pigs do not require special, lifetime aftercare facilities as individual chimpanzees do once they are of no further use in the lab (Cooper, Gollackner, and Sachs 2002; Niemann and Kues 2003). In terms of animal care protocols, pigs are categorized as farm rather than laboratory research animals, and so they fall under radically different—that is, less stringent—regulatory apparatuses. In the words of one medical ethicist whom I interviewed in 2002, "You can do a lot more to a pig than you can to a lab rat" because of such technical and legal distinctions (cf. Bayne 1999).

These sorts of utilitarian concerns play into assumptions about the sentient qualities of different animals. The specifics of the cultural worth of pigs allow many to farm, slaughter, and eat them with relatively little reproach. Finally, if pigs are considered distant in evolutionary terms, they bear far less cultural capital than do chimpanzees or even baboons. Few people lose sleep over sacrificing pigs to science, or pity them as much as dogs or apes that have, for instance, traveled to outer space and back, or been subjected to long-term deprivation experiments in the name of, say, developmental psychology. Pigs are also prolific, and thus easily replaceable. Just as American farm children raise them with care for 4-H projects, only to assist in their butchering later on to feed their own households, so, too, science farms and sacrifices pigs in the name of research in ways that remain forbidden for apes and monkeys.

My purpose here is not to inspire compassion for the pig; rather, I seek to underscore that in the end we are faced with a creature whose scientific value rests heavily on its devaluation in daily spheres of life. In the realm of xenotransplantation, swine are transformed into truly unusual and, thus, wondrous creatures. Experimental, transgenic piglets are delivered by cesarean section, reared out of reach of a nursing sow, and guarded within absolutely sterile conditions to eliminate chance exposure to porcine pathogens. They are also genetically part human, because their own DNA is spliced with very specific human material. The potential of the transgenic pig, then, lies in the fact that it is a viable alternative. These characteristics are what make it simultaneously such a valued and dangerous hybrid.

The Promise of the Pig

At present, xenotransplantation remains strictly experimental; nevertheless, it inspires a rich and imaginative genre of discourse employed by a range of involved parties. The hope that professionals invest in xenotransplantation's potential has persisted throughout the course of my research, and the topic was in fact first raised without prompting during two of my earliest interviews. On separate occasions in late 1991 and early 1992, two transplant social workers alerted me to the fact that surgeons on their respective wards were interested in the possibilities of this type of research, and one doctor was in the process of establishing a laboratory. As Tanya Ryder explained, for example, "We are all for it, anything that will keep you alive. But we've known about xenography for a long time. There is now a special kind of pig that is being bred for its kidneys."

Xenotransplantation, albeit still highly experimental, continues to define a realm of professional desire. It now has its own professional society, the International Xenotransplantation Association, which produces a bimonthly scientific journal and hosts professional conferences worldwide. I find especially that when I interview younger surgeons, some have already had direct experience with transpecies grafting. During his years of medical training, for example, Dr. Salvador experimented with perfusing rats with human blood and transferring organs from one rodent species to another. Also, the topic of xenotransplantation is raised regularly at transplant conferences and other similar gatherings. Without fail, at least one speaker will refer to xenotransplantation's remarkable possibilities. Most often the topic surfaces in presentations with titles such as "The History of Transplantation" or "The Future of Transplantation." Comments offered in 2003 by an East Coast

OPO director to a gathering of recipients and donor kin are exemplary. During a detailed PowerPoint presentation on fifty years of transplant history in the United States, he concluded by underscoring that current experimentation marked "the future" of organ transfer in a nation plagued by organ scarcity. Speaking specifically of baboons and pigs as potential donors, he put it thus: "Xenotransplantation means cross-species—remember Baby Fae [who received a baboon's heart]? It seems we're too close to baboons or something, so unfortunately the animal of choice is a pig. Well, maybe we don't identify with pigs? [Dr.] Starzl [the liver surgeon] says it's two years away [in terms of experimental trials]." The speaker then displayed a slide of pink baby pigs. "Those aren't little baby pigs [that will be used for xenotransplants]. If you've ever been on a farm—these pigs are *big*. Now, *that's* great science!"

This upbeat presentation style is driven by an incessant longing for an endless supply of organs, where xenografts are imagined as the great panacea for the national crisis. I frequently hear professionals comment, if only we could harvest organs from pigs, baboons, or chimpanzees, we would no longer need to ask kin for their consent, or what if we could perfect immunosuppression to the point that organs of animal origin would not matter? When asked where the future of transplantation lies, surgeons and other physicians, transplant nurses and social workers, and procurement specialists inevitably respond, in their own ways, that transplantation's "future hope" lies in xenotransplantation. As a leading transplant surgeon explained during a patient symposium at the 1992 Transplant Games in Los Angeles, "This may operate as a bridge—if you can't find a human liver, use a baboon until you can get the human liver. We need federal support for this research. It may be that this may be the next long-term solution." During a plenary address at a 1994 transplant conference, another aged surgeon spoke enthusiastically of xenotransplantation's possibilities: "We can think our way out of this! . . . When [in the future] you look back over twenty years, you'll see a different landscape." Together transplant and procurement professionals express this overwhelming preference for organs derived from living, nonhuman species, rather than mechanical devices, as the proper solution to the organ crisis.[8] This strong preference for xenografts over mechanical solutions was especially evident in the weeklong International Congress of the Transplantation Society in 2004, where xenotransplantation figured prominently as a focus for numerous research panels, plenary sessions, and general assembly meetings. The Transplantation Society's leadership barely uttered a word about artificial devices, even though a pediatric case was making headline news in the United States (Richter 2004). During professional conferences, discussions of mechanical organs typically take center stage only at events hosted by organizations whose members are more typically bioengineers and not surgeons or other clinicians.

For more than a decade, discussions and debates have focused persistently on the values and pitfalls of using simian versus porcine donors. The preference for each category of animal is shaped by ideological and pragmatic factors. Those who favor baboons or chimpanzees over swine embrace a Darwinian model of likeness, a common sentiment in our culture. That is, we think of nonhuman primates as our "cousins" (Dunbar and Barrett 2000), which, thus, define the most appropriate "match" for an ailing human body. For precisely the same reason, however, the scientific use of baboons and, even more so, chimpanzees, incites public outrage among those involved in protecting animals' rights. In laboratory circles, such public responses have shaped strict guidelines that dictate long-term and, ultimately, expensive care of simian creatures that outlive their laboratory potential. Thus, proponents of simian grafts recognize that their efforts may prove politically hazardous.

It is here where pigs enter: in spite of their internal anatomical similarity, pigs are not our cousins. They are domestic stock, a distinction that bears serious financial and political advantages. Within the realm of xenotransplantation, the pig has undergone a transformation of a very different sort from that of baboons and chimpanzees, emerging now as a lucrative category of *pharm* (from *pharmaceutical*) animal (Clark 1999: 146). No longer simply a source of bacon, the porcine body might also one day provide an unlimited supply of transplantable organs for dying human patients.

The Specter of Transgenesis

Whereas transplant and procurement professionals readily embrace the pig as a source of coveted organs, others who focus on larger, often global concerns underscore the dangers associated with gene-splicing technologies that generate a range of hybrid fauna and flora. Such hybrids inspire contempt and heated debate in the United States and beyond. Consider, for instance, the ongoing controversy over genetically altered crops, which currently define a focus for enormous outcry worldwide.[9] Specifically in reference to efforts that target the animal kingdom, truly peculiar chimeras are now emerging in the realm of the new genetics. A recently wondrous yet monstrous creature, for instance, is the spider goat, a genetically engineered animal whose milk bears tensile fibers previously generated only by orb-weaver arachnids (Christopher Helman 2001). Although benign in appearance, the spider goat nevertheless attracted much media attention because of its sheer perversity. The mere existence of this mismatched hybrid inevitably raises pointed questions about just how far science should go in altering the capabilities of a species.

Discussions of animal hybrids intended specifically for xenotransplantation are similarly highly polarized. On the one hand, scientists who work in partnership with biotechnology firms anticipate tremendous success and, ultimately, profits.[10] Among these parties, some transgenic creatures may well herald an exciting new world of hybrid possibilities (Haraway 1991a, 1992). The pig's potential is clearly expressed, for example, on the cover of the published proceedings from a conference on xenotransplantation, hosted by the New York Academy of Sciences (NYAS) in 1998. The NYAS hired Andy Levine, the artist who designed a stamp issued in 1998 by the U.S. Postal Service to promote organ donation (Ralph Brown, NYAS, personal communication, July 2005). Whereas the original image consisted of two merging human faces (figure 11), the one that graced the cover of *Xenotransplantation: Scientific Frontiers and Public Policy* featured a human merging with a pig (figure 12) (see Fishman, Sachs, and Shaikh 1998). Opponents, however (several of whom once engaged in such research themselves), are wary of efforts to tamper with nature in this way. These proponents view hybridity as heralding potentially disastrous outcomes as we disrupt what they see as the inherent balance of the natural world (Lindenbaum 2001: 375, citing Garrett 1994; cf. Soper 1995).

Clearly, then, the transgenic pig is a troublesome creature. Unlike the spider goat, the predicaments it engenders extend far beyond the desire to guard mammalian integrity. The transgenic pig's uniqueness lies in its genetic human qualities: partly human at the cellular level, it has been created solely as a source for replaceable human body parts. As a result, it pairs the hope of the medical miracle with that of lucrative rewards, while shadowed nonetheless by more sinister threats. Among the most troubling concerns is the very real possibility of transpecies contamination, a threat exemplified so clearly by the Beed rabies incident. Transgenic pigs are simultaneously wondrous and monstrous creatures because they bear the promise of an unending supply of transplantable parts, while also undermining the safety associated with species integrity.

Transgenesis defines a rich ground for anthropological analysis because it is fraught with these sorts of pragmatic and moral dilemmas. Of particular interest to me is how debates over the value of the transgenic pig figure in scientific and lay imaginings of the broader promises of xenotransplantation. If, as procurement professionals regularly argue, donor trends fail to climb because too many Americans remain suspicious of allotransplantation even after half a century of practice, what, then, of animal-to-human

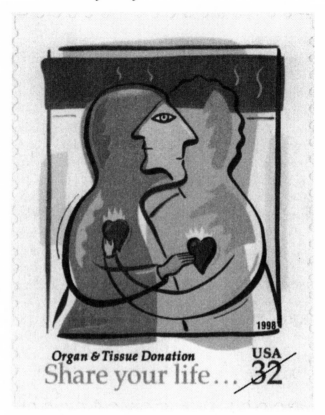

Figure 11. Postage stamp promoting organ donation, issued in 1998 by the United States Postal Service. The text reads: "Organ & Tissue Donation / Share your life . . . " (The full phrase that incorporates this phrase is "Donate Life. Share Your Life. Share Your Decision," a slogan promoted by the Coalition on Donation and used frequently on donor promotional materials of all types.) Artist: Andy Levine.

forms of organ transfer? As I will illustrate later, xenotransplantation, as a radical technology, jolts academic, clinical, and popular imaginations precisely because it so readily threatens the integrity of species, of humanity itself, and of individual bodies, too. Its transformative potential is what renders it so frightening: the success of xenotransplantation, as a hybrid technology, insists on transgressing body boundaries and on new, dangerous forms of sociality. Can, or should, we be melded with swine? What will become of the integrity of our species if we allow for such radical technological transgressions? Should we tamper in this way with what are assumed

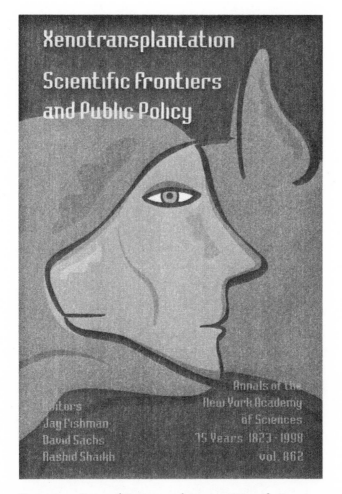

Figure 12. Cover of *Xenotransplantation: Scientific Frontiers and Public Policy,* Annals of the New York Academy of Sciences, vol. 862 (New York: New York Academy of Sciences, 1998). © 1998 New York Academy of Sciences, U.S.A. The NYAS hired Andy Levine, the same artist who designed the postage stamp promoting organ donation.

to be "natural" boundaries? What unseen dangers lurk in such forms of scientific tampering? As Paul Brodwin and others remind us, ethical questioning of new biotechnologies flags anxieties surrounding the manner in which they alter human bodies (Brodwin 2000a). As we shall see, the anxieties generated by xenotransplantation are hardly uniform, thus uncovering an intriguing array of comfort zones and fears.

Scientific Desire and Medical Hubris

Although transplant professionals might express some concern for hybridity and its ability to disrupt the integrity of the human body, they regularly embrace the promise of transgenic species. Still others, though, express outrage over xenotransplantation, viewing it as an illegitimate and dangerous attempt to tamper with nature. An especially pronounced source of alarm is the possibility that mammalian organ sources might transmit zoonotic or animal-derived infections to human recipients. When pigs are involved, among the most virulent pathogens identified to date are the porcine endogenous retroviruses (PERVs). Of particular concern is that such pathogens may remain undetected because swine carriers appear healthy and thus might transmit undetected yet lethal infections to organ recipients. Recipients could, in turn, infect their intimates. Recent zooepidemics affecting humans, including avian influenza (bird flu), severe acute respiratory syndrome (SARS), and mad cow disease (bovine spongiform encephalopathy [BSE] or new variant Creutzfeldt-Jakob disease [nvCJD] in humans), bolster such warnings of impending danger. "Epidemics are . . . lightning rods for eliciting the particular terrors that monitor the social forms and cultural values of different communities," writes Shirley Lindenbaum. In contemplating the cultural relevance of these perceived dangers, she underscores that "the shock of pestilence" (Lindenbaum 2001: 364) looms large in the minds of Americans, already unnerved by the specter of retrovirus and prion infections. As a brief introduction to such critiques, I turn to a published debate between medical anthropologist Margaret Clark (1999) and humanist and ethicist Harold Vanderpool (1999).

The human dangers of zoonotic pathogens define a central concern for Clark, who writes of the "startling and unnerving" speed at which "new biotechnologies [move] faster than our ability to monitor or regulate them" (1999: 137). Clark is especially concerned with the "formidable" (138) clinical, ethical, and policy risks associated with xenotransplantation research, and PERVs figure prominently. Clark's stance is bolstered by the work of Fritz Bach, a noted immunologist and established xenotransplant researcher who, a few years ago, called for a moratorium on clinical trials. Many of the dangers borne by PERVs remain unknown; thus, "the parade of horribles that can be imagined should be taken seriously and discussed openly," warned Bach and others (Bach, Ivinson, and Weeramantry 2001). Clark is also alarmed by the general absence of a social conscience in realms dominated by capitalist science. For example, she is wary of the current enthusiasm expressed by biotech firms to move ahead with attempts to implant xenografts in humans, regarding such desires as the mark of medical hubris. The desire for xenotransplantation's success hinges in large part on a newly configured form of body commodification, this time one dependent on an unusual human-animal hybrid.

Vanderpool, on the other hand, underscores the legitimacy of such scientific pursuits, even as they alter the course of nature. Unlike Clark (or Bach), Vanderpool expresses far greater trust in current laboratory projects. Instead of focusing on the threat of PERVs, Vanderpool celebrates the scientific ability to identify, screen, and avoid catastrophic dangers because legitimate, professional research is driven not simply by a desire for knowledge (or wealth) but by a mandate to protect our species, too. As he explains, simians bear more dangers for humans than do swine, and it is for this reason that the Food and Drug Administration (FDA) has declared a moratorium on transgenic chimpanzees. If transgenic swine in fact harbor lethal pathogens, such dangers will be identified and dealt with before xenotransplantation is attempted in human subjects. Vanderpool also stresses that knowledge of PERVs is more advanced than as described by Clark (and Bach, it seems). Furthermore, effective regulatory procedures and oversight committees already impose high standards of practice within this arena of experimental research (cf. Michaels 1998). Thus, whereas Clark views genetic manipulation as a form of immoral play, Vanderpool is wary of critiques hostile to experimental genetics. As Vanderpool underscores, science has long inspired fears of species tampering, and thus such reactions merely typify the evolution of new ideas. After all, medicine regularly "manipulate[s] nature toward human ends" (Vanderpool 1999: 155). Alarmist responses are unfortunate yet inevitable: the history of biomedicine is similarly marked by objections raised during the advent of anesthesia, invasive surgery, contraceptives, and heart transplants, all of which are now in regular medical use.

At the heart of these debates, whose participants include laboratory researchers, ethicists, and social scientists, are radically different perspectives on the human place in nature. Notably, both dominant pro and con arguments draw on various models of evolutionary progress. Clark, for example, embraces a gradual, plodding model of species evolution as inherently natural and thus morally sound (cf. Donnelley 1993, 1995, 1999). In essence, a world in balance is a safer world, rendered possible when humans leave other species well enough alone. An opposing stance, as exemplified by Vanderpool, celebrates human ingenuity and the scientific ability to transform nature deliberately, even at the cellular and molecular levels. A major source of contention is whether humans have the right to intervene in the paired processes of chance and change. Whereas Clark underscores the destructive tendency of our species to tamper with the natural world, Vanderpool rejoices in an ability to alter nature as quintessentially human. Both authors agree that science generates monsters: from Clark's perspective, xenotransplantation is a grave specter of scientific experimentation, whereas Vanderpool celebrates the healthy proliferation of chimeras as wonders of scientific inquiry and accomplishment.

A key factor that renders such oppositions irresolvable is that these two authors (and other theorists who share their opinions) are focused on very different realms of experience and scale. Both, in their own way, focus on individual lives: Vanderpool is especially concerned with how surgical and scientific experimentation might eventually save the lives of myriad patients. Clark's concerns, on the other hand, echo those voiced a decade earlier by Fox and Swazey (1992), two seasoned sociologists who tracked the effects the Jarvik-7 mechanical heart on recipients' lives and deaths. Clark underscores that patients who serve as experimental subjects will inevitably suffer severe emotional, medical, and social consequences. For example, xenotransplant patients would most likely have to endure intense media and medical scrutiny, their social relationships also monitored regularly by physicians and other scientific personnel intent on keeping them alive for as long as possible while also studying graft effects on the human body. If dangers to others arose, patients would most certainly be quarantined to protect the population at large from the threat of pandemics. Clark, who considers current regulatory procedures feeble at best, advocates careful pre- and posttransplant psychological counseling in anticipation of the hardships patients will face for the remainder of their lives.

As other ethicists and research scientists join the debate over the morality of transpecies grafting, professionals who currently work with organ recipients wait eagerly on the sidelines for news of laboratory breakthroughs. Assuming a stance not unlike Vanderpool's, most transplant professionals invest great faith in researchers to determine when it might be safe to test the melding of porcine and human bodies. We need only return, however, to the Beed rabies incident to realize that xenotransplantation harbors very real dangers that current regulatory procedures have failed to detect even when allografts are involved. Whereas professionals express widespread distaste for mechanical devices, they are nevertheless willing to test the potential success of xenotransplantation on human subjects, viewing this as a more "natural" solution than "artificial," mechanical devices of human design. Given such enthusiasm, and the assumption that xenotransplantation is inevitable (as I believe it is, too), an especially important question, posed originally by Fox and Swazey, remains pertinent today: "Who shall guard the guardians?" in this burgeoning experimental realm of the human "spare parts" industry (Fox and Swazey 1992: esp. 170–193).

DENATURED BODIES AND TRANSFORMED SELVES

In contrast to the hopes of transplant professionals that xenotransplantation could soon end the nation's organ crisis, and the sparring among research scientists and ethicists over the dangers of the hybrid porcine body, radically different concerns are expressed by organ recipients and other members of the lay public regarding mechanical and transgenic organs. Most strikingly, mechanical inventions tend to trigger fewer emotional responses or moral concerns than do organs of mammalian origin. As I will illustrate in this final section, when non–medically trained lay parties are asked to conceive of themselves as the recipients of experimental organs (something that professionals rarely ask themselves), their responses uncover broadly defined cultural (and nonmedical) understandings of what it means to be human, as well as how much private notions of selfhood hinge on our ability to inhabit a distinctly bounded body.

Embodying Difference

Echoing transplant and procurement professionals, organ recipients (and those awaiting transplants) worry incessantly about the scarcity of transplantable human parts. All are keenly aware that the demand outweighs the nation's supply and, especially where hearts, lungs, and livers are concerned, that they themselves might die before receiving the call from their transplant team announcing that a matching organ has been found. Patients readily fantasize about the deaths of strangers, such fantasies evolving in turn into a genre of gallows humor among those housed within the same hospital ward (see, for example, Siebert 2004: 170–73, 186). As detailed earlier, following their transplants, many recipients struggle with the sense that their survival is dependent on the deaths of anonymous strangers.

When asked about experimental alternatives, organ recipients are overwhelmingly supportive of such endeavors, although their technical knowledge is generally limited to what they might learn during abbreviated and sanitized presentations at conferences and support group meetings, or from offhand remarks made by medical personal from their respective transplant units. A common sentiment, as expressed by heart recipient Dale Sabrinski, is that "we should try anything—we're so short of organs right now, something's gotta give. My doc says this is the answer that might save many, many lives in the future. . . . Then we wouldn't have to wait for people to die anymore." The troubling question, though, of whether one would be willing to receive an organ from an animal, or be implanted with an artificial device, is a far more complicated one. Those who have already received organs of human origin express greater enthusiasm for current research; those who are still waiting typically fall silent when asked what they think, and then they cautiously weigh the consequences of mechanical and organically derived replacement parts. In the end, no solution proves as satisfactory as the human one.

In an attempt to gather preliminary data on how the lay public (and, thus, potential recipients) might perceive such options, in late 1992 I distributed a questionnaire to fifty undergraduate students attending the urban midwestern university where I taught. Their responses were complemented by an additional dozen responses gathered from faculty and university staff who expressed an interest in the study.[11] Xenotransplantation was already on the minds of many people in the United States, for by June of that same year surgeons in Pittsburgh had made two attempts to transplant baboon livers into adult recipients, one of whom lived for seventy days. As I learned through administering the questionnaire, the majority of student participants were also aware of experiments with "artificial hearts" (that is, the Jarvik-7) from the early 1980s, because they had been old enough to follow the news stories as children. Whereas my own childhood was marked by the breakthroughs of Christiaan Barnard's work in the 1960s, these college students had come of age during yet another phase of radical experimentation in the transplant arena.

When requested to choose and then rank their preferences for organs of baboon, human, or mechanical origin, 64 percent of the student respondents stated that they preferred organs from humans, and another 20 percent ranked mechanical as their first choice. None chose an organ from a baboon, and the remainder preferred to have no transplant at all. In terms of second and third choices, baboon and mechanical ranked evenly. Among those respondents who made only one choice, eight (out of a total of fifty) chose human and four chose mechanical; again, none chose baboon. In essence, human donors (or organs of human origin) were much preferred over baboon and mechanical parts, although these figured as alternative choices. Baboons, however, never figured as the first or only choice.

As a result of their exposure to a wide range of print and visual media, student respondents typically were familiar with science fiction depictions of the dehumanizing qualities of machines, yet the soulless, absolute efficiency of machines did not surface as a reason for concern with any great regularly. More often, if students expressed hesitation regarding machines, it was because the equipment could malfunction. Euro-American students in particular regularly stressed the superiority of artificial devices and the ingenuity of human inventors. As two wrote, "Nobody's used it before me and infected it," and "I would probably want the mechanical because by that time it would be much more advanced than the real thing." Another assumption was that fewer living creatures would be harmed if mechanical devices were used, although the possibilities embodied in such devices were more attractive in the abstract. As one student reflected, "It would not inflict loss of life on others . . . [it] would leave more human transplants for others. Exciting. If it could be properly connected with biofeedback sensors and a safety backup system . . . hell in time it might be better than the real thing. I would be scared of having one myself." The trust (albeit tentative at times) expressed by these participants (one that sometimes bordered on bravado) did not, however, characterize responses from African American and foreign students. As one African American woman put it, "God gave us hearts, who are we as humans to make our own for use?" I will return to the importance of such distinctions in my later discussion on organ recipients' responses.

The value of this preliminary survey is that it offers a glimpse into the thoughts of one segment of the lay population, one that is representative, at the very least, of an educated cohort of urban youth who reached young adulthood more than a decade ago and at the advent of a new period of experimentation in transplant medicine. These young people's responses must be understood as being framed by a shared sense that the development of organs of nonhuman origin may well define an inevitable medical development in their lifetimes. Their answers have helped shape questions I have subsequently posed to transplant patients over the years, too. As I will illustrate later, recipients' responses parallel students' answers in many respects, although recipients more quickly imagine how such unusual meldings would reshape their private sense of self or of being in the world.

The Mechanized Body

As reflected in earlier chapters, machine imagery abounds in the transplant arena, employed by surgeons and other transplant personnel as a means to dehumanize organs of human origin. These metaphors are employed by recipients in still other ways as a strategy for depersonalizing their donors. Recall, for instance, Dale Sabrinski's elaborate description of his body as a race car, a metaphor employed by yet another male heart recipient of similar age who reported, "I held the record in [my hospital]—I was out in seven days. I told [my surgeon] 'You can't get a new transmission put in right and your car fixed in seven days, but you can get a new heart!'" Whereas transplant professionals express anxiety over the melding of mechanical parts with human bodies, recipients (like the undergraduates just mentioned) are far more willing to embrace such possibilities. Among the most striking aspects of recipients' answers is their assumption that mechanical devices are relatively benign in terms of their potential to transform the self into something new, different, and thus fearful. Of greater concern to them are the pragmatics of machine use. In the words of Tina Zim, a Euro-American kidney recipient in her fifties, "Machines are bound to break," and malfunctions could easily occur when one is far from those who possess repair skills. If, then, artificial devices are to define the future of transplant medicine, skilled mechanics must be as readily available as, say, those familiar with pacemakers are today.[12]

Transplant patients are well aware of the dehumanizing consequences of being tethered to a machine. After all, many have already undergone months or years of hemodialysis; joined the legions of "pole pushers" who walk the halls of the nation's cardiac units connected to portable, computerized telemetry boxes that monitor (and stimulate) their hearts (Siebert 2004: 169–72); or endured mechanical support for their ailing lungs, either in bedridden states or by carrying backpack-sized portable units wherever they go. All, too, have found themselves connected to a host of devices that track their postsurgical progress, attached, for instance, to ventilators, an experience generally considered so irksome that a common sign of patients' recovery is that they will attempt to yank the tube from their mouths. Among the most basic frustrations associated with medical machinery is that it restricts mobility and renders patients dependent on medical personnel for their care (Bea 2003; Murphy 1987: 245).

Recipients are nevertheless far less threatened by these machines' cyborgic tendencies than are the professionals who manage their care. At issue here are different concerns about body boundaries. Whereas ethicists debate threats to species integrity, and transplant professionals express concern for patient autonomy or the loss of one's humanity through cyborgic couplings, transplant recipients are far more disturbed by xenotransplantation's potential to undermine one's *personal* sense of self as intact or whole, defined specifically in reference to the body's invasion by a foreign species. After all, all implants, whether human, mechanical, or mammalian, can well require that patients "lose" their natural or "native hearts." Machinery, as artifice, is considered both inert and benign, thus posing far less of a threat than do parts derived from animals. These nonhuman yet fleshy organs are truly strange things that threaten to undermine an already shaky, and very private, sense of self.

Hybrid Anxiety

As was true with the student respondents, organ recipients express great ambivalence regarding organs taken from baboons. As my research has progressed, I find that some, too, now struggle to imagine the possibility of porcine implants. Although they are well aware of the current scientific fascination with xenotransplantation, recipients may resist engaging in serious discussions on the topic. In support group settings, talk about xenotransplantation quickly degenerates into ribald joking or attempts to change the subject. These sorts of reactions are shaped by two key factors. First, the vast majority of recipients I encounter lack detailed training in the laboratory sciences, medicine, or genetics; thus xenotransplantation defines an esoteric body of knowledge about which they are uncomfortable expressing opinions. As a result, my attempts to breach the topic of organs of simian and porcine origins most often provoke responses of puzzlement and wonder. Recipients find it easier to grasp—or at least imagine—what a mechanical device might do. Nevertheless, most of them are deeply troubled by any mention of the scientific desire to graft whole organs from animals to human bodies because they worry that they themselves might one day be offered such an option. The silent response that so often follows my questions signals a deep-seated discomfort with these sorts of monstrous couplings.

Objections to xenotransplantation are multifaceted, and students' questionnaire responses provided important clues for understanding subsequent data generated from interviews with recipients. A common concern voiced by students focused on the humane treatment of animals. Those students who self-identified as vegetarians or as participants in the animal rights movement found the shedding of blood for humans especially abhorrent. As one explained, "I strongly disagree with killing animals to provide organs for humans. Would you kill people from the Third World to provide organs for the first world? It's the same thing."[13] Another put it thus: "I prefer the natural to the machine. But then again, I wouldn't take the baboon's heart without his informed consent!" Still others wrote of the dangers of difference, or the natural hierarchy of species. In the words of one, "As much as I hate to put the animal last, deep down I would have to be honest with myself. As Americans we think we are superior creatures and a baboon's heart isn't suitable." Yet another mused on the polluting nature of nonhuman species: "[I would prefer] a human heart because it was created to operate in our bodies and probably would operate best; the mechanical heart would be next just because, although the stereotype may be wrong, when I think of animals you think of an inferior being and you think it's dirty."

Organ recipients also express great concern over the taking of another creature's life. Unlike the students, however, their responses inevitably track back to their current predicament: Is it better to sacrifice animals deliberately or to wait for a human being to die accidentally? In short, both sources of organs generate their own forms of guilt and responsibility, weighed in terms of the level of one's desperation and how one values different life-forms. Unlike students, however, recipients are more concerned with a natural order, so to speak, of human-animal difference, and the manner in which xenografts will alter who they themselves are. Recipients (and their intimates) are thus apt to think more carefully than students about the psychological and social consequences of such strange bodily meldings. After all, many recipients of human organs already struggle on a daily basis to make sense of the fact that their bodies now house parts from other human beings, and many go to great lengths to incorporate their donors as an integral component of their new private sense of self. In light of this, they perceive xenotransplantation as triggering even more troubling existential crises than do allographs or organs of human origin.

A key anxiety concerns the dangers associated with taking on the characteristics of the creature whose organ might be implanted within one's body. Sid Rodke, a forty-two-year-old Euro-American man whose brother had received a cadaveric kidney two years earlier, put it thus: "If all worked equally well, I wouldn't care. Though it would be a little strange to have a baboon heart. Would I start baring my teeth and bottom?" Howard Turner, a fifty-six-year-old Euro-American liver recipient, joked in a support group meeting, "Imagine that: maybe we'd all be grunting and rooting around like pigs!"—a response that made two other recipients laugh so hard that it brought tears to their eyes.

A sentiment voiced repeatedly by recipients throughout the course of my research is the desire to avoid, whenever possible, the sense of alienation from one's own body; thus, animal sources are especially troubling in this regard. It is one thing to deny the origin of an organ from an anonymous human donor while still integrating it as part of oneself; it is altogether another to do so with a newly grafted part that came from a baboon or a pig. One possibility would be to embrace simians as our natural "cousins," or swine as so anatomically "similar" as to be indistinguishable from us. Although such sentiments dominate expressions of scientific and professional longing, I have yet to encounter any recipient comfortable with such ideas.

Most striking in this regard are responses offered specifically by African Americans.[14] Whereas all recipients are uneasy about integrating nonhuman parts into their bodies, African Americans more readily underscore the dangers associated specifically with human and animal experimentation. As a result, the majority I have interviewed typically display more visceral and even angry responses to the mention of xenographs. Arnie Popper, a man who was in his forties when I met him in 1992 during the Los Angeles Transplant Games, had received a kidney transplant four years previously and was now on the waiting list for a second. A large and muscular man, he had won a medal the day before in the men's shot put competition. As he put it, "My kidney's not a very good one, though, and so I'm back on the waiting list hoping I'll get another one. The one I have has scar tissue in it and it doesn't work well. But they put it in me anyway. I had been on dialysis for [nearly two years]." As the son of a biochemistry professor, Arnie found the subject of xenotransplantation especially intriguing, explaining his stance as follows: "I prefer not to kill animals. It's better to harvest organs that don't kill life. It reminds me too much of the experiments in *Planet of the Apes*. Do you remember that? Remember how the humans were kept in cages and the apes experimented on them? This is the same thing but the other way around. I don't think it's right."

In 1997, during another transplant event, I shared a lunch table with two men, both of whom were kidney recipients from the same hospital in Washington, D.C. When I asked Joe Dillon, an African American man in his forties, if he would be willing to accept an organ from a baboon or a pig, he replied immediately and emphatically, "No!" When his friend Russell Arnold, a Euro-American man ten years his junior, insisted that Joe's stance was illogical, Joe put down his fork, leaned over to me, and said: "Look, I already have enough trouble knowing who I am normally; I don't need something like this in my life. It would be too complicated. . . . It's unnatural. I don't really know why I don't like the idea, but it just doesn't feel right. . . . I don't want animal parts in me. If I had them, I wouldn't tell anyone." Both Arnie and Joe emphasize the strangeness of such hybrid couplings, where xenotransplantation is inherently undignified and debases one's human qualities. Echoing the responses of many recipients, they underscore the troublesome quality of boundary breakdowns. The critiques offered by Arnie and Joe expose in turn an especially strong sense of the unnatural dangers associated with the melding of human and animal bodies. Both men nevertheless present a clearer vision of the ethical dilemmas surrounding experimentation than do the majority of Euro-American recipients whom I encounter.

These two men's responses are certainly shaped by quotidian experiences with racism, as well as a pronounced familiarity with the unequal distribution of quality health care in America. This issue of equity is a source of widespread concern for transplant and procurement professionals, who, on the one hand, strive to refine organ distribution policies, yet who nevertheless may seem clueless when approaching patients whose backgrounds are radically different from their own (Sharp 2002). Structural problems inherent in our society affect minorities in specialized ways (Baker 1999; McGary 1999), rendering African Americans particularly suspicious of pronouncements of brain death (Stell 1999). African American research participants also regularly sense that they occupy the bottom portion of the nation's waiting lists for kidneys because of long-term practices that, until very recently, have privileged histocompatibility and, thus, essentially racial matching between donors and recipients (Davidson and Devney 1991; Hall et al. 1991; Johannes 2004; Roberts 1988). African Americans are also apt to be wary of human experimentation, their resistance due in part to their knowledge of the appalling Tuskegee syphilis experiments that spanned 1930–73 (Jones 1981; Reverby 2000; Sharp in press [a]). In turn, little funding may be available for ailments specific to this population (Rouse forthcoming; Wailoo 2001). Finally, as Joe Dillon's terse response makes all too clear, men such as he are keenly aware of the deep psychological and social damage caused by comparing dark-skinned people to animals. I offer these reflections, first, to underscore that African American informants regularly offer more sophisticated insights into the ethical dangers of transpecies grafting and, second, to inspire other researchers to delve deeper into the relevance of race to conversations about hybridity and, more broadly, experimental transplant research.

Among recipients as a more general social category, there appears to be little hope at present, at least, for newly invented forms of sociality with baboons or pigs. How are future patients to maintain a strong sense of self when their transformations or "rebirths" are owed to a foreign species? Although I can only hypothesize here, perhaps professionals believe that recipients will regard animal parts as so foreign that they will dispense with current attempts to cross the guarded divide of donor anonymity to establish kinship ties with surviving donor kin. I wonder, though, too, about the shame and embarrassment that at least the first generation of recipients might experience when their bodies successfully integrate, on an immunological level, simian or porcine parts (cf. Clark 1999). Clues about potential social and psychological resistance to xenotransplantation might lie in some patients' responses to the current use of pig heart valve implants. Cardiologists report that observant Jewish and Muslim patients regularly seek counseling from their religious leaders before accepting such implants, and I find that patients of an array of backgrounds more typically leave out references to pig origins when speaking of their valve surgeries. Full organs from other species will inevitably engender objections among an even wider array of patients. Animal parts unquestionably raise concerns about monstrous couplings with human bodies: simian species because, although considered inferior creatures, they are too close for comfort, and pigs because they are not human enough.

NATURE'S BODY

In 1991, the year I began my research, Donna Haraway argued in *Simians, Cyborgs and Women: The Reinvention of Nature* that practices inherent in late twentieth-century capitalist medicine were characterized by "critical boundary breakdowns" that bore great potential for reshaping humanity. Emergent forms of hybridity included "intensified machine-body relations"; in yet other contexts, boundaries "between human and animal" were "thoroughly breached" (Haraway 1991b: 151, 171). In the face of widespread concerns over the morality of such couplings, Haraway urged her readers instead to celebrate certain hybrid bodies as bearing remarkable potential for subverting entrenched forms of social oppression. Such celebrations are indeed widespread in the realm of transplant medicine, although enthusiasm for hybridity is hardly uniform. Ambivalence reigns in many quarters, even among those who favor at least one of these dominant hybrid possibilities. As the data presented within this chapter reveal, professional and lay opinions concerning implants of mechanical versus mammalian origin exhibit a range of preferences and fears. Hybridity is, ultimately, disturbing; yet, as ethicist Leon Kass emphasizes, there is often "wisdom [in] repugnance" (1998). Sentiments are shaped by the manner in which involved parties imagine and value nature and the ability of millennial medicine to define what is natural while it refashions the human body.

The concept of "nature," writes Kate Soper, bears a host of meanings in our culture, "yet . . . its complexity is concealed by the ease and regularity with which we put it to use" (1995: 1). Attempts to define nature, and related questions over what is "natural," frequently degenerate into dualistic models and even polemical disputes. Within American cultural contexts, contrasts are drawn regularly between human and inhuman, humanity and animality, and natural and artifice, and even nature itself may be broken down into categories of "friend or foe." In attempts to assign qualities to *human* nature, we regularly assert our uniqueness as a species, where the world's inhabitants (be they human or animal) fall into contrasting categories of self/same and other/different. Nonhuman species are ultimately valued in terms of their evolutionary proximity to human beings (Soper 1995).

This tendency to adopt dualistic modes of thinking about the world is most certainly at work within the curious realm of organ transfer. Of particular interest to me is that all involved parties are committed on some level to guarding the boundaries of the human body. A range of discrete groups, including laboratory scientists, ethicists and other theorists, transplant professionals, and organ recipients, all grapple with the pragmatic and moral consequences of human hybridity, yet they vary widely in the definitions they offer for what is inherently natural or unnatural about experimental transplant medicine. With careful probing, it becomes clear that clinical settings are particularly troubled by such conflicts. Whereas transplant professionals invest great hope in transgenic species, the very individuals whose bodies might one day incorporate grafts of nonhuman origin express a range of anxieties over such imagined couplings. It is one thing to celebrate, on an abstract level, the transformative possibilities engendered by such wildly experimental hybrid forms; it is altogether another to accept unquestionably the breaching of the boundaries of one's own body.

Bodies Familiar and Strange

All involved parties recognize on some level the debasing qualities of implanting mechanical or animal parts in the bodies of human beings. The question of what, precisely, is being debased is answered very differently according to one's level of involvement with organ transfer. Ethicists, immunologists, and social scientists who specifically challenge current experimental initiatives argue passionately for the need to guard species integrity, flagging the dangers that may well arise when one deliberately tampers with an assumed natural, evolutionary progression. Such critics view scientific tampering as a form of reckless hubris that not only threatens the assumed delicate balance of nature but also debases us as a species. Within this framework, we, as human beings, are so intent on change that we might well destroy ourselves in the process. Still others within these same disciplinary camps celebrate current experimental efforts as evidence of human ingenuity. The uniqueness of our species is marked by our ability to transform nature and, in the process, either save or radically improve the lives of those who suffer terribly from the consequences of organ failure. As such advocates argue, the decision to abort current research initiatives is cowardly, shortsighted, and heartless. Our failure to utilize scientific findings to alleviate suffering ultimately debases us as inhumane creatures.

Unlike laboratory scientists and moral theorists, transplant professionals are more unified in their responses. Those engaged in developing new mechanical devices most certainly invest their greatest hopes in these prototypes; overall, however, the majority share the opinion of many laboratory researchers that xenografts are superior to machines. These same transplant professionals are nevertheless preoccupied with altogether different concerns that ultimately shape their preferences. As specialists who work directly and daily with organ recipients, they often must make concerted efforts to uncouple patients from machines. As a result, xenotransplantation garners greater support within these ranks; it bears the promise of granting patients autonomy by freeing them from the dehumanizing effects of technological dependence.

Transplant professionals consider xenografts inherently natural because their origins can be traced to mammalian bodies. These same professionals also value the simplicity and natural elegance embedded in corporal origins, in contrast to the clumsiness they associate with bulky machines. Organs of animal origin—as flesh and blood—are understood as offering far better solutions than do, say, battery-operated hydraulic pumps fashioned from titanium and polyurethane plastic (CHFpatients.com 2004; Rowland 2001).[15] The naturalization of the chimera in laboratory settings similarly heralds the possibility that, in the near future, xenografts can be so carefully disguised immunologically as to be recognized as "self" by the host recipient body, rendering immunosuppressants unnecessary.[16] These are truly wondrous dreams.

Recipients, however, do not share such visions. Instead, when patients imagine themselves as the potential recipients of experimental grafts, they reject xenotransplantation in favor of mechanical implants. As they embrace the mechanical, recipients subvert professionals' understandings of the natural. Although they, too, long for a potentially unlimited supply of replacement organs, recipients favor those of flesh and blood, as long as they are of human origin. Recipients recoil from the possibilities borne by xenografts, expressing various levels of discomfort (ranging from puzzlement to disgust) when asked to consider melding their own bodies with parts derived from animals. The beauty of the mechanical solution is that it is fully inert and, thus, devoid of any origin, save for the medical engineer's laboratory. A mechanical implant has never been harbored in another body, and thus it bears an aura of purity. Finally, the crises that engender new forms of sociality with once living donors make no sense here. Thus, mechanical prototypes bear an altogether different promise unimagined by transplant professionals and researchers: one day, recipients might incorporate artificial parts and be done with the agony of knowing that their own lives are so heavily dependent on the deaths of strangers.

The Debasement of Humanity

In a comparative project that explores American versus cosmopolitan Greek reactions to xenotransplantation, Eleni Papagaroufali exposes an American commitment to the preeminence of humans within a species hierarchy. As she explains, Americans regularly assert their place within nature as framed by a model of evolutionary progression, and this ultimately shapes how we respond to other species. Greeks, on the other hand, express little interest in dominating nature; instead, Greek identity is strongly Hellenocentric and it is one's Greek heritage that defines one as quintessentially human. Thus, whereas Americans are most concerned with their biological origins, Greeks think in terms of their cultural history. In addition, Greeks do not share the American fascination for simian species. Chimpanzees, for instance, are not regarded as "close cousins" of human beings but, rather, as truly exotic creatures whom many Greeks have never even viewed, in the wild, in zoos, or in laboratories (Papagaroufali 1996). Americans, Papagaroufali continues, are also deeply committed to what others label the technological imperative (Brodwin 2000a; Davis-Floyd 1994; Koenig 1988; Lock, Young, and Cambrosio 2000; M. Lynch and Woolgar 1990; Volti 1995). In reference to xenotransplantation, she is struck especially by how readily Americans embrace biotechnological answers as solutions to human suffering. Greeks, in contrast, are far less committed to this paradigm, given that their nation remains peripheral to the scientific realm, one whose values are otherwise deeply entrenched in American society. As a result, Greeks care far less about dominating, harnessing, or transforming nature; they are more concerned with guarding the completeness specifically of the Greek body (Papagaroufali 1996).

A shortcoming of Papagaroufali's argument is that it glosses over variations in opinion within the American context (and perhaps the Greek one, too) that ultimately uncover a wider range of cultural interpretations of human hybridity. For instance, whereas Papagaroufali chooses to limit Greek sentiments to those expressed by cosmopolitans, Americans are inevitably lumped into one category. A nagging suspicion that dogged my work as I surveyed midwestern undergraduates was that perhaps at least some students' responses would be shaped by the fact that the university where I taught lay within the Bible Belt. Furthermore, the city itself was surrounded by expansive farms (some of which raised hogs) from which some students hailed. Although a significant proportion of students were deeply religious Protestants (a number of whom rejected a Darwinian model of evolution), this appeared to have little effect on how they did in fact respond overall to the possibility of melding parts from apes and monkeys with their own bodies. Papagaroufali's comparative insights are helpful nevertheless because they expose American transplant professionals' deep-seated (and often unquestioned) commitment to experimental nonhuman species and technological innovations as logical solutions to the nation's transplant crisis.

As my data reveal, the sentiments toward—and the values assigned to—nature are indeed multifaceted within the American context. Laboratory scientists, ethicists and other theorists, transplant professionals, and recipients frame the promises and dangers of hybridity in radically different terms. Whereas researchers' actions are driven by a deep commitment to enhance medicine by transforming the human body, transplant professionals' arguments seem driven by a Marxian logic of sorts, where the human, in embodying technology, literally succumbs to and thus risks becoming the machine itself. These professionals thus recoil from such body enhancements because they ultimately herald artificiality. Not so with recipients, for whom mechanical forms of body melding might once and for all seal the body's boundaries and eliminate the current dependency on fleshy parts that bear the weight of too much history.

A Strangely Disordered World

The experimental territory of organ transfer heralds truly unusual dangers. The language of risk employed by those who oppose xenotransplantation on moral grounds underscores the already permeable quality of our bodies' boundaries (Martin 1994). Transplanted, transpecies organs thus define an immunological Trojan horse of sorts: implanted willfully in individual bodies, they nevertheless bear the potential for wreaking havoc on patients, on their intimates and communities, and even on our species as a whole. Such nightmarish visions expose collective fears of the perils of a "world out of balance" (Garrett 1994; cf. Lindenbaum 2001), where porcine bodies and their parts appear particularly menacing.

Alongside such global concerns lie murkier, private responses that lead recipients to reject swine as the postmillennial solution to our nation's organ crisis. Indeed, all parties struggle to articulate why they find particular forms of hybridity more repulsive than others; pigs nevertheless inspire the most pronounced, visceral responses among those whose bodies may ultimately be melded with them. This repulsion is rooted, argues Papagaroufali, in the struggle to "subordin[ate] the 'other' to the same.' When the 'other' is 'altered,' 'developed,' 'domesticated,' 'protected,' even 'received' into one's own body—so as to become same/familiar—something else is excluded, evaluated as not natural/familiar/same" (1996: 251). In essence, when organs are made of flesh and blood, recipients find it impossible to forget where they came from. This is especially evident in the forceful responses offered by African American research participants, who refuse to embrace celebrations of human-animal hybrid forms. Such boundary crossings are unnatural because they resonate all too clearly with racist threats in other spheres of daily life. Others likewise guard bodily integrity on the grounds that new experiments might well jar our humanity or deeply private sense of self.

My fear is that, in learning of such responses, some readers (particularly transplant professionals) might well interpret these as still another set of irrational behaviors that warrant educational campaigns to instill reform. Yet as Mary Douglas argued so long ago, our talk of contamination, impurity, and filth out of place provides valuable clues for understanding a critical (that is, comprehensive) view of the world and how we think it should in fact be ordered. Embedded in the language of risk lies a profound cultural wisdom concerning how we distinguish ourselves as humans from those creatures we currently study, nurture, farm, butcher, and eat (Douglas 1966, 1970; Douglas and Wildavsky 1982; cf. Kass 1998).

CONCLUSION

And so I end with this aversion to monsters or, perhaps more appropriately put, the fear of becoming a monster. The intertwined themes of strangeness, monstrousness, and hybridity are indeed central to shaping current reactions to the imagined possibilities borne by xenotransplantation as an emerging, experimental biotechnology. It is too early to determine the fate of this experimental realm, given that it currently inspires repugnance in some quarters. Only a few years ago, for instance, the head of the patent office in England raged, "There will be no patents on monsters, at least while I am commissioner!" (Clark 1999: 143). In response, Margaret Clark urges us to consider that xenotransplantation "may tap deep emotions that no one really understands. Mythologies of all cultures are full of creatures who are part human, part animal. . . . Sharing a body with another being is not in our experience" (140). We have yet to witness the fate of such peculiar hybrid solutions whose dangers lie in the ease with which they denature human bodies.

Epilogue

The researcher who endeavors to study organ transfer in America must accept and even anticipate the inevitability of change. The surgical replacement of organs requires radical forms of medical intervention, where extraordinarily complex clinical skills undergo constant refinement. A single visit to any relevant professional conference quickly reveals that surgeons and related medical personnel are driven by a persistent desire to perfect their craft. Recent innovations include, for instance, graceful sternal retractors that lock into position like the quick release of a bicycle wheel, a design that eliminates the need for more than one set of hands; the perfection of laparoscopic nephrectomy, such that surgeons can now harvest donor kidneys more rapidly than is possible through older, standard surgical techniques; and a range of still other devices that can be slipped into, around, and over the body's cavities, arteries, and organs to sustain, correct, or subvert their purpose and function. Pharmaceutical corporations in turn compete fiercely to produce and market new immunosuppressants that replace those that now qualify as generic drugs. Alongside such developments, medical professionals at some transplant centers hope to wean their patients altogether from their hefty (and exorbitantly expensive) drug regimens.

The social marketing of organ transfer defines yet another domain of change and innovation: labels, rhetorical phrases, and attitudes shift every few years as procurement professionals rethink strategies designed to encourage a hesitant public to embrace organ donation as an important, compassionate endeavor. Even the criteria that determine whether one qualifies as a donor shift over time, such that "extended" or "marginal" markers of the sociomedical worth of dead and dying patients rapidly assume ordinary status. The terminology employed—including the corporate names of OPOs, the expressions for procurement and bereavement work, or the descriptives applied to donors and their body parts—changes regularly. For the ethnographer set on accurately recording techniques, behaviors, and beliefs, there can be no sense of an ethnographic present—that is, any attempt to offer representative, yet ultimately ahistorical description (Clifford 1988: 31–32), remains futile.

In 1992, Renée Fox and Judith Swazey concluded their remarkable book *Spare Parts* by publicly declaring their decision to leave this field of study. Fox and Swazey were already seasoned fieldworkers, having published several other related, groundbreaking works that together encompassed more than three decades of involvement (Fox 1959; Fox and Swazey 1978, 1992). They had, by this point, tracked the history of surgical innovation from the onset of kidney transplants in the 1950s through the experimental trials with the artificial Jarvik-7 heart in the 1980s. Their reasons for ending their work included the following:

> Our decision to leave the field has been a complex one and a long time in the making. Over the past decade or so, we gradually recognized in ourselves the signs and symptoms of what we diagnosed as "participant-observer burnout"—akin to what we have witnessed over the years in some of the medical professionals immersed in the world of organ replacement efforts. Our burnout has its roots in the fact that there have been aspects of these efforts that we always have found especially troubling. Prominent among them have been some components of the "courage to fail" value system prevalent among transplantation and artificial organ pioneers. This ethos includes a classically American frontier outlook: heroic, pioneering, adventurous, optimistic, and determined. It also involves, however, a bellicose, "death is the enemy" perspective; a rescue-oriented and often zealous determination to maintain life at any cost; and a relentless, hubris-ridden refusal to accept limits. It is disturbing to witness, over and over, the travail and distress to which this outlook can subject patients. (Fox and Swazey 1992: 199)

I suspect that over time I might well experience similar fatigue. The problems identified by these authors persist and have even intensified since the early 1990s. If we expand the field to include the full range of activities that define organ transfer, we encounter still other developments that challenge the researcher's ability to maintain the impartiality assumed central to ethnographic inquiry. Work of this sort is frequently emotionally draining, too, and requires at least temporary withdrawal from time to time. Organ transfer is indisputably a life-and-death matter, and all involved parties— be they transplant personnel, organ recipients, OPO employees, or donor kin—have borne witness to the untimely deaths of intimates and strangers.

Also troubling are the ethics of the work involved, as the criteria for declaring death are expanded, and as larger pools of patients—extending from newborns to the aged—qualify for either recipient or donor status. Of particular concern for me is the escalation of organ scarcity anxiety and its consequences.

I have profited from resources that were not readily available to Fox and Swazey when they officially declared their departure. Among the more helpful developments has been a growing interest in the intersection between anthropology and bioethics, in which Fox herself has played a significant role. Another, related trajectory has been the assertion voiced by some practicing anthropologists that we should challenge dominant yet dangerous clinical assumptions and insist on radical change (Brodwin 2000a; Crigger 1995; Hoffmaster 1992; Illich 1976; Kleinman, Fox, and Brandt 1999; Koenig 1988; Kunstadter 1980; Lock 1997, 2001, 2003; Marshall 1992; Marshall and Koenig 1996; Muller 1994; Scheper-Hughes 1995; Sharp 2002a; Slomka 1995). It is, in fact, difficult to dodge requests from those most intimately involved with organ transfer for personal reflections, advice, and even, sometimes, criticism. Over time, I have learned to temper my own concerns such that I might help identify, redirect, or alter some of the more disturbing practices I encounter (Sharp 1999, 2000a, 2000b, 2001, 2002b).

Yet another consequence of long-term research is a desire to anticipate the future trajectory of organ transfer. Already, youthful (and alive) organ donors are being recruited from among the ranks of healthy kin to supply kidneys to ailing grandparents (Kaufman, Russ, and Shim 2006); a semi-clandestine market in body parts, culled from the living, now defines a crisis (L. Cohen 1999; Scheper-Hughes 1998a, 1998b); and, simultaneously, professionals now openly propose a range of incentives that could encourage the most desperate to sell parts of themselves legally for cash or for other essential goods and services in nations where such practices are currently illegal and are considered unethical (AMA 2003; Arnold et al. 2002; Delmonico et al. 2002; Goldberg 2003; Radcliffe-Richards et al. 1998). Such current realities expose the fact that the bedrock of an assumed gift economy has already eroded. A shared clinical and lay commitment to saving and extending lives, at any cost, means that we are quick to accept organ replacement as a legitimate medical right rather than, as I argue at various junctures within this book, a strangely wondrous corner of American life.

An intriguing (and, simultaneously, perplexing) development involves the search for nonhuman alternatives as sources that might extend human life without relying on the deaths of or injuries to other human beings. I have watched, for instance, attempts at xenotransplantation shift from renegade and even fantasy status to a seriously considered alternative within laboratories and during medical conferences. Xenotransplantation now competes neck and neck with mechanical prototypes, and the competition is fierce, particularly in response to desires to replace entire organs. As I write this, experts in transgenic research have set their sights squarely on the liver as a patch of experimental terrain they might declare as their own, fully aware that biomechanical expertise is currently most interested in heart replacement. The fact that at least one recipient has survived comfortably for more than five years with a fully portable heart assist device spurs the activities of specialists focused on human alternatives. There is, nevertheless, surprisingly little written from the perspective of patients who must endure the trials associated with often horrifically painful procedures, not to mention the short- and long-term social consequences of serving as an experimental object (see Bea 2003; Clark 1999; Fox and Swazey 1992; Houghton 2001).

Amid this clamor for new sources of replacement parts, I am fascinated by the assumptions that drive such concerns, as well as the sociomedical consequences of an ethos that insists on further perfecting the human organism. Nevertheless, there are many other moments when I wonder why we seem so reluctant to accept death as a natural consequence of life. The answers can be found, of course, in the very data culled for the purposes of this study: so many of us long for a second chance, which is why transplantation is so widely conceived of as a form of rebirth. Still others, now faced with horrific, tragic personal losses, embrace the opportunity to rebalance the world and, perhaps, even witness the effects of the transmigration of human body parts.

In concluding this study, then, I am tempted to offer predictions of organ transfer's experimental future. Instead, I close on this note: medicine is fully committed to full-scale organ replacement as a means for extending human life. Furthermore, technical expertise will most certainly experience further refinement. I cannot say whether an incessant longing for replacement parts will find its answer in expanded criteria for human donor pools, the organogenesis of full organs from cell cultures, the genetic transformation of nonhuman species, or the invention of finely tuned mechanical prototypes. My fear, as an anthropologist alert to socioethical concerns, is that we may be so captivated by seemingly miraculous pursuits that we disregard or discredit the associated social dangers. As I illustrate throughout this book, the practices that define organ transfer in this country are directed by a powerful ethos, one dominated nevertheless by a set of paradoxical premises. Practicing anthropologists and researchers from related fields would do well to focus squarely on the anxieties surrounding innovation if we are to offer productive counsel in a medical realm so wondrous and so strange.

Notes

1. To avoid the tedium that accompanies the repetition of the expression "in the United States," I have opted to speak at times of "American" transplant trends. I trust that readers will forgive me for using this to the exclusion of other nations in the Americas; it is not an ethnocentric slip but rather is a convenient stylistic choice.

2. For work on living related kidney donors in Mexico, see Crowley-Matoka (in press).

3. A danger associated with the long-term consequences of living donation is that living donors have no second, or backup, kidney, should they themselves suffer from kidney failure later in life. In response, a national policy currently in place (and employed by the United Network for Organ Sharing [UNOS]) is that those who give kidneys to others when healthy should move to the top of the national waiting list if they themselves later require a kidney transplant.

In response to the scarcity associated with other organs, numerous transplant centers are now attempting to perfect the transfer of single lungs and sectioned livers from living donors to patients experiencing organ failure. Most frequently these surgeries involve transfers from parents to their children. These procedures are far more complicated (and thus life-threatening) for both donor and recipient than are living kidney donations. For more details, see Barr et al. (1998); Kirchner (1991); Mack et al. (2001); Miller et al. (2001).

4. L. Cohen (1999); Marshall, Thomasma, and Daar (1996); Rothman et al. (1997); Rothman (1998); Scheper-Hughes (1996, 1998b, 1998c, 2000).

5. In this sense, at least, cadaveric donation bears some similarity to adoptees' searches for their birth mothers. I will explore this theme in chapter 3.

6. For discussions of the cultural relevance of visual technologies, readers should consult the following: Cartwright (1992, 1995); Downey (1992); Dumit (1997); M. Lynch and Woolgar (1990); Petchesky (1987); Taylor (1998, 2005).

7. Rejection is a continuous process marked by immediate (acute) and long-term (chronic) forms that occur at the immunologic, histopathologic and vascu-

lar, and cellular levels. Responses to each of these range from a few hours to days or weeks following transplantation. Thus, patient well-being (and survival) is dependent on immunosuppressants, which recipients must take for the remainder of their lives (or for as long as they have their transplanted organs). Prior to the development of cyclosporine, patients could survive surgery, but the vast majority would die within a few weeks. Today, transplant recipients are in a constant state of rejection, a state managed through the expert administration of powerful pharmaceuticals. A lively folklore circulates among recipients about patients who have stopped their medications without telling their doctors. Some transplant centers are now experimenting with weaning long-term patients from their drug regimens. A current goal is to eliminate dependence on steroids and then, hopefully someday, immunosuppressants, too.

8. The European countries included in these surveys were Austria, Belgium, Luxembourg, Denmark, Czech Republic, Finland, France, Germany, Greece, Hungary, Italy, Netherlands, Norway, Poland, Portugal, Spain, Sweden, Switzerland, the United Kingdom, and Ireland.

9. Here I refer only to the legal offering of a kidney; as explained by a colleague who worked in a specialized transplant ward that typically serviced patients of international origins, patients would sometimes arrive from abroad with a supposed close relative in tow as a donor. At times transplant staff suspected that the donor was only posing as such and was being paid for the kidney. Staff found it impossible to verify this, however, and typically proceeded with the surgery.

10. See www.unos.org (consulted October 13, 2003).

11. For various proposals concerning donor incentives, see AMA (2003); Arnold et al. (2002); Buxton (1997); Goldberg (2003). For critiques, see AMA (2003); Delmonico et al. (2002); Joralemon and Cox (2003); Siminoff and Leonard (1999). For an earlier rendering of recommendations published in the *Journal of the American Medical Association,* see Peters (1991); also Prottas (1992).

12. Pennsylvania Department of Health and Human Services, personal communication, October 2003.

13. Traffic fatality figures for the year 2002 for America's youth read as follows: for auto fatalities, ages 16–20 account for just under 20 percent and ages 0–20 as a whole for just under 24 percent of a total of 20,416 deaths. Contrary to assumptions expressed by procurement professionals, the largest number of motorcycle fatalities occur in the 25–54 age bracket; nevertheless, ages 0–20 also account for approximately 19 percent of a total of 3,244 deaths. Ages 0–20 account for nearly 27 percent of a total of 444 bicycle fatalities (U.S. Department of Transportation 2002). Recent drops in road fatalities among America's young have had a direct effect on the size of the organ donor pool (Perez-Pena 2003).

14. Rafael Matesanz, in describing the "Spanish model" and its relevance to other programs that replicate its approaches, writes, however, that "Spain theoretically has a presumed consent law, but from a practical point of view, fam-

ily consent is always solicited, and the wishes of the relatives are always respected, as it is practised in almost all EU countries" (2003: 737–38). See also Michelsen (1991) on Belgium.

15. Remarkably, even brain death criteria work this way, for the diagnostic tests applied to potential donors vary not only from state to state but even among hospitals located in the same city. I will return to this later.

16. As Reynolds (2005) reports, in the 1980s the number was even lower, with the upper age limit set around sixty years.

17. This procedure is sometimes referred to as the Cleveland Protocol because it was initially conceived of by the Cleveland Clinic in partnership with the local procurement agency LifeBanc; elsewhere it is called the Pittsburgh Protocol because it is now in use at this location, which stands as one of the largest—and most prestigious—transplant centers in the country.

18. I have encountered one instance where a handful of staff members in one procurement office were said to have offered as an incentive partial funeral cost compensation to a few donor families. They were later fired from their jobs under a new director who was brought in to clean house. Based on the repugnance procurement staff show for blatant forms of body commodification, I believe this is an isolated incident. More publicized examples involve the transmission of undetected infections of HIV, West Nile virus, and rabies from deceased donors to organ and tissue recipients (Altman 1991; AP 2004b; Iwamoto 2003). I will discuss this in more detail in chapter 4.

19. In fact, a few years ago a kidney was offered for sale on eBay; within a few hours it had generated offers of more than a million dollars. It later turned out to be a hoax.

20. See, for instance, Crigger (1995); Hoffmaster (1992); Kleinman (1999); Kunstadter (1980); Marshall (1992); Marshall and Koenig (1996); Muller (1994); Sharp (2000b).

21. An entirely different picture emerges on the international front. For a chilling account of the merging of fiction (or film) with the realities of global kidney trafficking, see Scheper-Hughes (2004).

22. It thus strikes me as a humorous coincidence that I now teach at Barnard College.

23. Maman'i'Annie was also a truly great *bavarde;* she died from congestive heart failure during the year in which I was writing this book. Transplantation was never even a remote possibility for her in Madagascar, although under radically different circumstances in the United States this might very well have prolonged her wonderfully rich life. I dedicate this chapter in her memory.

24. These were the Annual Meeting of the North American Transplant Coordinators Organization (NATCO) in Boston, Massachusetts (1995); the First International Symposium on Transplant Recipient Compliance in Arlington, Virginia (1998); and the Eighth Annual National Kidney Foundation Clinical Nephrology Meetings in Washington, D.C. (1999).

1. WE ARE THE DEAD MEN

I wish to note that the poetry of T. S. Eliot inspired the title for this chapter.

1. The art of distinguishing the brain from the mind is a tricky affair: neurologists, for instance, may draw little if any distinction between the two and may rarely use the term *mind* at all. Some, such as Antonio Damasio, equate mind with consciousness and emotions, stressing nevertheless that both are inevitably rooted in the organic neurological complex known as the brain (Damasio 1999; Plum and Posner 1966). Cognitive psychologists are similarly most concerned with brain function as evidence of mind. Within psychoanalysis (as rooted especially in the Freudian paradigm), the mind presumes an elevated status in the study of conscious versus unconscious action and thought, such that the brain disappears altogether. As a medical anthropologist I am especially taken with the manner in which the categories of brain and mind play off one another within the realm of organ transfer. As will become clear throughout this chapter, in organ transfer the brain is understood as a complex organ whose dysfunction proves destructive to both bodily functions and the social and emotional attributes that define who we are. To preserve the distinction between the organic and abstract aspects of our selves, I employ *brain* to refer to the organ itself, whereas I associate *mind* (which is recognized in organ transfer as dwelling within the brain) with social personhood and the private self or psyche. The mind, then, should be understood within this study as encompassing the abstract, symbolic aspects of our selves: our emotions, thoughts, dreams, tastes, and desires. If the brain keeps us alive and human, it is the mind that allows others to sense us as unique persons who can be loved and mourned by others.

2. Events include the biannual Transplant Olympic Games, held in various cities within the United States; celebratory affairs hosted by transplant units and hospitals; and annual commemorative services staged primarily by OPOs that honor a region's donors for that year. I will discuss the significance of such events in greater detail in chapters 2 and 3.

3. Readers interested in more detailed accounts should see HMS and Beecher (1968); Annas (1983); Cowan et al. (1987); Fox and Swazey (1978, 1992); *Life* (1967); Lock (2002); Plough (1986); Rothman (1991); and Starzl (1992).

4. For a systematic review of amendments and drafted revisions, see CUSL 1988.

5. Cyclosporine's success is marked by the fact that it has remained the immunosuppressant of choice for more than a decade, although now an array of other drugs—from established to experimental—are regularly prescribed instead for transplant recipients.

6. For more details, see the Web site maintained by the Department of Health and Human Services: organdonor.gov/opo.htm (consulted February 22, 2004).

7. See www.aopo.org (consulted February 22, 2004).

8. Whereas long-standing federal legislation renders it illegal to commod-

ify organs (that is, buy and sell them for profit), human tissues are exempt from such restrictions. Thus, bone, skin, corneas, and a range of other body parts define highly profitable commodities in the United States, as do the cadavers and body parts that individuals have willed for medical research purposes. For a succinct and lively treatment of this topic, see Roach (2003); recent exposés include AP (2004a), Broder (2004), Cheney (2004), Newman (2004), and Saranow (2003). An even more troubling and recent trend in the United States involves relying increasingly on *any* living donors rather than only on living *related* donors, especially for kidney transplants. A concern voiced (albeit quietly) by some physicians I have encountered who are involved with such surgeries is that some of their wealthy patients in the United States may in fact be paying members of the underclass, or employees beholden to them, to provide kidneys. It is unclear to what extent this may already be an established practice in this country, and thus it warrants careful investigation by future researchers (Rohter 2004).

9. Sources here include www.unos.org/helpSaveALife (consulted April 22, 2004), as well as a fact sheet prepared by the Musculoskeletal Transplant Foundation (acquired May 2004). Others have gone so far as to place the number at 150, a figure often cited by speakers at transplant events. My sense is this larger number of parts hinges on the number of body repair procedures involved, as well as the breakdown of categories (e.g., specific bones or tendons rather than listing these generally).

10. The realm of procurement is rife with references to life, not death. UNOS's current slogan, for instance, is "Donate Life," and a range of OPOs and tissue banks have adopted such names as LifeCenter (in both Alabama and Washington), Life Choice (Connecticut), Gift of Life (Delaware and Michigan), Life Link, Life Alliance, TransLife, and LifeQuest (Florida), LifeCenter (Idaho), LifeSource (Minnesota), LifeShare (North Carolina), LifeNet (Virginia), LifeBanc, Life Connection, and Lifeline (Ohio).

11. Much has been written on the reasons for why kin refuse to consent to donation, an issue I will address in greater detail later. The reasons most commonly cited by staff within this OPO were "religious beliefs" and "distrust of the medical system." For more detailed discussions of these themes, see DeJong et al. (1998); Etienne et al. 1991; Ford and Smith (1991); Franz et al. (1997); Hessing and Elfers (1986–87); Lewis and Snell (1986); Parisi and Katz (1986); Pearson et al. (1995); Portmann (1999); and Sanner (1994).

12. Coded language and derogatory slang are very much a part of emergency medical work; again, see Coombs et al. (1993).

13. There is no mention of the hardships that many organ recipients endure after transplant. These include complications stemming from surgery, mild and severe forms of organ rejection, and a lifetime course of potent immunosuppressants and steroids, alongside a host of other medications designed to counteract many of the side effects of the other two categories of drugs. Transplant recipients live in a constant state of rejection and suffer the serious consequences of long-term immunosuppressant and steroid use, ranging from rare cancers to painful osteoporosis. In addition, some of the standard medications

they take are toxic to the kidneys and liver, though these may be the very organs they have acquired through transplantation. Organ recipients may also struggle to fend off infections that present only mild problems in individuals whose immune systems are not compromised. Posttransplant care is typically very expensive, and some recipients find they are unable to afford the medications necessary to keep them alive (which can cost the uninsured several thousand dollars per month). Many remain on disability for the rest of their lives, and they may suffer from depression because they had hoped to return to full-time employment after being healed. Also, divorce is not uncommon: a once supportive spouse, for instance, may feel he or she can move on now that the patient has survived surgery. In a word, the "medical miracle" of transplantation evolves into a long-term clinical, emotional, and/or financial nightmare for some recipients (House 1999; Sharp 1999).

14. J. Wace and M. Kai, for instance, writing as recently as 2000, described brain death as "unsurvivable coma" (Wace and Kai 2000).

15. This language is derived from the Uniform Determination of Death Act, which states that "the entire brain must cease to function, irreversibly," involving "the brain stem, as well as the neocortex" (CUSL 1980).

16. In addition to field interviews, I consulted the following written sources: Kerridge et al. (2002); Plum and Posner (1966); University of North Dakota (1998); Wijdicks (1995a); Wijnen and van der Linden (1991); P. Young and Matta (2000). I also wish to thank Dr. Z., a neurologist, who read this passage for errors. Any discrepancies that remain are my fault alone.

17. Noteworthy exceptions include LifeBanc (1994); LifeCenter Northwest (n.d.).

18. The Association of Organ Procurement Organizations (AOPO) has compiled an especially comprehensive list of "frequently asked questions" and their answers (www.aopo.org, consulted February 22, 2004). For a long list of religions and their official attitudes toward organ donation, see DCIDS (2004).

19. No pun (in reference to donors dying in car collisions) was intended here.

20. For an example of the unforeseen consequences of this policy, see Reynolds (2005). I will discuss this and related cases in more detail in chapter 4.

21. This passage is derived from www.aopo.org (consulted February 22, 2004). As noted earlier, tissue and blood samples are removed from the patient during the assessment period in the ICU. Also, interviews with surgical personnel confirm that the ventilator is turned off a bit earlier. I will address this last point and other discrepancies later.

22. Technically this is referred to as a "midline incision," made "from the suprasternal notch to the pubis" after which "the sternum is split" (Gelb and Robertson 1990: 807).

23. Surgeons first remove the heart and lungs, followed by the liver, then the kidneys and pancreas and, finally, tissue. The order is determined primarily by the length of time different organs remain viable, once they are no longer supplied with oxygenated blood, while being kept moist, cool, and sterile. Kidneys can survive the longest outside the body, their "life" extended even fur-

ther if connected to a mechanical filtering device designed specifically for this purpose.

24. For data sources, see Sharp (1994); www.unos.org (consulted May 3, 2004). These figures do not include living donors, of which there were an additional 3,102 in 1994 and 7,004 in 2004 (www.optn.org/latestData/npt.Data.asp, consulted July 8, 2005). In contrast, the United Kingdom witnessed a decline in cadaveric organ donors between 1991 and 1998 (with the exception of the year 1995) while the demand for organs (and number of surgeries) increased (Morgan 1999).

25. Most OPOs still speak of "the seven-organ donor" (two kidneys, two lungs, and one liver, heart, and pancreas). I have nevertheless encountered surgeons who stress that there are, in fact, nine transplants possible; these doctors include the large intestine, and they count the transected liver twice. The latter is possible because the liver is capable of regeneration and thus can be divided and shared by two patients.

26. The domino procedure involves transplanting a pair of lungs with a heart into a recipient who needs only a set of lungs. His or her diseased lungs are discarded and the removed, healthy heart is preserved so that it may be transplanted in another patient in need of a heart only (see the example in chapter 3). Some surgical teams prefer this technique because it proves easier than suturing a new set of lungs to an already existing heart.

27. As noted by William Ritchie in this same online discussion, these drugs were already being used by some procurement agencies, but "only after death has occurred," meaning after brain death was declared. Hogle (1999) reports this as well.

28. Thomas Starzl lobbied hard for the introduction of new DCD protocols in Pittsburgh.

29. In some states, designated donors must update their intent: in Arizona, for instance, licensed drivers must contact the division of motor vehicles and respecify their desire to be donors. Their license then becomes imprinted with a small heart. Some states, such as New York, have also instituted tissue and donor registries that accomplish the same goal.

30. My cousin Porter, whom I knew as an elderly, avuncular man, loved to recount tales from his experiences as an assistant to his stepfather, a mortician based in the Deep South. One of his favorite stories concerned a corpse that sat up spontaneously in the back of the hearse and appeared to stare at the two men in the front seat.

31. This fact was underscored, for instance, during an interview with Octavia Zamora, a procurement professional with long-term experience with Native American groups in the Southwest.

32. For a striking exception from Germany, see Hogle (1999: 166–67), where staff were repulsed by a surgeon's rough handling of a donor's body as he employed techniques more vulgar than even those characteristic of an autopsy.

33. For other ingenious (although still hypothetical) forms of human recycling, see T. Lynch (1997: 77–99); Roach (2003: chaps. 10 and 11).

34. I would like to thank a reviewer who read an earlier version of the manuscript for this observation.

35. In bioethics, see Andrews (1992); Bailey (1990); Blumstein (1992, 1993); Bowden and Hull (1993); Brecher (1994); Caplan (1992); Chadwick (1989); Childress (1992); Delmonico et al. (2002); Dossetor (1992); Hansmann (1989); Land and Dossetor (1991); Prottas (1992); Sells (1992); Siminoff and Leonard (1999);G. Smith (1993); Zutlevics (2001). Classics in science fiction include Cook (1977); Harrison (1964); and Niven (1968, 1980).

2. MEMORY WORK

1. Although as a rule I employ pseudonyms for many organizations throughout this study, LifeNet, NKF, NDFC, the Transplant Games, Transweb, TRIO, and UNOS are well-known, high-profile organizations or events in the realm of organ transfer, and so it is difficult to justify altering their names when speaking of their public memorial projects. I have nevertheless obscured the identities of employees, as is common practice in anthropology, and as I promised throughout my interviews.

2. For more information on the Donor Quilt, see www.kidney.org/recips/donor/quiltHistory.

3. I have found that recipients and professionals are unaware of the origins of the testimonial. The pervasiveness of this narrative form is, I believe, indicative of the mainstream use of language derived from twelve-step and other self-help groups and, as I illustrate later, of Christian testimonial forms of "witnessing" or declaring one's faith.

4. Only a handful of interviewees who follow other non-Christian faiths expressed distaste for the Christian overtones of transplant events. Their objections tended to focus on a heavy reliance on chaplains with Christian leanings who regularly serve as public speakers, and who invariably ask audience members to bow their heads in prayer. Another concern was the regular staging of donor services in church settings. As one informant, an older Jewish woman, reflected, however, Christian ideological principles and rituals are pervasive in American culture, and thus the task at hand is much larger than targeting transplant professionals. Yet another Buddhist informant, who herself is a chaplain with hospital and OPO experience, described her amazement upon returning from a meeting hosted by a local chapter of the American Red Cross. She found the religious references so pervasive that she assumed for some time afterward that it was a Christian-based organization. What such a reaction implies is that those who embrace other faiths, or who are put off by Christian references and rituals, may altogether avoid participating in the public realm of organ transfer.

5. For an additional ethnographic account of recipients' experiences with "the call" see Chillag (1997: 131–39).

6. For a personal account that details the battle to acquire health insurance that would pay for a heart transplant, see Bea (2003: 212–15).

7. This is not unusual: transplant professionals regularly speak of the necessity of donation to those who have already granted their consent. See Sharp (2002b).

8. For more information on TRIO, see www.Trioweb.org. This story is recounted in a speech delivered by Mary Reames, wife of Brian Reames, who together founded TRIO. See Reames (1997).

9. When I visited this site in June 2004, although it was nearly complete, heavy rains had delayed construction by several months, and the project was still short of its funding goal. My description here draws on firsthand observation, descriptions offered by UNOS staff directly involved with the project, and the virtual tour available on UNOS's Web site www.donormemorial.org (consulted May and June 2004). Unless stated otherwise, phrases in quotation marks are drawn from this source.

10. This was not functioning during my visit.

11. One reviewer who read an earlier version of this text asked what might be the effect of straying from the designated order of the tour and whether such an act might be viewed as subversive. It should be understood that there are no arrows or other markers designating how one should tour this site (although the online visual tour is more clear-cut in this regard). Instead, the architects appear to have left the space open to allow visitors to wander throughout as they please. The effect of doing so, however, is that one might miss the largely subtle "story" told by the flow of water throughout the various "rooms" of the Memorial. A more striking aspect of the project overall is its invocation of contemplative space, with benches in each area that invite visitors to sit and reflect on their surroundings. Benches are common in donor gardens throughout the country.

12. Occasionally this label is applied to recipients, too. In one instance, a rehabilitation specialist addressed a group of recipients attending a conference in this manner: "You're all experiencing the miracle, the gift of life . . . you find [yourself walking] around feeling endeared to another. You don't owe anything to anyone. You are all heroes in your own way."

13. When I visited this grove in mid-2004, there were in fact two damaged stones devoid of plaques; further, there were five empty spots where, clearly, trees had once stood. For more details see the Web site www.homestead.com/prosites_johnrcotter/lost_battalion_museums_307.html.

14. Of course, in other settings where donors are *philanthropists*, host institutions may not hesitate to leave room for future names.

15. These first three examples are derived from Cowherd (2003); those that follow are drawn from my field notes.

16. Although the subject lies beyond the purview of this research project, it is worth noting that discussions with relief workers who have responded to airplane crashes report similar long-term effects on surviving kin. What both contexts share is that the sense of loss is especially traumatic and open-ended when triggered by an unexpected and (as for numerous donor kin) horrific event. Further, in both contexts bodies, when retrieved, are no longer whole. Such is

often the case with the wartime dead as well, although one always knows upon entering battle zones that one might very well die there.

17. For a discussion of the gendered nature of quilt making as grief work, see Sturken (1997: 202–06).

18. I will explore in greater detail the significance of the public involvement of donor mothers in the following chapter.

19. See www.kidney.org/recips/donor/quiltHistory.cfm.

20. Transweb, currently based at the University of Michigan, was founded in late 1994 by Michigan Transplant, when the World Wide Web was just becoming a site for mounting information for public readers. The Web site was established in large part as a response to a general paucity of Web-based information on organ transfer, when the only other existing site focused exclusively on recipients' experiences. Subsequent activities have included webcasts of events at the Transplant Games, an educational Web site for youth, informative postings on recipient and donor experiences, and survey research funded by external sources. For more information, see www.Transweb.org/about_tw/about_tw.htm.

21. Popular books include the personal account by heart recipient Gene Bea titled *A Heart Full of Life* (2003); the collection edited by Pat Helmberger, whose sister received a transplant, published by the mail-order pharmacy CHRON-IMED, Inc. (Helmberger 1992); and Kathy Eldon and Amy Eldon's *Angel Catcher* (1998).

22. Cindy's explanation bears much in common with the metaphor of the decorated house offered by Dr. Lazarre in chapter 1. The similarity could spring from the fact that the body-as-house offers evidence of a dominant cultural understanding of brain death, or perhaps that neurologists themselves rely on this sort of image when training other medical personnel, such as EMTs.

3. PUBLIC ENCOUNTERS AS SUBVERSIVE ACTS

1. I would like to thank the members of several audiences for their comments on earlier presentations based on this chapter. They are the Lifelong Learning Seminar at Columbia University; the Metropolitan Medical Anthropology Association of New York; Shirley Lindenbaum and her students at the CUNY Graduate Center; David Valentine and his students at Sarah Lawrence College; and my colleagues at the Russell Sage Foundation during my residency there in 2003–4.

2. Yet another such innovative response has come from an East Coast–based procurement office. After its staff witnessed warm encounters between recipients and donor kin at the Transplant Games, this OPO decided to host its own local event, which it sponsors every other year when the Games are held outside of the United States. All workshops are open to both recipients and donor kin, who mingle freely during workshops, meals, and less formal moments of the day.

3. For a compelling contrast, see Kaufman (2000) on the care of patients who lie in a persistent vegetative state (PVS).

4. As I report elsewhere, however, they are more likely to do so if the recipient is African American (Sharp 2001, 2002b).

5. See www.Transweb.org; in addition, UNOS now sponsors online donor tributes as a component of the National Donor Memorial, as described in chapter 2.

6. Anecdotal evidence suggests that the Northwest is an exception: the oldest stories I have collected on communication, when facilitated by professional intervention, are from this part of the country. European policies appear to stand in contrast to those implemented in the United States up until the mid-1990s. Following a presentation I made at a transplant conference, I was approached by a procurement coordinator from England who explained that communication, as well as face-to-face encounters, occurred regularly where she worked. It had never occurred to her that communication would be problematic, and she wondered if perhaps this was because she worked in a rural area where everyone knew each other, and thus local inhabitants could easily match the dates of donor deaths and transplants with one another. I heard a similar story from a coordinator from the Netherlands. Such data are, however, purely anecdotal and clearly call for in-depth comparative research.

7. The label of "communications coordinator" is one of my own design. Personnel who fit this category go by a host of titles, including director or coordinator of donor family services, grief counselor, and others.

8. The NDFC's Donor Family Bill of Rights was subsequently updated in 2004.

9. As explained in chapter 2, donor parents always include the deceased child in their tabulation of their children, and they often speak of the deceased child in the present tense.

10. Here Sara actually means the parents of the recipient; the recipient was only an infant at the time.

11. By this point Jules would actually be a six-year-old child.

12. Transplant recipients take large doses of immunosuppressants to stave off graft rejection and consequently, are rendered susceptible to a host of infections that their immune system struggles to combat. For this they regularly take powerful steroids such as prednizone. Hirsuitism and overgrown gums are common side effects of long-term use of this medication.

13. Note that here she actually means Jules—she is in effect confusing the two children.

14. During the course of his own story Larry spoke primarily of the difficulties he experienced prior to transplantation (some of which have persisted following surgery). These include the humiliation of forced retirement, the depression that accompanied his disabled status, his fear of transplant surgery, and his suicidal thoughts. Such experiences are all too familiar to many organ recipients.

15. A shortfall of Schneider's arguments is his disregard for cultural variability. Schneider himself raised this point in later editions, stressing nevertheless that assimilated groups quickly embrace such concepts. My own findings

confirm this, and this may very well be because biological thinking dominates our society. As noted, Schneider argued that this concept was so pervasive that it quickly shaped the thinking of assimilated immigrant groups as well. This assertion is borne out in my classes of undergraduates whose cultural backgrounds are highly heterogeneous. I frequently make use of a kinship assignment, and the charts this generates display clearly at which point immigrant kin arrived in the United States, with the kinship terminology shifting from, say, a lineage system to bilateral forms of reckoning.

16. As Rabinow explains elsewhere, his concept of biosociality is akin to what Michel Foucault referred to as bio(-technico-)power; see Rabinow's comment in Marcus (1995: 449), as well as Rabinow (1992: 234); cf. Foucault (1978: 139).

17. As noted by a reviewer who read an earlier version of this manuscript, the stitching together of memory squares and quilts in honor of donors might even be read as a symbolic act of recomposing donors' lives (and bodies).

18. The institution of blood siblinghood, or the mixing of blood from two people to create social bonds with specific obligations attached, offers other interesting parallels; see Tegnaeus (1952).

19. As Silverman et al. (1988) report, adoptees are frequently the offspring of underage, and often unwed, mothers who succumb to pressures from elders to surrender their infants. Such mothers may endure significant emotional trauma for decades, even when they have married and had other children. Such factors frequently transform birth mothers into searchers.

20. This process is not unlike the experiences of successful spirit mediums in other cultural contexts, whose spirits may define aspects of restructured selfhood. As I have argued elsewhere (Sharp 1995), this process can generate for mediums more reflexive understandings of themselves than is possible under regular circumstances within their societies.

21. As Campbell et al. report from their own research, 69 percent of the adoption reunions they documented (where $n = 114$) involved contact with birth mothers. In those involving other blood kin (such as birth fathers or siblings), the birth mother generally was deceased. As noted, too, birth mothers (rather than birth fathers) are far more likely to seek out reunions with surrendered children (Campbell, Silverman, and Patti 1991; Howe and Feast 2000; Silverman et al. 1988).

22. I am drawing exclusively from the example provided by gestational surrogacy, and not from those cases where the surrogate's ovum was fertilized. Precisely because such fetal origins may lead a surrogate to claim a newborn as her own, traditional surrogacy has given way exclusively in recent years to gestational surrogacy. Under the latter arrangement, the contracting mother need not officially adopt the child, as is true under the former.

23. Procured organs, prior to transplant, are washed thoroughly in a saline solution and thus actually retain few traces of the donor's blood. Blood (and at times tissue) matching nevertheless defines an important part of the process when placing organs with appropriate recipients. Mistakes made in matching blood types can prove fatal to the recipient, as illustrated by the infamous story

involving Jesica Santillan, who died at Duke University Hospital in February 2003 following the transplant of a mismatched set of lungs and heart (Kirkpatrick and Shamp 2003; Sharp in press [a]; Wailoo, Guarnaccia, and Livingston in press).

24. In gestational surrogacy the social mother is so threatened by this that she must deliberately destabilize this bond to assert her own presence in the surrogate's womb.

25. My data, though limited, also suggest that male recipients may be more likely to seek out donor mothers than are female recipients. This trend stands in contrast to the adoption literature, where female offspring most frequently become searchers (Howe and Feast 2001; Silverman et al. 1988). The reasons for this are unclear. Perhaps male transplant recipients are more likely to long for forms of nurturing they associate with mothers. Yet another factor may simply be the gendered nature of transplantation in this country. Between 1991 and 2003, 72 to 78 percent of all transplanted hearts went to male recipients (OPTN 2003). As I have shown, this is the most symbolically charged organ. Men predominate as heart recipients in part because heart disease is still perceived as a greater health hazard for men than women of middle or advanced age. This then means that men are more likely to end up on transplant waiting lists. As Ralph Needham's story reveals, however, wives may in fact be the party who initially responds to correspondence from donor kin.

4. HUMAN HYBRIDITY

1. The heart was deemed unsuitable for transplantation.

2. This patient received a transplanted liver taken from another donor.

3. As reported by Gretchen Reynolds (2005), who later interviewed staff and family, transplant surgeons at Baylor assumed that Beed's brain hemorrhage was caused by recent use of crack cocaine; traces of cocaine and marijuana were found in his urine at the time of death. I will address the significance of this assumption later.

4. The patient who received the artery from Beed had not yet been identified.

5. For extensive personalized musings on such dominant metaphors, see Siebert (2004).

6. I take up a more detailed discussion on mechanical parts in Sharp (in press [b]).

7. The Chimera was a monster in Greek mythology that preyed upon humans. Part goat, part serpent, and part lion, it was slain by Bellerophon, who rode the winged horse Pegasus. Within contemporary biomedicine, the term *chimerism* is used to describe the successful integration within a particular body of other cells of non-host origin. As Antin et al. explain, there are varying degrees of chimerism, ranging from microchimerism to split, mixed, and full chimerism. See Antin et al. (2001); Quaini et al. (2002); van den Bergh and Holley (2002).

8. It seems that procurement professionals stand to lose their jobs if xenotransplantation does in fact prove successful; nevertheless, their steadfast ded-

ication to relieving the nation's organ shortage apparently overrides a desire to guard their profession. The lack of protest from this corner may spring in part, of course, from the fact that, whereas clinical trials could perhaps begin again in earnest in a few years, most surgeons believe that regular use of transgenic organs is most likely a decade or more away.

9. For recent discussions see Cayford (2004); Ten Eyck, Gaskell, and Jackson (2004); van den Bergh and Holley (2002).

10. For a marvelous (and often tongue-in-cheek) critique of experimental mechanical implants versus xenotransplantation written for venture capitalists, see Maeder and Ross (2002). These authors find "mech" solutions to be "much sexier" and inherently safer for investors than "orgo" (that is, organic) substitute organs. I discuss the implications of this article in more detail in Sharp (in press [b]). See also Frontline (2001).

11. The questionnaire itself required students to write brief answers to a set of fifteen open-ended questions. All fifty students completed and returned the forms. Student respondents consisted of thirty-two females and twenty-two males, of whom 88 percent were Euro-American, 10 percent African American, and 8 percent foreign born (I exclude sample responses from the last category because of my interest in reporting dominant American cultural values within this chapter). Nearly all respondents were Protestant (if they claimed a faith); the remainder were Catholic (four), Christian Scientist (one), Jewish (one), and Hindu (one). Questions targeted attitudes on being a donor and recipient. In reference to my discussion here, I sought their opinions on receiving an organ from a human or an animal, or a mechanical device, and I asked them to rank their preferences and explain their reactions. I also asked if the organ they needed mattered.

12. I thank Maureen Hickey for this observation.

13. Ethicist Pierre Effa, from Cameroon, makes a similar argument (Effa 1998).

14. According to UNOS, blacks defined 17 percent of all transplants performed between 1988 and 2005 (58,861 of a total of 345,537). Whites represent the largest number (235,858, or a little more than 68 percent) when recipients are categorized by ethnicity. Among the 93,847 deceased donors for the same period, blacks constitute just under 12 percent (10,884) and whites 71,114, or just under 75 percent. Blacks define the largest minority group in both categories. Counts are also available for Hispanic, Asian, American Indian/Alaskan Native, Pacific Islander, multiracial, and unknown. See www.optn.org/latestData/rptData.asp (consulted July 22, 2005).

15. See also www.CHFpatients.com, entry on "Artificial Hearts" (consulted January 14, 2004).

16. It is worth noting that the experimental Jarvik 2000 LVAD (left ventricular assist device), an auxiliary pump that is attached to the heart, makes no detectable noise exterior to the recipient's body and requires only a fully portable rechargeable battery to run. Because the device is made of metal and inert plastic, fewer medications are required than with allografts: the implanted

patient takes no immunosuppressants or steroids, for instance. Because it is a continuous flow device, the recipient has no pulse (P. Houghton, personal communication, July 2005). The strangely unnatural quality of a heart with no altering pace has its precursor in the realm of organ transfer: a "denervated" transplanted heart runs at a steady pace (set at, say, ninety-nine beats per minute by the surgeon) and does not respond to exercise or emotions because it lacks the nerve connections triggered by the brain (Clough 1990). Professionals I have interviewed have never made this comparison with mechanical devices (but see Siebert 2004). I believe this springs from larger professional concerns that mechanical devices as complicated as artificial hearts ultimately dehumanize patients, as argued throughout this chapter.

Glossary

allograft   An organ and/or tissue transferred between members of the same species; within the realm of organ transfer the term refers to instances involving human donors and recipients.

allotransplantation   The surgical act of organ and/or tissue replacement between members of the same species; human-to-human transplantation.

AOPO   Association of Organ Procurement Organizations, a national consortium of American procurement organizations; its central office is based near Washington, D.C.

cadaveric donor   A body from which organs and/or tissues may be procured; most often such donors have been declared brain dead. *Compare:* living (related) donor.

CDC   Centers for Disease Control and Prevention, a division of the U.S. Department of Health and Human Services. Based in Atlanta, the CDC monitors human health and safety issues in the United States. Founded originally in the 1940s to combat malaria, its purview today includes tracking epidemics, workplace and environmental hazards, and disabilities.

chimera   Originally a creature from Greek mythology composed of parts of a serpent, lion, and goat. Within contemporary biomedicine, the term *chimerism* is used to describe the successful integration, within a particular body, of other cells of non-host origin, thus potentially reducing or eliminating the need for immunosuppression.

clinical coordinator   An employee of an organ procurement organization responsible for monitoring the medical status of patients who might become, or who have already been identified as, organ donors. The clinical coordinator often remains in charge of the patient-donor until the moment he or she enters surgery for procurement purposes.

CPR   Cardiopulmonary resuscitation, a widespread technique used by emergency medical technicians and hospital personnel to stimulate lung and heart function in a traumatized patient.

cyclosporine   Also spelled *cyclosporin,* a potent immunosuppressant drug derived from a fungus. It was approved for clinical use in the early 1980s, radicalizing the medical ability to sustain patients long-term who had received organ transplants. Without the support of this or similar medications, patients are certain to die from the effects of acute graft rejection.

DCD   Donation after cardiac death, a term applied to organ donors who did not qualify for brain death status. Instead, organ retrieval follows the cessation of a detectable heartbeat, often in contexts where cardiac arrest was anticipated. *See also* NHBD.

decoupling   A communication technique developed in the 1990s by several organ procurement organizations as a means to generate better outcomes following requests for organ donation from the kin of hospitalized patients who might soon die or who have already been declared dead. Decoupling is a two-step process involving the delivery of two messages: the first concerns brain death criteria (its cause and irreparable qualities); once kin show signs of accepting that the diagnosed patient is dead, the second message is delivered, one focused on a request to donate tissue and organs.

DNR   Do not resuscitate, generally an advanced order placed on a patient's medical chart, following instructions from the patient or from next of kin, in anticipation of cardiopulmonary crisis. A DNR order instructs medical personnel to desist in using CPR or a respirator to revive such patients if and when they are in crisis and, thus, near death.

donor kin   The surviving family members of a deceased organ donor. It is they who grant consent to organ donation at the time of death.

EMT   Emergency medical technician; EMTs typically staff ambulances in the United States.

family counselor   An organ procurement organization employee whose primary duty is to comfort the kin of potential donors in hospitals and to encourage them to consent to organ and tissue donation when faced with a sudden or imminent death.

FDA   Food and Drug Administration, the U.S. government agency whose duties include the approval of pharmaceuticals for human use.

fictive kinship   The incorporation of other people as kin who previously bore no relation by marriage or blood.

ICU   Intensive care unit, the ward within a hospital where patients who have experienced severe trauma, or who require special postsurgical monitoring, are cared for.

Jarvik-7 heart   A cumbersome mechanical device developed in the 1980s in the United States that was designed to fully replace the human heart.

living (related) donor   A living and presumably healthy person who offers an entire or part of an organ, or tissues (such as bone marrow), to another person in need. Although most often this is a kidney, it is possible to harvest one lung or part of a liver (which regenerates). Living donors have long been relatives of recipients; increasingly, however, friends and strangers are offering kidneys as well. *Compare:* cadaveric donor.

LVAD Left ventricular assist device, a surgically implanted mechanical device that helps a failing heart pump blood more efficiently. Contemporary prototypes are fully portable and run on battery power. The Jarvik-7 was the precursor of one such LVAD, the Jarvik-2000.

NDFC National Donor Family Council, a grassroots organization currently housed in the national headquarters of the National Kidney Foundation. The NDFC is an advocacy group that represents the interests of organ donor kin.

NHBD Non-heartbeating donor, an organ donor who has been declared dead following cardiac, rather than brain, death. *See also* DCD.

NKF National Kidney Foundation, a volunteer organization whose origins can be traced to the 1950s. The NKF, whose national headquarters are in New York City, focuses on preventing kidney and urinary tract diseases, assisting those affected by such medical conditions, and promoting kidney donation and transplantation within the United States. It hosts the Transplant Olympics and also houses the National Donor Family Council.

NOTA National Organ Transplant Act, passed by the U.S. Congress in 1984, a law that provided guidelines to ensure safe matching and equitable distribution of organs. It established the Organ Procurement and Transplantation Network, which oversees the nation's waiting list of organ recipients, in conjunction with the United Network for Organ Sharing.

OPO Organ procurement organization, an agency that oversees organ transfer within a particular territory or state of the United States. Staff duties include mounting educational campaigns designed to promote organ donation; identifying potential donors in local hospitals; monitoring the clinical status of such patients; working with local transplant units and the United Network for Organ Sharing to place viable organs; and working alongside surgical teams when they arrive to remove organs for use in patients elsewhere. OPO staff may also conduct the procurement themselves, especially in cases where kidneys or tissues are involved.

OPTN Organ Procurement and Transplantation Network, a nonprofit organization created by the U.S. Congress in 1984 to direct the sharing and allocation of organs. The OPTN is a consortium of the nation's transplant and procurement centers. Its current board of directors is the same as that for UNOS, and in many ways the two organizations are indistinguishable.

Patches of Love Project A donor memorial quilt coordinated by the National Donor Family Council.

Perfusionist A clinical specialist who monitors the flow of fluid through tissue; for instance, during open-heart surgery the perfusionist oversees the operation of the heart-lung machine.

PERVs Porcine endogenous retroviruses, a significant barrier to xenotransplantation because of the potential for transmission to humans of these zoonotic diseases harbored within pigs' bodies.

pressor short for *vasopressor;* a medication administered to control blood pressure, especially drops in pressure.

presumed consent The assumption that one is willing to be an organ donor unless specified otherwise in writing (say, within a national registry, in an advanced medical directive, or in one's will). Although presumed consent is characteristic of the policies of several European countries, professionals there generally ask kin if they can procure organs before doing so. The long-standing policy within the United States assumes instead that an individual and his or her kin must designate that one is an organ donor; recent legislation passed by various states marks a move toward presumed consent, however.

procurement professional An employee of an organ procurement organization.

recipient An individual who has received an organ transplant.

TAH Total artificial heart, a fully implantable (and, to date, highly experimental) device designed to replace the functions of an excised human heart. A range of prototypes are now under development and are being implanted on an experimental basis within patients.

Transplant Olympics Also referred to as the Transplant Games. An event hosted every other year within the United States by the National Kidney Foundation; in alternating years there are international games based overseas. Spanning several days, the Transplant Olympics include a wide spectrum of events in which organ (and some tissue) recipients of all levels of athletic competency and ages compete; a range of symposia and other similar gatherings also take place that involve nonathletes, their families, and the kin of organ donors.

TRIO Transplant Recipients International Organization, a grassroots organization founded in 1983 to represent the needs of organ recipients. The national headquarters is currently based in Washington, D.C.

Uniform Anatomical Gift Act An act passed in 1968 by the U.S. Congress and ratified by all fifty states. Its original purpose was to establish uniform and comprehensive laws concerning anatomical gifts. It was subsequently revised in 1987. The law designates, for example, the order of priority of kin who may determine the granting of anatomical gifts; it also defines the language used subsequently to describe organs as "gifts" rather than as marketable commodities.

UNOS The United Network for Organ Sharing. Based in Richmond, Virginia, UNOS is the national headquarters for the organization that oversees the allocation and distribution of organs throughout the United States. UNOS personnel maintain computerized waiting lists for recipients awaiting transplants throughout the country; they also oversee all procurement and placement activities of organ procurement organizations and transplant centers in the country. An organ procurement organization, for example, must alert UNOS that it has identified a potential donor, and it is UNOS that determines the placement of procured organs from a cadaveric donor. Alongside the activities of the Organ Procurement Transplant Network, UNOS also maintains a comprehensive statistical database on the numbers and categories of the nation's donors, organs transplanted, and recipients who have received organs.

xenograft   An organ or tissue that is transferred between disparate species; for example, a liver derived from a baboon that is implanted in a human patient is a xenograft.

xenotransplantation   The process of transferring organs from one species to another; current efforts focus on the development of simian and porcine species that might one day supply organs for human use.

zoonoses   Diseases of animal origin; they are of particular concern within the context of transplantation because of the dangers associated with grafts from animals that might transmit diseases of animal origin to human patients who receive such grafts. PERVs are one such example.

References

AAP (American Academy of Pediatrics).

1987 Report of Special Task Force: Guidelines for the Determination of Brain Death in Children. *Pediatrics* 80:298–300.

ABC (Australian Broadcasting Corporation).

1996 Artificial Hearts. In *The Health Report, Radio National Transcripts*. Australia: ABC Radio National.

Agar, Michael.

1996 *The Professional Stranger: An Informal Introduction to Ethnography.* San Diego: Academic Press.

Agich, George J.

1999 From Pittsburgh to Cleveland: NHBD Controversies and Bioethics. *Cambridge Quarterly of Healthcare Ethics* 8:269–74.

Alliance for Health Reform.

2003 *Covering Health Issues: A Sourcebook for Journalists* [online sourcebook]. Washington, DC: Alliance for Health Reform.

Altman, Lawrence K.

1984a Baby Fae, Who Received a Heart from a Baboon, Dies after 20 Days. *New York Times,* November 16.

1984b Baby with Baboon Heart Better; Surgeons Defend the Experiment. *New York Times,* October 30.

1984c Confusion Surrounds Baby Fae. *New York Times,* November 6.

1991 Three Transplant Recipients Get AIDS—Same Donor; Officials Seek Others with Dead Man's Tissues. *San Francisco Chronicle.*

AMA (American Medical Association).

2003 AMA Testifies before Congress on Organ Donation Motivation: Encourages Study of Financial Incentives [press release], June 3.

AMA Council on Ethical and Judicial Affairs.

1994 Strategies for Cadaveric Organ Procurement: Mandated Choice and Presumed Consent. *Journal of the American Medical Association* 272:809–12.

Andrews, Lori.
1992   The Body as Property: Some Philosophical Reflections—A Response to J. F. Childress. *Transplantation Proceedings* 24:2149–51.

Andrews, Lori, and Dorothy Nelkin.
2001   *Body Bazaar: The Market for Human Tissue in the Biotechnology Age.* New York: Crown.

Annas, George J.
1983   Defining Death: There Ought to Be a Law. *Hastings Center Report* 13 (1): 20–21.

Antin, Joseph H., et al.
2001   Establishment of Complete and Mixed Donor Chimerism after Allogeneic Lymphohematopoietic Transplantation: Recommendations from a Workshop at the 2001 Tandem Meetings. *Biology of Blood and Marrow Transplantation* 7:473–85.

AP (Associated Press).
2000   Donated Human Body Parts Are Being Sold Overseas. *San Diego Union-Tribune*, May 22.
2004a   Donated Bodies Used in Land Mine Tests. *New York Times*, March 11.
2004b   Identities of Three Rabies Transplant Victims Released. *Houston Chronicle*, July 3.

Arnold, R., et al.
2002   Financial Incentives for Cadaver Organ Donation: An Ethical Reappraisal. *Transplantation* 73:1361–67.

Ashwal, Stephen
2001   Clinical Diagnosis and Confirmatory Testing of Brain Death in Children. In *Brain Death,* edited by E. F. M. Wijdicks, 91–114. Philadelphia: Lippincott Williams and Wilkins.

Ayres, B. Drummond.
1998   Missouri May Spare Inmate Organ Donors. *New York Times*, March 23.

Bach, Fritz H., Adrian J. Ivinson, and H. E. Judge Christopher Weeramantry.
2001   Ethical and Legal Issues in Technology: Xenotransplantation. *American Journal of Law and Medicine* 27:283–300.

Bailey, Ronald.
1990   Should I Be Allowed to Buy Your Kidney? *Forbes,* May 28, 365–72.

Baker, Robert.
1999   Minority Distrust of Medicine: A Historical Perspective. *Mount Sinai Journal of Medicine* 66:212–22.

Barr, M. L., et al.
1998   Recipient and Donor Outcomes in Living Related and Unrelated Lobar Transplantation. *Transplantation Proceedings* 30:2261–63.

Bartz, Clifford Earle.

2003   Operation Blue, ULTRA: DION—The Donation Inmate Organ Network. *Kennedy Institute of Ethics Journal* 13:37–43.

Bateson, Gregory.

1958   *Naven: A Survey of the Problems Suggested by a Composite Picture of the Culture of a New Guinea Tribe Drawn from Three Points of View.* Stanford, CA: Stanford University Press.

Bayne, Kathryn.

1999   Developing Guidelines on the Care and Use of Animals. In *Xenotransplantation: Scientific Frontiers and Public Policy.* Annals of the New York Academy of Sciences, vol. 862, edited by J. Fishman, D. Sachs, and R. Shaikh, 105–10. New York: New York Academy of Sciences.

BBC (British Broadcasting Corporation).

1999   Doctors Back Organ Donation Reform. BBC News, online Health Section, July 8.

Bea, Gene.

2003   *A Heart Full of Life: The Powerful but Wonderfully Warm and Whimsical Journey of a Heart Transplant Recipient.* Bloomington: AuthorHouse.

Beidel, Deborah C.

1987   Psychological Factors in Organ Transplantation. *Clinical Psychology Review* 7:677–94.

Bell, Kim.

1998   House Committee Appears Unlikely to Pass Bill on Death-Row Organ Donors. *St. Louis Post-Dispatch,* March 26.

BioTransplant, Inc., and Massachusetts General Hospital (MGH).

1999   MGH and BioTransplant Scientists to Lead Discussions on Key Topics at International Xenotransplantation Association Conference [press release], October 25, Nagoya, Japan on the PRNewswire.

Birmingham, Karen.

1999   WHO Hosts Web Discussion on Xenotransplantation Policy. *Nature Medicine* 5:595.

Bloch, Maurice.

1971   *Placing the Dead: Tombs, Ancestral Villages, and Kinship Organization in Madagascar.* New York: Seminar Press.

Bloch, Maurice, and Jonathan Parry.

1982   *Death and the Regeneration of Life.* Cambridge: Cambridge University Press.

Blumstein, J. F.

1992   The Case for Commerce in Organ Transplantation. *Transplantation Proceedings* 24:2190–97.

1993   The Use of Financial Incentives in Medical Care: The Case of Commerce in Transplantable Organs. *Health Matrix* 3:1–30.

Bowden, A. Bruce, and Alan R. Hull.

1993   *Controversies in Organ Donation: A Summary Report.* New York: National Kidney Foundation.

Branton, M., and E. Snider.

1990   *The Right to Know: America's Adoption Crisis* (videotape). Alhambra, CA: Two Peasa Production.

Brecher, Bob.

1994   Organs for Transplant: Donation or Payment? In *Principles of Health Care Ethics,* edited by R. Gillon. New York: Wiley.

Broder, John.

2004   In Science's Name, Lucrative Trade in Body Parts. *New York Times,* March 11.

Brodwin, Paul E., ed.

2000a   *Biotechnology and Culture: Bodies, Anxieties, Ethics.* Bloomington: Indiana University Press.

2000b   Biotechnology on the Margins: A Haitian Discourse on French Medicine. In *Biotechnology and Culture: Bodies, Anxieties, Ethics,* edited by P. E. Brodwin, 264–84. Bloomington: Indiana University Press.

2000c   Introduction. In *Biotechnology and Culture: Bodies, Anxieties, Ethics,* edited by P. E. Brodwin, 1–23. Bloomington: Indiana University Press.

Buell, J. F., et al.

2003   Donors with Central Nervous System Malignancies: Are They Truly Safe? *Transplantation* 76:340–43.

Butler, Declan.

1999a   Europe Is Urged to Hold Back on Xenotransplant Clinical Trials. *Nature* 397:281–82.

1999b   FDA Warns on Primate Xenotransplants. *Nature* 398:549.

Buxton, M. J.

1997   Economics of Transplantation in the 21st Century: New Scientific Opportunities but Greater Economic Problems. *Transplantation Proceedings* 29:2723–24.

Campbell, Lee H., Phyllis R. Silverman, and Patricia B. Patti.

1991   Reunions between Adoptees and Birth Parents: The Adoptees' Experience. *Social Work* 36:329–35.

Campion-Vincent, Véronique.

1992   Bébés en pièces détachées: Une nouvelle "légende" latino-américaine. *Cahiers Internationaux de Sociologie* 93:299–319.

1997   *La légende des vols d'organes.* Paris: Les Belles Lettres.

Caplan, Arthur L.

1992   *If I Were a Rich Man Could I Buy a Pancreas? And Other Essays on the Ethics of Health Care.* Bloomington: Indiana University Press.

Cartwright, Lisa.
1992 Women, X-Rays, and the Public Culture of Prophylactic Imaging. *Social Science and Medicine* 29:19–54.
1995 *Screening the Body: Tracing Medicine's Visual Culture.* Minneapolis: University of Minnesota Press.

Cayford, Jerry.
2004 Breeding Sanity in the GM Food Debate. *Issues in Science and Technology* 20 (2): 49–56.

CDC (Centers for Disease Control and Prevention).
2004 Investigation of Rabies Infections in Organ Donor and Transplant Recipients—Alabama, Arkansas, Oklahoma, and Texas, 2004. *MMWR* (Dispatch), July 1.

CE (Council of Europe).
2003 *Report on the State of the Art in the Field of Xenotransplantation.* Strasbourg: Working Party on Xenotransplantation under the Steering Committee on Bioethics and European Health Committee.

Chadwick, R.
1989 The Market for Bodily Parts: Kant and the Duties to Oneself. *Journal of Applied Philosophy* 6:129–39.

Cheney, Annie.
2004 The Resurrection Men: Scenes from the Cadaver Trade. *Harper's,* March, 45–54.

CHFpatients.com.
2004 Artificial Hearts. January 14.

Childress, James F.
1992 The Body as Property: Some Philosophical Reflections. *Transplantation Proceedings* 24:2143–48.

Chillag, Kata.
1997 Defining "Normal": Representations of Patients' and Families' Experiences after Liver Transplantation. Ph.D. diss., University of Pittsburgh.

Clark, Margaret.
1993 Medical Anthropology and the Redefining of Human Nature. *Human Organization* 52:233–42.
1999 This Little Piggy Went to Market: The Xenotransplantation and Xenozoonose Debate. *Journal of Law, Medicine and Ethics* 27:137–52.

Clifford, James.
1988 *The Predicament of Culture: Twentieth-Century Ethnography, Literature, and Art.* Cambridge, Mass.: Harvard University Press.

Clough, Peggy.
1990 The Denervated Heart. *Clinical Management* 10 (4): 14–17.

Cohen, C.
1992   The Case for Presumed Consent to Transplant Human Organs after Death. *Transplantation Proceedings* 24:2168–72.
Cohen, Jeffrey Jerome.
1996   *Monster Theory: Reading Culture.* Minneapolis: University of Minnesota Press.
Cohen, Lawrence.
1999   Where It Hurts: Indian Material for an Ethics of Organ Transplantation. *Daedalus* 128 (4): 135–64.
Cook, Robin.
1977   *Coma.* Boston: Little Brown.
Coombs, Robert H., Sangeeta Chopra, Debra R. Schenk, and Elaine Yutan.
1993   Medical Slang and Its Functions. *Social Science and Medicine* 36:987–98.
Cooper, David K. C., Bernd Gollackner, and David H. Sachs.
2002   Will the Pig Solve the Transplantation Backlog? *Annual Review of Medicine* 53:133–47.
Corr, Charles A., Margaret B. Coolican, Lucy G. Nile, and Nancy R. Noedel.
1994   What Is the Rationale For or Against Contacts between Donor Families and Transplant Recipients? *Critical Care Nursing Clinics of North America* 6:625–32.
Cowan, Dale H., Jo Ann Kantorowitz, Jay Moskowitz, and Peter H. Rheinstein.
1987   *Human Organ Transplantation: Societal, Medical-Legal, Regulatory, and Reimbursement Issues.* Ann Arbor: Health Administration Press (in cooperation with the American Society of Law and Medicine).
Cowherd, Robin.
2003   *Healing the Spirit: Inspirational Stories of Organ and Tissue Donors and Their Families.* Lenexa, KS: Applied Measurement Professionals, Inc. for LifeNet Donor Memorial Foundation.
Crigger, Bette-Jane.
1995   Bioethnography: Fieldwork in the Lands of Medical Ethics (review). *Medical Anthropology Quarterly* 9:400–417.
Crowley-Matoka, Megan.
In press   *Producing Transplanted Bodies: Life, Death, and Value in Mexican Organ Transplantation.* Durham, NC: Duke University Press.
CUSL (Commissioners on Uniform State Laws).
1980   Uniform Determination of Death Act. Annual Conference of Commissioners on Uniform State Laws, Kauai, Hawaii, 1980.
1988   Uniform Anatomical Gift Act (1987) (draft). Annual conference, National Conference of Commissioners on Uniform State Laws, Newport Beach, CA, 1988.
Damasio, Antonio.
1994   *Descartes' Error: Emotion, Reason, and the Human Brain.* New York: Avon Books.

1999   *The Feeling of What Happens: Body and Emotion in the Making of Consciousness.* San Diego: Harcourt.

Davidson, M. N., and P. Devney.

1991   Attitudinal Barriers to Organ Donation among Black Americans. *Transplantation Proceedings* 23:2531–32.

Davis-Floyd, Robbie.

1994   The Technocratic Body: American Childbirth as Cultural Expression. *Social Science and Medicine* 38:1125–40.

Davis-Floyd, Robbie, and Joseph Dumit.

1998   *Cyborg Babies: From Techno-Sex to Techno-Tots.* New York: Routledge.

Davis-Floyd, Robbie, and Gloria St. John.

1998   *From Doctor to Healer: The Transformative Journey.* New Brunswick, NJ: Rutgers University Press.

DCIDS (DCI Donor Services–New Mexico).

2004   Religious Views.

DeJong, William, et al.

1998   Requesting Organ Donation: An Interview Study of Donor and Nondonor Families. *American Journal of Critical Care* 7 (1): 13–23.

Delmonico, Francis L., Robert Arnold, Nancy Scheper-Hughes, Laura Siminoff, Jeffrey Kahn, and Stuart Youngner.

2002   Ethical Incentives—Not Payment—for Organ Donation. *New England Journal of Medicine* 346:2002–5.

Descartes, René.

1999 [1637]   *Discours de la méthode* [Discourse on Method and Related Writings]. Trans. D. M. Clarke. London: Penguin.

DeVita, M. A.

1993   Development of the University of Pittsburgh Medical Center Policy for the Care of Terminally Ill Patients Who May Become Organ Donors after Death following the Removal of Life Support. *Kennedy Institute of Ethics Journal* 3:131–43.

di Leonardo, Micaela.

1998   *Exotics at Home: Anthropologists, Others, American Modernity.* Chicago: University of Chicago Press.

Donnelley, Strachan.

1993   The Ethical Challenges of Animal Biotechnology. *Livestock Production Science* 36:91–98.

1995   The Art of Moral Ecology. *Ecosystem Health* 1:171–76.

1999   How and Why Animals Matter. *ILAR Journal* 40 (1): 22–28.

Doss, Erika.

2002   Death, Art, and Memory in the Public Sphere: The Visual and Material Culture of Grief in Contemporary America. *Mortality* 7:63–82.

In progress.   Memorial Mania: Self, Nation, and the Culture of Commemo-
ration in Contemporary America. Manuscript.

Dossetor, J. B.

1992   Rewarded Gifting: Is It Ever Ethically Acceptable? *Transplantation Proceedings* 24:2092–94.

Douglas, Mary.

1966   *Purity and Danger: An Analysis of Concepts of Pollution and
Taboo.* New York: Praeger.

1970   *Natural Symbols: Explorations in Cosmology.* New York:
Pantheon.

Douglas, Mary, and Aaron Wildavsky.

1982   *Risk and Culture: An Essay on the Selection* of Technological
and Environmental Dangers. Berkeley and Los Angeles: University of California Press.

Downey, Gary.

1992   Human Agency in CAD/CAM Technology. *Anthropology Today*
8 (5): 2–6.

Downey, Gary, Joe Dumit, and Sharon Traweek.

1997   *Cyborgs and Citadels: Anthropological Investigations in Emerging Sciences and Technology.* Santa Fe, NM: School of American
Research Press.

DuBois, James M.

1999   Non-Heart-Beating Organ Donation: A Defense of the Required Determination of Death. *Journal of Law, Medicine and
Ethics* 27:126–36.

Dumit, Joe.

1997   A Digital Image of the Category of the Person: PET Scanning
and Objective Self-Fashioning. In *Cyborgs and Citadels: Anthropological Investigations in Emerging Science and Technology,*
edited by G. Downey, J. Dumit, and S. Traweek, 83–102. Santa
Fe, NM: School of American Research Press.

Dunbar, Robin, and Louise Barrett.

2000   *Cousins: Our Primate Relatives* [Based on a television program
broadcast by BBCI and the Discovery Channel]. London: DK
Publishers.

Eastland, Lynette S., Sandra L. Herndon, and Jeanine R. Barr.

1999   *Communication in Recovery: Perspectives on Twelve-Step Groups.*
Cresskill, NJ: Hampton Press.

Effa, Pierre.

1998   Transplantation and Xenotransplantation: Legal Perspectives
for Third World Countries. In *Xenotransplantation: Scientific
Frontiers and Public Policy.* Annals of the New York Academy of
Sciences, vol. 862, edited by J. Fishman, D. Sachs, and R. Shaikh,
234–36. New York: New York Academy of Sciences.

Eldon, Kathy, and Amy Eldon.
1998   *Angel Catcher: A Journal of Loss and Remembrance.* San Fran-
            cisco: Chronicle Books.

Emmrich, M.
1994   Wenn der Butdruck der Leiche dramatisch steigt. *Frankfurter
            Rundshau,* June 27, 18.

Etienne, T., et al.
1991   Increases in Organ Donation Refusals and the Efficiency of a
            Transplant Program. *Transplantation Proceedings* 23:2558–59.

Evers, Sandra.
2002   *Constructing History, Culture and Inequality: The Betsileo in
            the Extreme Southern Highlands of Madagascar.* Leiden: Brill.

Feast, J., M. Marwood, S. Seabrook, and E. Webb.
1998   *Preparing for Reunion: Experiences from the Adoption Circle.*
            London: Children's Society.

Feeley-Harnik, Gillian.
1984   The Political Economy of Death: Communication and Change
            in Malagasy Colonial History. *American Ethnologist* 11:1–19.
1991   *A Green Estate: Restoring Independence in Madagascar.* Wash-
            ington, DC: Smithsonian Institution Press.

Fehar, M., R. Naddaff, and B. Tazi, eds.
1989   *Fragments for a History of the Human Body.* Vol. 3. New York:
            Zone.

Fishman, J., D. Sachs, and R. Shaikh, eds.
1998   *Xenotransplantation: Scientific Frontiers and Public Policy.* An-
            nals of the New York Academy of Sciences, vol. 862. New York:
            New York Academy of Sciences.

Flye, M. Wayne.
1995   Atlas of Organ Transplantation. Philadelphia: Saunders.

Ford, Leigh Arden, and Sandi W. Smith.
1991   Memorability and Persuasiveness of Organ Donation Strategies.
            American Behavioral Scientist 34:695–711.

Foucault, Michel.
1978   *The History of Sexuality,* vol. 1, *An Introduction.* Trans. R. Hur-
            ley. New York: Pantheon.

Fox, Renée C.
1959   *Experiment Perilous.* Glencoe, IL: Free Press.
1993   An Ignoble Form of Cannibalism: Reflections on the Pittsburgh
            Protocol for Procuring Organs from Non-Heart-Beating Donors.
            Kennedy Institute of Ethics Journal 3:231–39.

Fox, Renée C., Michael A. DeVita, and William Ritchie.
1998   The Waiting Game: Organ Transplant Controversy. In Online
            NewsHouse Forum, PBS.

Fox, Renée C., and Judith P. Swazey.

1978   The Courage to Fail: A Social View of Organ Transplants and Dialysis. Chicago: University of Chicago Press.

1992   Spare Parts: Organ Replacement in Human Society. Oxford: Oxford University Press.

Franklin, Sarah.

1997   Embodied Progress: A Cultural Account of Assisted Conception. New York: Routledge.

Franklin, Sarah, and Heléna Ragoné.

1998   Reproducing Reproduction: Kinship, Power, and Technological Innovation. Philadelphia: University of Pennsylvania Press.

Franz, Holly, et al.

1997   Explaining Brain Death: A Critical Feature of the Donation Process. Journal of Transplant Coordination 7 (1): 14–21.

Freud, Sigmund.

1974   Remembering, Repeating and Working-Through (Further Recommendations on the Technique of Psycho-Analysis II). In The Standard Edition of the Complete Psychological Works of Sigmund Freud, edited by J. Strachey and A. Freud, 12:145–56. London: Hogarth Press.

Frontline, PBS.

2001   Organ Farm: The Business of Xenotransplantation, Past and Present.

Fung, J. J.

2000   Use of Non-Heart-Beating Donors. Transplantation Proceedings 32:1510–11.

Garrett, L.

1994   The Coming Plague: Newly Emerging Diseases in a World Out of Balance. New York: Penguin.

Gean, Alisa D.

1994   Imaging of Head Trauma. New York: Raven Press.

Geertz, Clifford.

1973   The Interpretation of Cultures. New York: Basic Books.

1983   Local Knowledge: Further Essays in Interpretative Anthropology. New York: Basic Books.

1988   Works and Lives: The Anthropologist as Author. Stanford, CA: Stanford University Press.

Gelb, Adrian W., and Kerri M. Robertson.

1990   Anaesthetic Management of the Brain Dead for Organ Donation. Canadian Journal of Anaesthesia 37:806–12.

Gil, Gideon.

1989   The Artificial Heart Juggernaut. Hastings Center Report 19 (2): 24–31.

Ginsburg, Faye D., and Rayna Rapp.

1995   *Conceiving the New World Order: The Global Politics of Reproduction.* Berkeley and Los Angeles: University of California Press.

Goldberg, Carey.

2003   Fiscal Incentive Weighed to Boost U.S. Organ Supply. *Boston Globe,* October 8.

Grady, Denise.

2004   Fourth Rabies Death Reported from a Single Organ Donor. *New York Times,* July 9.

Gray, C. H.

1995   *The Cyborg Handbook.* New York: Routledge.

Gray, John.

1992   *Men Are from Mars, Women Are from Venus: A Practical Guide for Improving Communication Skills and Getting What You Want in Your Relationships.* New York: HarperCollins.

Greenberg, Gary.

2001   As Good as Dead: Is There Really Such a Thing as Brain Death? *New Yorker,* August 13, 36–41.

Griffin, C. J. G.

1990   The Rhetoric of Form in Conversion Narratives. *Quarterly Journal of Speech* 76:152–63.

Gutkind, L.

1988   *Many Sleepless Nights.* New York: Norton.

Guttmann, Ronald D.

1992   On the Use of Organs from Executed Prisoners. *Transplantation Reviews* 6:189–93.

Hall, L. E., C. O. Callender, C. L. Yeager, J. B. Barber Jr., G. M. Dunston, and V. W. Pinn-Wiggins.

1991   Organ Donation in Blacks: The Next Frontier. *Transplantation Proceedings* 23:2500–4.

Hamilton, Anita.

2001   Inventions of the Year; Your Health; Abiocor Artificial Heart. *Time,* November 19.

Hansmann, Henry.

1989   The Economics and Ethics of Markets for Human Organs. *Journal of Health Politics, Policy, and Law* 14 (1): 57–85.

Haraway, Donna.

1989   The Biopolitics of Postmodern Bodies: Determinations of Self in Immune System Discourse. *Differences* 1 (1): 3–43.

1991a   A Cyborg Manifesto. In *Simians, Cyborgs, and Women: The Reinvention of Nature,* 149–91. New York: Routledge.

1991b   *Simians, Cyborgs, and Women: The Reinvention of Nature.* New York: Routledge.

1992   The Promises of Monsters: A Regenerative Politics for Inappropriate/d Others. In *Cultural Studies*, edited by L. Grossberg, C. Nelson, and P. Treichler, 295–337. New York: Routledge.

Harris, Marvin.

1985   *The Sacred Cow and the Abominable Pig. Riddles of Food and Culture.* New York. Simon and Schuster.

Harrison, Harry.

1964   *Make Room! Make Room!* New York: Bantam Spectra.

Hedges, Stephen J., and William Gaines.

2000   Donated Tissue Used for Profit. *Times Union*, May 21.

Helman, Cecil.

1988   Dr. Frankenstein and the Industrial Body. *Anthropology Today* 4 (3): 14–16.

1992   *The Body of Frankenstein's Monster: Essays in Myth and Medicine.* New York: Norton.

Helman, Christopher.

2001   Charlotte's Goat. *Forbes Global* (online), February 19.

Helmberger, Pat Stave.

1992   *Transplants: Unwrapping the Second Gift of Life. The Inside Story of Transplants as Told by Recipients and Their Families, Donor Families, and Health Professionals.* Minneapolis, MN: CHRONIMED Publishing.

Hessing, Dick J., and Henk Elfers.

1986–87   Attitude toward Death, Fear of Being Declared Dead Too Soon, and Donation of Organs after Death. *Omega* 17:115–26.

Hill, David J.

1999   Issues in Organ Donation and Transplantation [letter]. *Journal of the Royal Society of Medicine* 92:493–94.

HMS (Harvard Medical School "Ad Hoc" Committee) and Henry K. Beecher (chair).

1968   A Definition of Irreversible Coma. In *Updating Life and Death*, edited by D. R. Cutler, 55–63. Boston: Beacon Press.

Hoffmaster, Barry.

1992   Can Ethnography Save the Life of Medical Ethics? *Social Science and Medicine* 35:1421–31.

Hogle, Linda F.

1995a   Standardization across Non-standard Domains: The Case of Organ Procurement. *Science, Technology, and Human Values* 20:482–500.

1995b   Tales from the Cryptic: Technology Meets Organism in the Living Cadaver. In *The Cyborg Handbook*, edited by C. H. Gray, 203–16. New York: Routledge.

1999   *Recovering the Nation's Body: Cultural Memory, Medicine, and the Politics of Redemption.* New Brunswick, NJ: Rutgers University Press.

2001 Chemoprevention for Healthy Women: Harbinger of Things to Come? *Health* 5:299–320.

2002 Claims and Disclaimers: Whose Expertise Counts? *Medical Anthropology* 21:275–306.

Hogshire, Jim.

1992 Sell Yourself to Science. Port Townsend, WA: Loompanics Unlimited.

Houghton, Peter.

2001 *On Death and Not Dying.* London: Jessica Kingsley.

House, Robert M.

1999 Psychiatric Complications of Organ Transplantation. In *Neurologic Complications in Organ Transplant Recipients,* edited by E. F. M. Wijdicks, 91–106. Boston: Butterworth Heinemann.

Howe, David, and Julia Feast.

2000 *Adoption, Search and Reunion: The Long Term Experience of Adopted Adults.* London: Children's Society.

2001 The Long Term Outcome of Reunions between Adult Adopted People and Their Birth Mothers. *British Journal of Social Work* 31:351–68.

Hunkeler, David, Alan Cherrington, Ales Prokop, and Ray Rajotte, eds.

2001 *Bioartificial Organs III: Tissue Sourcing, Immunoisolation, and Clinical Trials.* Annals of the New York Academy of Sciences, vol. 944. New York: New York Academy of Sciences.

Hunkeler, David, Ales Prokop, Alan Cherrington, Ray Rajotte, and Michael Sefton, eds.

1999 *Bioartificial Organs II: Technology, Medicine, and Materials.* Annals of the New York Academy of Sciences, vol. 875. New York: New York Academy of Sciences.

Huyssen, Andreas.

1994 Monument and Memory in a Postmodern Age. In *The Art of Memory: Holocaust Memorials in History,* edited by J. E. Young, 9–17. New York: Prestel.

Illich, Ivan.

1976 *Medical Nemesis.* New York: Pantheon.

Institute of Medicine.

1997 *Non-Heart-Beating Organ Transplantation: Medical and Ethical Issues in Procurement.* Washington, DC: National Academy Press.

ITCS (International Transplant Coordinators Society).

1997 *Europe: 1997 Transplant Statistics, per Country, in Alphabetical Order.* Linden, Belgium: ITCS.

Iwamoto, M., et al.

2003 Transmission of West Nile Virus from an Organ Donor to Four Transplant Recipients. *New England Journal of Medicine* 348: 2196–2203.

Jankowski, Renee, and Suzanne T. Ildstad.
1997   Chimerism and Tolerance: From Freemartin Cattle and Neonatal Mice to Humans. *Human Immunology* 53:155–61.
Jensen, George H.
2000   *Storytelling in Alcoholics Anonymous: A Rhetorical Analysis.* Carbondale: Southern Illinois University Press.
Johannes, Laura.
2004   In Kidney Quest, New Rules Boost Chances for Blacks. *Wall Street Journal,* June 18.
Jonasson, Olga, and Mark A. Hardy.
1985   The Case of Baby Fae. *Journal of the American Medical Association* 254:3358–59.
Jones, James H.
1981   *Bad Blood: The Tuskegee Syphilis Experiment.* New York: Free Press.
Joralemon, Donald, and Phil Cox.
2003   Body Values: The Case against Compensating for Transplant Organs. *Hastings Center Report* 33 (1): 27–33.
Kass, Leon.
1998   The Wisdom of Repugnance. In *The Ethics of Cloning Humans: A Reader,* edited by G. Pence, 13–37. Boulder, CO: Rowman and Littlefield.
Kauffman, Myron H., Maureen A. McBride, and Francis L. Delmonico.
2000   First Report of the United Network for Organ Sharing Transplant Tumor Registry: Donors with a History of Cancer. *Transplantation* 70:1747–51.
Kaufman, Sharon R.
2000   In the Shadow of "Death with Dignity": Medicine and Cultural Quandaries of the Vegetative State. *American Anthropologist* 102:69–83.
2005   *—And a Time to Die: How American Hospitals Shape the End of Life.* New York: Scribner.
Kaufman, Sharon R., Ann J. Russ, and Janet K. Shim.
2006   Aged Bodies and Kinship Matters: The Ethical Field of Kidney Transplant. *American Ethnologist* 33(1): 81–99.
Kerridge, I. H., P. Saul, M. Lowe, J. McPhee, and D. Williams.
2002   Death, Dying, and Donation: Organ Transplantation and the Diagnosis of Death. *Journal of Medical Ethics* 28:89–94.
Kimbrell, Andrew.
1993   *The Human Body Shop: The Engineering and the Marketing of Life.* San Francisco: Harper and Row.
Kirchner, Sandra A.
1991   Living Related Lung Transplantation. *AORN Journal* (Association of Operating Room Nurses) 54:703–9.

Kirkpatrick, C. D., and Jim Shamp.

2003   Jesica's Ordeal Ends. Teen Dies at Duke after Transplant Efforts Fail. Girl's Life Support Pulled; Focus Now on Errors. *Durham (NC) Herald-Sun*, February 22.

Kleinman, Arthur.

1999   Moral Experience and Ethical Reflection: Can Ethnography Reconcile Them? A Quandary for "The New Bioethics." *Daedalus* 128 (4): 69–97.

Kleinman, Arthur, Veena Das, and Margaret Lock.

1997   *Social Suffering*. Berkeley and Los Angeles: University of California Press.

Kleinman, Arthur, Renée Fox, and Allan M. Brandt.

1999   Introduction [special volume on Bioethics and Beyond]. *Daedalus* 128 (4): v–x.

Koenig, Barbara.

1988   The Technological Imperative in Medical Practice: The Social Creation of a "Routine" Treatment. In *Biomedicine Examined*, edited by M. Lock and D. Gordon, 465–96. London: Kluwer Academic.

Kopytoff, Igor.

1986   The Cultural Biography of Things: Commoditization as Process. In *The Social Life of Things: Commodities in Cultural Perspective*, edited by A. Appadurai, 64–91. Cambridge: Cambridge University Press.

Kübler-Ross, Elisabeth.

1969   *On Death and Dying*. New York: Macmillan.

1975   *Death: The Final Stage of Growth*. Englewood Cliffs, NJ: Prentice-Hall.

1981   *Living with Death and Dying*. New York: Macmillan.

Kunstadter, Peter.

1980   Medical Ethics in Cross-Cultural and Multi-cultural Perspectives. *Social Science and Medicine* 14B:289–96.

Kushner, Thomasine, and Raymond Belliotti.

1985   Baby Fae: A Beastly Business. *Journal of Medical Ethics* 11: 178–83.

LaCapra, Dominick.

1999   Trauma, Absence, Loss. *Critical Inquiry* 25 (Summer): 696–727.

Land, W., and J. B. Dossetor.

1991   *Organ Replacement Therapy: Ethics, Justice, Commerce*. Berlin: Springer-Verlag.

Latour, Bruno.

1993   *We Have Never Been Modern*. Trans. C. Porter. Cambridge, MA: Harvard University Press.

Layne, Linda L.
1999   *Transformative Motherhood: On Giving and Getting in Consumer Culture.* New York: New York University Press.
Leach, Edmund.
1964   Anthropological Aspects of Language: Animal Categories and Verbal Abuse. In *New Directions in the Study of Language,* edited by E. Lenneberg, 23–64. Cambridge, MA: MIT Press.
Leder, Drew.
1990   *The Absent Body.* Chicago: University of Chicago Press.
Ledoux, Denis.
1993   *Turning Memories into Memoirs: A Handbook for Writing Lifestories.* Lisbon Falls, ME: Soleil Press.
Levinson, Mark M., and Jack G. Copeland.
1987   The Organ Donor: Physiology, Maintenance, and Procurement Considerations. *Contemporary Anesthesia Practice* 10:31–45.
Lewis, Alan, and Martin Snell.
1986   Increasing Kidney Transplantation in Britain: The Importance of Donor Cards, Public Opinion and Medical Practice. *Social Science and Medicine* 22:1075–80.
Life.
1967   The Gift of a Heart. December 15, 24–27.
LifeBanc.
1994   *Understanding Brain Death: Commonly Asked Ques*tions [pamphlet], June. Cleveland, OH: LifeBanc.
LifeCenter Northwest.
N.d.   Understanding Brain Death [informational card from packet prepared for donor families]. Bellevue, WA: LifeCenter Northwest.
Lifton, B. J.
1975   *Twice Born: Memoirs of an Adoptive Daughter.* New York: McGraw-Hill.
1988   *Lost and Found: The Adoption Experience.* New York: Harper and Row.
Lindenbaum, Shirley.
2001   Kuru, Prions, and Human Affairs: Thinking about Epidemics. *Annual Review of Anthropology* 30:363–85.
2004   Thinking about Cannibalism. *Annual Review of Anthropology* 33:475–98.
Lock, Margaret.
1995   Contesting the Natural in Japan: Moral Dilemmas and Technologies of Dying. *Culture, Medicine, and Psychiatry* 19 (1): 1–38.
1997   Culture, Technology, and the New Death: Deadly Disputes in Japan and North America. *Culture* 17 (1–2): 27–48.
2001   The Tempering of Medical Anthropology: Troubling Natural Categories. *Medical Anthropology Quarterly* 15:478–92.

2002   *Twice Dead: Organ Transplants and the Reinvention of Death.*
              Berkeley and Los Angeles: University of California Press.
2003   On Making Up the Good-as-Dead in a Utilitarian World. In *Remaking Life and Death: Toward an Anthropology of the Biosciences,* edited by S. Franklin and M. Lock, 165–92. Santa Fe: School of American Research Press.

Lock, Margaret, and Christina Honde.
1990   Reaching Consensus about Death: Heart Transplants and Cultural Identity in Japan. In *Social Science Perspectives on Medical Ethics,* edited by G. Weisz, 99–119. Philadelphia: University of Pennsylvania Press.

Lock, Margaret, Allan Young, and Alberto Cambrosio.
2000   *Living and Working with the New Medical Technologies: Intersections of Inquiry.* Cambridge: Cambridge University Press.

Luhrmann, Tanya M.
2000   *Of Two Minds: The Growing Disorder in American Psychiatry.* New York: Knopf.

Lynch, J., and M. K. Eldadah.
1992   Brain-Death Criteria Currently Used by Pediatric Intensivists. *Clinical Pediatrics* 31:457–60.

Lynch, Michael, and Steve Woolgar.
1990   *Representation in Scientific Practice.* Cambridge, MA: MIT Press.

Lynch, Thomas.
1997   *The Undertaking: Life Studies from the Dismal Trade.* New York: Penguin.

Lynn, J.
1993   Are the Patients Who Become Organ Donors under the Pittsburgh Protocol for "Non-Heart-Beating Donors" Really Dead? *Kennedy Institute of Ethics Journal* 3:167–78.

Machado, Nora.
1998   *Using the Bodies of the Dead: Legal, Ethical and Organisational Dimensions of Organ Transplantation.* Aldershot, Hampshire, UK: Ashgate.

Mack, Cara L., Mario Ferrario, Michael Abecassis, Peter F. Whitington, Riccardo A. Spuperina, and Estella M. Alonson.
2001   Living Donor Liver Transplantation for Children with Liver Failure and Concurrent Multiple Organ System Failure. *Liver Transplantation* 7:890–95.

Maeder, Thomas, and Philip E. Ross.
2002   Machines for Living. Red Herring 113:41–46.

Malinowski, Bronislaw.
1961 [1922]   Introduction: The Subject, Method and Scope of This Inquiry. In *Argonauts of the Western Pacific,* 1–25. Prospect Heights, IL: Waveland.

Maloney, Raelynn, and Alan D. Wolfelt.

2001   *Caring for Donor Families Before, During, and After: How to Communicate with and Support Families Before, During, and After the Decision to Donate Organs, Tissues, and Eyes.* Fort Collins, CO: Companion Press.

Mandell, M. S., G. J. Taylor, A. D'Alessandro, L. J. McGaw, and E. Cohen.

2004   Executive Summary from the Intraoperative Advisory Council on Donation after Cardiac Death of the United Network for Organ Sharing: Practice Guidelines. *Liver Transplantation* 9:1120–23.

Marcus, George E.

1995   *Technoscientific Imaginaries: Conversations, Profiles, and Memoirs.* Chicago: University of Chicago Press.

Marshall, Patricia A.

1992   Anthropology and Bioethics. *Medical Anthropology Quarterly* 6:49–73.

Marshall, Patricia A., and Barbara A. Koenig.

1996   Bioethics in Anthropology: Perspectives on Culture, Medicine, and Morality. In *Medical Anthropology: Contemporary Theory and Method,* edited by T. M. Johnson and C. F. Sargent, 349–73. Westport, CT: Praeger.

Marshall, Patricia A., David C. Thomasma, and Abdallah S. Daar.

1996   Marketing Human Organs: The Autonomy Paradox. *Theoretical Medicine* 17 (1): 1–18.

Martin, Emily.

1992   The End of the Body? *American Ethnologist* 19:121–40.

1993   Histories of Immune Systems. *Culture, Medicine, and Psychiatry* 17:67–76.

1994   *Flexible Bodies: Tracking Immunity in American Culture from the Days of Polio to the Age of AIDS.* Boston: Beacon Press.

Matesanz, Rafael.

2003   Factors Influencing the Adaptation of the Spanish Model of Organ Donation. *Transplant International* 16:736–41.

Matta, A.

2000   Reply [correspondence]. *Anaesthesia* 55:695–96.

McGary, Howard.

1999   Distrust, Social Justice, and Health Care. *Mount Sinai Journal of Medicine* 66:236–40.

Metcalf, Peter, and Richard Huntington.

1991   *Celebrations of Death: The Anthropology of Mortuary Ritual.* Cambridge: Cambridge University Press.

Michaels, Marian.

1998   Xenozoonoses and the Xenotransplant Recipient. In *Xenotransplantation: Scientific Frontiers and Public Policy.* Annals of the New York Academy of Sciences, vol. 862, edited by J. Fishman,

D. Sachs, and R. Shaikh, 100–104. New York: New York Academy of Sciences.

Michelsen, P.
1991   Three Years of Experience with "Presumed Consent" Legislations in Belgium: Its Impact on Multi-organ Donation in Comparison with Other European Countries. *Transplantation Proceedings* 23:903–4.

Miller, Charles M., et al.
2001   One Hundred Nine Living Donor Liver Transplants in Adults and Children: A Single-Center Experience. *Annals of Surgery* 234:301–12.

Modell, Judith.
2002   *A Sealed and Secret Kinship: The Culture of Policies and Practices in American Adoption.* New York: Berghahn Books.

Morgan, Vanessa.
1999   Issues in Organ Donation and Transplantation. *Journal of the Royal Society of Medicine* 92 (July): 356–58.

Morioka, Masahiro.
2001   Reconsidering Brain Death: A Lesson from Japan's Fifteen Years of Experience. *Hastings Center Report* 31 (4): 41–46.

Muller, Jessica H.
1994   Anthropology, Bioethics, and Medicine: A Provocative Trilogy. *Medical Anthropology Quarterly* 8:448–67.

Murphy, Robert F.
1987   *The Body Silent.* New York: Norton.

Murray, T. H.
1987   Gifts of the Body and the Needs of Strangers. *Hastings Center Report* 17 (2): 30–38.

Nathan, Howard M.
2000   Late Gov. Casey Made Sure Others Could Benefit from Organ Donors [obituary]. *Morning Call*, June 4.

NDFC (National Donor Family Council).
1994   *Bill of Rights for Donor Families.* New York: National Kidney Foundation.
1997   *National Communication Guidelines.* New York: NDFC.

Nelkin, Dorothy, and Lori Andrews.
1998   Homo Economicus: The Commercialization of Body Tissue in the Age of Biotechnology. *Hastings Center Report* 28 (5): 30–39.

Neumann, Peter I., and Milton C. Weinstein.
1991   The Diffusion of New Technology: Costs and Benefits to Health Care. In *The Changing Economics of Medical Technology,* edited by Institute of Medicine, 1–20. Washington, DC: National Academies Press.

Newman, Andy.
2004   The Logistics of the Cadaver Supply Business. *New York Times,* March 12.

Niemann, H., and W. A. Kues.

2003   Progress in Xenotransplantation Research Employing Trans-
              genic Pigs. *Transplantationsmedizin* 15:3–14.

Niven, Larry.

1968   *A Gift from Earth.* New York: Ballantine.

1980   *The Patchwork Girl.* New York: Ace Science Fiction.

Nuland, Sherwin B.

1993   *How We Die: Reflections on Life's Final Chapter.* New York:
              Knopf.

OPTN (Organ Procurement and Transplantation Network).

2003   *Transplants in the U.S. by Recipient Gender; January 1, 1998–*
              September 30, 2003. Richmond, VA: OPTN.

Otte, J. B., et al.

1989   Organ Procurement in Children: Surgical, Anaesthetic and Lo-
              gistic Aspects. *Intensive Care Medicine* 15:S67–S70.

Pallis, C., and D. H. Harley.

1996   *ABC of Brainstem Death.* London: BMJ Publishing Group.

Pantagraph.

1991   Organ Transplants Cause AIDS Deaths. May 18.

Papagaroufali, Eleni.

1996   Xenotransplantation and Transgenesis: Im-moral Stories about
              Human-Animal Relations in the West. In *Nature and Society:*
              Anthropological Perspectives, edited by P. Descola and G. Páls-
              son, 240–55. New York: Routledge.

Parisi, Nina, and Irwin Katz.

1986   Attitudes toward Posthumous Organ Donation and Commit-
              ment to Donate. *Health Psychology* 5:565–80.

PBS (Public Broadcasting Service).

2002   Sparing No Expense. Online newsletter, August 22.

Pearson, I. Y., P. Bazeley, T. Pencer-Plane, J. R. Chapman, and P. Robertson.

1995   A Survey of Families of Brain Dead Patients: Their Experiences,
              Attitudes to Organ Donation and Transplantation. *Anesthesia*
              and Intensive Care 23 (1): 88–95.

Percy, W.

1958   Symbol, Consciousness, and Intersubjectivity. *Journal of Phi-*
              losophy 55:631–42.

Perez-Pena, Richard.

2003   Downside to Fewer Violent Deaths: Transplant Organ Shortage
              Grows. *New York Times,* August 19.

Petchesky, Rosalind P.

1987   Fetal Images: The Power of Visual Culture in the Politics of Re-
              production. *Feminist Studies* 13:263–92.

Peters, Thomas J.

1991   Life or Death: The Issue of Payment in Cadaveric Organ Dona-
              tion. *Journal of the American Medical Association* 265:1302–5.

Plomin, R.

1994   *Genetics and Experience: The Interplay between Nature and Nurture.* Newbury Park, CA: Sage.

Plough, Alonzo L.

1986   *Borrowed Time: Artificial Organs and the Politics of Extending Lives.* Philadelphia: Temple University Press.

Plum, Fred, and Jerome B. Posner.

1966   The Pathological Physiology of Signs and Symptoms of Coma. In *The Diagnosis of Stupor and Coma,* 1–42. Philadelphia: F. A. Davis.

Portmann, John.

1999   Cutting Bodies to Harvest Organs. *Cambridge Quarterly of Healthcare Ethics* 8:288–98.

Poulton, B., and M. Garfield.

2000   The Implications of Anaesthetising the Brainstem Dead: 1 [correspondence]. *Anaesthesia* 55:695.

Powdermaker, Hortense.

1966   *Stranger and Friend: The Way of an Anthropologist.* New York: Norton.

Prottas, J. M.

1992   Buying Human Organs—Evidence That Money Doesn't Change Everything. *Transplantation* 53:1371–73.

Proulx, E. Annie.

1993   *The Shipping News.* New York: Maxwell Macmillan International.

Quaini, Federico, Carlo A. Beltrami, Bernardo Nadal-Ginard, Jan Kajstura, Annarosa Leri, Piero Anversa.

2002   Chimerism of the Transplanted Heart. *New England Journal of Medicine* 346:5–15.

Rabinow, Paul.

1992   Artificiality and Enlightenment: From Sociobiology to Biosociality. In *Incorporations: Zone 6,* edited by J. Crary and S. Kwinter, 234–52. New York: Urzone.

Radcliffe-Richards, J., A. S. Daar, R. D. Guttmann, R. Hoffenberg, I. Kennedy, M. Lock, R. A. Sells, N. Tilney.

1998   The Case for Allowing Kidney Sales. *Lancet* 351:1950–52.

Ragoné, Heléna.

1994   *Surrogate Motherhood: Conception in the Heart.* Boulder, CO: Westview Press.

1996   Chasing the Blood Tie: Surrogate Mothers, Adoptive Mothers and Fathers. *American Ethnologist* 23:352–65.

1999   The Gift of Life: Surrogate Motherhood, Gamete Donation and Constructions of Altruism. In *Transformative Motherhood: On Giving and Getting in a Consumer Culture,* edited by L. Layne, 65–87. New York: New York University Press.

Ramsey, Paul.
1968   On Updating Death. In *Updating Life and Death*, edited by D. R. Cutler, 31–54. Boston: Beacon Press.
Rapp, Rayna.
2000   *Testing Women, Testing the Fetus: The Social Impact of Amniocentesis in America*. New York: Routledge.
Reames, Mary.
1997   Speech by Mary Reames, wife of TRIO founder, Brian Reames. Conference presentation, TRIO "Celebration of a Decade of Caring," October 23, 1997. www.trioweb.org/97conference/maryreames_c.html (consulted July 2004).
Reverby, Susan M., ed.
2000   *Tuskegee's Truths: Rethinking the Tuskegee Syphilis Study*. Chapel Hill: University of North Carolina Press.
Reynolds, Gretchen.
2005   Will Any Organ Do? *New York Times Magazine*, July 10, 36–41.
Rhodes, Lorna.
1991   *Emptying Beds: The Work of an Emergency Psychiatric Unit*. Berkeley and Los Angeles: University of California Press.
Richardson, Ruth.
1996   Fearful Symmetry: Corpses for Anatomy, Organs for Transplantation? In *Organ Transplantation: Meanings and Realities*, edited by R. Fox, L. O'Connell, and S. Youngner, 66–100. Madison: University of Wisconsin Press.
Richter, Ruthann.
2004   Baby's Successful Heart Transplant Causes Parents to Celebrate and to Mourn. *Stanford Report*, September 22.
Roach, Mary.
2003   *Stiff: The Curious Life of Human Cadavers*. New York: Norton.
Roberts, Karen Y.
1988   Black American Attitudes towards Organ Donation and Transplantation. *Journal of the National Medical Association* 80: 1121–26.
Robson, Simon, Jan Schulte Am Esch II, and Fritz H. Bach.
1999   Factors in Xenograft Rejection. In *Bioartificial Organs II: Technology, Medicine, and Materials*. Annals of the New York Academy of Sciences, vol. 875, edited by D. Hunkeler, A. Prokop, A. Cherrington, R. Rajotte, and M. Sefton, 261–76. New York: New York Academy of Sciences.
Rohter, Larry.
2004   The Organ Trade: A Global Black Market; Tracking the Sale of a Kidney on a Path of Poverty and Hope. *New York Times*, May 23.
Rollin, Bernard E.
1995   *The Frankenstein Syndrome: Ethical and Social Issues in the Ge-*

netic Engineering of Animals. Cambridge: Cambridge University Press.

Rothman, D. J.

1991   *Strangers at the Bedside: A History of How Law and Bioethics Transformed Medical Decision Making*. New York: Basic Books.

1997   Body Shop. *The Sciences* 37 (6): 17–21.

1998   The International Organ Traffic. *New York Review of Books*, March 26.

Rothman, D. J., E. Rose, T. Awaya, B. Cohen, A. Daar, S. L. Dzemeshkevich, C. J. Lee, et al.

1997   The Bellagio Task Force Report on Transplantation, Bodily Integrity, and the International Traffic in Organs. *Transplantation Proceedings* 29:2739–45.

Rouse, Carolyn.

Forthcoming The Politics of Uncertain Suffering, Race, and Medicine: Racial Health Disparities and Sickle Cell Disease. Berkeley: University of California Press.

Rowland, Rhoda.

2001   Patient Gets First Totally Implanted Artificial Heart. CNN.com/ Health, July 3.

Sachdev, P.

1989   *Unlocking the Adoption Files*. Lexington, MA: Lexington Books.

Sacks, Oliver.

1973   *Awakenings*. New York: Vintage.

1985   *The Man Who Mistook His Wife for a Hat and Other Clinical Tales*. New York: Simon and Schuster.

1998   *A Leg to Stand On*. New York: Touchstone.

Sangaramoorthy, Thurka.

1998   Myths, Monsters, and Medicine: Towards an Anthropology of Xenotransplantation. Senior thesis, Barnard College.

Sanner, Margareta.

1994   Attitudes toward Organ Donation and Transplantation: A Model for Understanding Reactions to Medical Procedures after Death. *Social Science and Medicine* 8:1411–52.

Saranow, Jennifer.

2003   What Is Your Body Worth? Putting Prices on the Pieces. *Wall Street Journal*, May 6.

Sarti, Armando.

1999   Organ Donation [review article]. *Paediatric Anaesthesia* 9:287–94.

Savulescu, J.

2002   Two Deaths and Two Lessons: Is It Time to Review the Structure and Function of Research Ethics Committees? *Journal of Medical Ethics* 28:1–2.

Sawday, Jonathan.
1995   The Body Emblazoned: Dissection and the Human Body in Re-
             naissance Culture. New York: Routledge.
Scheper-Hughes, Nancy.
1992   Death without Weeping: The Violence of Everyday Life in Brazil.
             Berkeley and Los Angeles: University of California Press.
1995   The Primacy of the Ethical: Propositions for a Militant Anthro-
             pology [including commentaries and reply]. Current Anthro-
             pology 36:409–40.
1996   Theft of Life: The Globalization of Organ Stealing Rumours.
             Anthropology Today 12 (3): 3–11.
1998a   Bodies of Apartheid: Witchcraft, Rumor, and Racism Confound
             South Africa's Organ Transplant Program. Worldview, Fall, 47–53.
1998b   The New Cannibalism: International Traffic in Human Organs.
             New Internationalist 300 (April).
1998c   Truth and Rumor on the Organ Trail. Natural History 107 (8):
             48–57.
2000   The Global Traffic in Human Organs. Current Anthropology
             41:191–211, 218–24 (reply).
2004   Parts Unknown: Undercover Ethnography on the Organs-
             Trafficking Underworld. Ethnography 5 (1): 29–72.
Scheper-Hughes, Nancy, and Margaret Lock.
1987   The Mindful Body: A Prolegomenon to Future Work in Med-
             ical Anthropology. Medical Anthropology Quarterly 1:6–41.
Scheper-Hughes, Nancy, and Loïc J. D. Wacquant.
2003   Commodifying Bodies. Thousand Oaks, CA: Sage.
Schneider, David M.
1972   What Is Kinship All About? In Kinship Studies in the Morgan
             Centennial Year, edited by P. Reining, 42–63. Washington, DC:
             Anthropological Society of Washington.
1980 [1965] American Kinship A Cultural Account. Chicago: University of
             Chicago Press.
1984   A Critique of the Study of Kinship. Ann Arbor: University of
             Michigan Press.
Schusky, Ernest L.
1965   Manual for Kinship Analysis. New York: Holt, Rinehart, and
             Winston.
Sells, Robert A.
1992   The Case against Buying Organs and a Futures Market in Trans-
             plants. Transplantation Proceedings 24:2198–2202.
Selzer, Richard.
1974   Mortal Lessons: Notes on the Art of Surgery. New York: Touch-
             stone.
1990   Whither Thou Goest. In Imagine a Woman and Other Tales,
             1–28. New York: Random House.

Sharp, Lesley A.

1993   *The Possessed and the Dispossessed: Spirits, Identity, and Power in a Madagascar Migrant Town.* Berkeley and Los Angeles: University of California Press.

1994   Organ Transplantation as a Transformative Experience: Anthropological Insights into the Restructuring of the Self. *Medical Anthropology Quarterly* 9:357–89.

1995   Playboy Princely Spirits of Madagascar: Possession as Youthful Commentary and Social Critique. *Anthropological Quarterly* 68:75–88.

1997   Royal Difficulties: A Question of Succession in an Urbanized Sakalava Kingdom. *Journal of Religion in Africa* 27:270–307.

1999   A Medical Anthropologist's View of Posttransplant Compliance: The Underground Economy of Medical Survival. *Transplantation Proceedings* 31 (Suppl. 4A): 31S–33S.

2000a   Comment on "The Global Traffic in Human Organs," N. Scheper-Hughes. *Current Anthropology* 41:216–17.

2000b   The Commodification of the Body and Its Parts. *Annual Review of Anthropology* 29:287–328.

2001   Commodified Kin: Death, Mourning, and Competing Claims on the Bodies of Organ Donors in the United States. *American Anthropologist* 103:1–21.

2002a   Bodies, Boundaries, and Territorial Disputes: Investigating the Murky Realm of Scientific Authority. *Medical Anthropology* 21:371–81.

2002b   Denying Culture in the Transplant Arena: Technocratic Medicine's Myth of Democratization. *Cambridge Quarterly of Healthcare Ethics* 11:142–50.

2002c   *The Sacrificed Generation: Youth, History, and the Colonized Mind in Madagascar.* Berkeley and Los Angeles: University of California Press.

In press (a)   Babes and Baboons: Jesica Santillan and Experimental Pediatric Transplant Research in America. In *A Death Retold: Jesica Santillan, the Bungled Transplant, and the Paradoxes of Medical Citizenship,* edited by K. Wailoo, P. Guarnaccia, and J. Livingston. Chapel Hill: University of North Carolina Press.

In press (b)   *Bodies, Commodities, and Biotechnologies.* New York: Columbia University Press.

Shildrick, Margrit.

2002   *Embodying the Monster: Encounters with the Vulnerable Self.* London: Sage.

Shrader, Douglas.

1986   On Dying More Than One Death. *Hastings Center Report* 16 (1): 12–16.

Siebert, Charles.

2004   *A Man after His Own Heart: A True Story.* New York: Crown.

Silverman, Phyllis R., Lee H. Campbell, Patricia B. Patti, and Carolyn Briggs Style.

1988   Reunions between Adoptees and Birth Parents: The Birth Parents' Experience. *Social Work,* November–December, 523–28.

Siminoff, L. A.

2004   Death and Organ Procurement: Public Beliefs and Attitudes. *Kennedy Institute of Ethics Journal* 14:217–34.

Siminoff, L. A., N. Gordon, J. Hewlett, and R. M. Arnold.

2001   Factors Influencing Families' Consent for Donation of Solid Organs for Transplantation. *Journal of the American Medical Association* 286:71–77.

Siminoff, L. A., and M. D. Leonard.

1999   Financial Incentives: Alternatives to the Altruistic Model of Organ Donation. *Journal Transplant Coordination* 9:250–56.

Simpson, M., H. Timm, and H. I. McCubbin.

1981   Adoptees in Search of Their Past: Policy Induced Strain on Adoptive Families and Birth Parents. *Family Relations* 30:427–34.

Slomka, Jacquelyn.

1995   What Do Apple Pie and Motherhood Have to Do with Feeding Tubes and Caring for the Patient? *Archives of Internal Medicine* 155:1258–63.

Smith, Brian D.

1994   The Gift of Life. *Indianapolis Monthly,* February, 86–91, 131–35.

Smith, G. P. II.

1993   Market and Non-market Mechanisms for Procuring Human and Cadaveric Organs: When the Price Is Right. *Medical Law International* 1:17–32.

Snider, Elizabeth Ann.

1997   The Female Adoptee's Identity and the Post-reunion Relationship with Her Birth Mother. Manuscript. California School of Professional Psychology.

Solomon, Steven.

1978   Spare Parts for Humans. *Forbes,* May 29, 52–54.

Soper, Kate.

1995   *What Is Nature?* Oxford: Blackwell.

Starzl, Thomas E.

1992   *The Puzzle People: Memoirs of a Transplant Surgeon.* Pittsburgh: University of Pittsburgh Press.

Starzl, Thomas E., et al.

1993   Baboon-to-Human Liver Transplantation. *Lancet* 341:65–71.

Stell, Lance K.

1999   Diagnosing Death: What's Trust Got to Do with It? *Mount Sinai Journal of Medicine* 66:229–35.

Stoller, Kenneth P.

1990 Baby Fae: The Unlearned Lesson. *Perspectives on Medical Research* (online journal). Vol. 2. Published by Americans/ Europeans/Japanese for Medical Advancement. www.curedisease .com/perspectives.

Strathern, Marilyn.

1992a The Meaning of Assisted Kinship. In *Changing Human Reproduction: Social Science Perspectives,* edited by M. Stacey, 148–69. London: Sage.

1992b *Reproducing the Future: Anthropology, Kinship, and the New Reproductive Technologies.* New York: Routledge.

Sturken, Marita.

1997 *Tangled Memories: The Vietnam War, the AIDS Epidemic, and the Politics of Remembering.* Berkeley and Los Angeles: University of California Press.

Taylor, Janelle S.

1998 Image of Contradiction: Obstetrical Ultrasound in American Culture. In *Reproducing Reproduction: Kinship, Power, and Technological Innovation,* edited by S. Franklin and H. Ragoné, 15–45. Philadelphia: University of Pennsylvania Press.

2005 Surfacing the Body's Interior. *Annual Review of Anthropology* 34:741–56.

Tegnaeus, Harry.

1952 *Blood-Brothers: An Ethno-sociological Study of the Institutions of Blood-Brotherhood with Special Reference to Africa.* Stockholm: Ethnographic Museum of Sweden.

Ten Eyck, Toby A., George Gaskell, and Jonathan Jackson.

2004 Seeds, Food, and Trade Wars: Public Opinion and Policy Responses in the USA and Europe. *Journal of Commercial Biotechnology* 10:258–67.

Triseliotis, J.

1973 *In Search of Origins: The Experience of Adopted People.* Boston: Beacon Press.

Turner, M.

2000 The Implications of Anaesthetising the Brainstem Dead: 2 [correspondence]. *Anaesthesia* 55:695.

University of North Dakota.

1998 Brain Death and Organ Donation [videotaped training session]. Ralston Lecture Series, North Dakota School of Medicine and Health Sciences, Health Education Network, produced by MedStar.

UNOS (United Network for Organ Sharing).

2000 *Organ and Tissue Donation: A Reference Guide for Clergy.* 4th ed. Richmond, VA: UNOS.

2003a Special National Donor Memorial Edition: Honoring America's Organ and Tissue Donors. *UNOS Update.*

2003b   U.S. Transplants by Organ and Donor Type: January, 1992–May, 2003. Richmond, VA: UNOS/OPTN.

2004a   *Donation after Cardiac Death: A Reference Guide.* Richmond, VA: UNOS.

2004b   OPTN/UNOS Statement Regarding Rabies Transmission via Organ Transplantation [press release]. Richmond, VA.

2004c   Organ Transplantation and Donation Facts at a Glance (Newsroom Fact Sheet). Richmond, VA: UNOS. www.unos.org.

U.S. Department of Transportation.

2002   Traffic Safety Facts 2002. *A Compilation of Motor Vehicle Crash Data from the Fatality Analysis Reporting System and the General Estimates System,* early edition. Washington, DC: National Highway Traffic Safety Administration, National Center for Statistics and Analysis.

van den Bergh, J. C. J. M., and J. M. Holley.

2002   An Environmental-Economic Assessment of Genetic Modification of Agricultural Crops. *Futures* 34:807–22.

Van Wolputte, Steven.

2004   Hang On to Your Self: Of Bodies, Embodiment, and Selves. *Annual Review of Anthropology* 33:251–69.

Vanderpool, Harold Y.

1999   Commentary: A Critique of Clark's Frightening Xenotransplantation Scenario. *Journal of Law, Medicine and Ethics* 27:153–57.

Veatch, R. M.

1997   Non-Heart-Beating Cadaver Organ Procurement: Two Remaining Issues. *Transplantation Proceedings* 29:3339–40.

Verdery, Katherine.

1999   *The Political Lives of Dead Bodies: Reburial and Postsocialist Change.* New York: Columbia University Press.

Vesalius, Andreas.

1973   The Illustrations from the Works of Andreas Vesalius of Brussels. Ed. and trans. J. B. de C. M. Saunders and Charles D. O'Malley. New York: Dover.

Volti, Rudi.

1995   *Society and Technological Change.* 3rd ed. New York: St. Martin's Press.

Wace, J., and M. Kai.

2000   Anaesthesia for Organ Donation in the Brainstem Dead [correspondence]. *Anaesthesia* 55:590.

Wailoo, Keith.

2001   *Dying in the City of the Blues: Sickle Cell Anemia and the Politics of Race and Health.* Chapel Hill: University of California Press.

Wailoo, Keith, Peter Guarnaccia, and Julie Livingston.
In press   *A Death Retold: Jesica Santillan, the Bungled Transplant, and the Parodoxes of Medical Citizenship.* Chapel Hill: University of North Carolina Press.

Waldby, Catherine.
2000   Virtual Anatomy: From the Body in the Text to the Body on the Screen. *Journal of Medical Humanities* 21 (2): 5–107.

Weisbard, A. J.
1993   A Polemic on Principles: Reflections on the Pittsburgh Protocol. *Kennedy Institute of Ethics Journal* 3:217–30.

Wetzel, R. N., N. Setzer, J. Stiff, and M. Rogers.
1985   Hemodynamic Responses in Brain Dead Organ Donor Patients. *Anesthesia and Analgesia* 64:125–28.

White, Luise.
2000   *Speaking with Vampires: Rumor and History in Colonial Africa.* Berkeley and Los Angeles: University of California Press.

Wijdicks, Eelco F. M.
1995a   Determining Brain Death in Adults. *Neurology* 45:1003–11.
1995b   In Search of a Safe Apnea Test in Brain Death: Is the Procedure Really More Dangerous Than We Think? *Archives of Neurology* 52:338.
2001   *Brain Death.* Philadelphia: Lippincott Williams and Wilkins.
2002   Brain Death Worldwide: Accepted Fact but No Global Consensus in Diagnostic Criteria. *Neurology* 58 (1): 20–25.

Wijnen, R. M. H., and C. J. van der Linden.
1991   Donor Treatment Pronouncement of Brain Death: A Neglected Intensive Care Problem. *Transplant International* 4:186–90.

Wolfelt, Alan D.
2002   *Healing Your Traumatized Heart: 100 Practical Ideas after Someone You Love Dies a Sudden, Violent Death. For Those Who Grieve after a Homicide, Suicide or Accidental Death.* Fort Collins, CO: Companion Press.

Young, Allan.
1997   *The Harmony of Illusions: Inventing Post-traumatic Stress Disorder.* Princeton, NJ: Princeton University Press.

Young, James E.
1993   Introduction: The Texture of Memory. In *The Texture of Memory: Holocaust Memorials and Meaning,* edited by J. E. Young, 1–15. New Haven, CT: Yale University Press.

Young, P. J., and B. F. Matta.
2000   Anesthesia for Organ Donation in the Brainstem Dead—Why Bother? [editorial]. *Anaesthesia* 55:105–6.

Youngner, Stuart.
1990   Organ Retrieval: Can We Ignore the Dark Side? *Transplantation Proceedings* 22:1014–15.

1996   Some Must Die. In *Organ Transplantation: Meanings and Re-alities,* edited by S. Youngner, R. C. Fox, and L. J. O'Connell, 32–55. Madison: University of Wisconsin Press.

Youngner, Stuart J., Robert M. Arnold, and Michael A. DeVita.
1999   What Is "Dead"? *Hastings Center Report* 29 (6): 14–21.

Youngner, S. J., C. S. Landefeld, C. J. Coulton, B. W. Juknialis, and M. Leary.
1989   "Brain Death" and Organ Retrieval. A Cross-Sectional Survey of Knowledge and Concepts among Health Professionals. *Journal of the American Medical Association* 261:2205–10.

Zola, Irving K.
1978   Medicine as an Institution of Social Control. In *The Cultural Crisis of Modern Medicine,* edited by J. Ehrenreich, 80–100. New York: Monthly Review Press.

Zutlevics, T. L.
2001   Markets and the Needy: Organ Sales or Aid? *Journal of Applied Philosophy* 18:297–302.

Index

Text: 10/13 Aldus
Display: Aldus
Compositor: Integrated Composition Systems
Illustrator: Bill Nelson